Pharmacoepidemiology

Volume I

Edited by Stanley A. Edlavitch

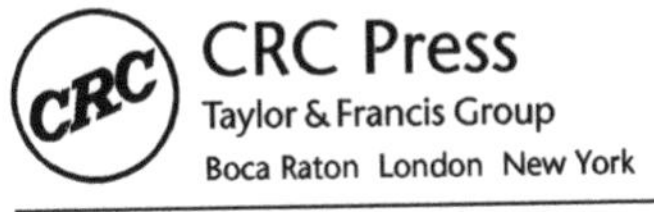

CRC Press
Taylor & Francis Group
Boca Raton London New York

CRC Press is an imprint of the
Taylor & Francis Group, an **informa** business

Published 1989 by CRC Press
Taylor & Francis Group
6000 Broken Sound Parkway NW, Suite 300
Boca Raton, FL 33487-2742

First issued in paperback 2019

ISBN-13: 978-0-367-45102-8 (pbk)
ISBN-13: 978-0-87371-129-6 (hbk)

Visit the Taylor & Francis Web site at
http://www.taylorandfrancis.com

and the CRC Press Web site at
http://www.crcpress.com

Introduction

This volume contains work presented (sometimes expanded for publication) at the 3rd International Conference on Pharmacoepidemiology, held September 9–11, 1987, in Minneapolis, Minnesota.

This book is published with two major objectives in mind. The first is to document the state of the science of pharmacoepidemiology as evidenced by presentations at the 3rd International Conference. The second is to provide a reference for day-to-day use and for classroom teaching. It has certainly been a pleasure and privilege to work with the contributors to this compendium. I hope you find this volume useful.

As Dr. Tilson points out in the insightful preface which follows, pharmacoepidemiology has progressed far from its scientific infancy. There is general consensus that the field was born as scientists, legislators, and regulators reacted to the public and professional outcry following the thalidomide disaster of the late 1960s. Today it is a maturing discipline making a significant impact on drug regulation and public health practice.

The International Conferences on Pharmacoepidemiology reflect the growth and importance of this discipline. The Division of Epidemiology of the University of Minnesota and its Director, Dr. Henry Blackburn, invested in the concept of a scientific forum for pharmacoepidemiologists at a time when most academic institutions were unwilling to consider the need. The first Minnesota Conference attracted only 75 attendees and I considered not continuing the series. However, the enthusiasm of the attendees, the support of leaders in the pharmaceutical industry, and the support of this University convinced me to continue with a second Conference. Attendance doubled, enthusiasm increased, sponsorship increased, and the Conferences became established as the important scientific forum this discipline.

The planning committee for the early conferences consisted of just a handful of colleagues. I would like to take this opportunity to thank them for taking a chance with me. They were Hugh Tilson, MD, DrPH, Burroughs Wellcome Co.; David Lilienfeld, MD, MS Engin, MPH, Mt. Sinai Medical School; and, from the University of Minnesota, David Lane, PhD, Tom Rector, PharmD, PhD, Albert Wertheimer, PhD, and Barry Garfinkle, MD, FRCP(C).

The 3rd International Conference and hence this volume are the result of the commitment of effort by a larger number of colleagues. Abstracts were peer-reviewed by a committee of volunteers. Nineteen persons contributed their time and energy to planning the 3rd Conference. Their names are listed in the Appendix. Members of this committee represented the pharmaceutical industry, academia, medical practitioners, and regulators. A subgroup of this committee met to select papers for inclusion in the program and in the proceedings.

As those of you have attempted to institute annual conferences of this nature are painfully aware, this effort is time-consuming and requires substantial support. Underwriting for this has come from the University of Minnesota, the pharmaceutical industry, and attendees. The University of Minnesota made the largest initial and continued investment. The pharmaceutical industry generously provided essential financial support. A list of those companies who contributed to the 3rd International Conference on Pharmacoepidemiology are listed in the Appendix. Finally, most important has been the support of the attendees and speakers. Speakers and attendees contribute to these Conferences by their scientific input. The program committee, speakers, and attendees alike pay their own registration and travel expenses.

The 3rd Conference and its published proceedings also owe a great deal to the people behind the scenes. Nola Fortner organized and handled the many details involved, including management of the main desk during the Conference itself; Carolyn Kurtz assisted at the desk and performed the major task of editing all 27 scientific papers from international authors; and Janet Tarolli of Lewis Publishers guided us gently and carefully, with unstinting good humor, through the lengthy maneuvers of the book publishing business.

Stanley A. Edlavitch, PhD

Preface

The papers in this book reflect the four themes of the 3rd International Conference on Pharmacoepidemiology: legal aspects, social impact, drug surveillance, and reports on specific studies. Authors contribute perspectives from academia, practice, government, industry, and the law.

The field of pharmacoepidemiology has, at last, come of age. Whether this maturity is marked by the twenty-five years since the public outcry for more careful postapproval monitoring following the thalidomide tragedy, the seven years since the issuance of the Melmon Commission Report, or the three years of the existence of these International Conferences is of little importance—the field has now blossomed. No longer are we talking about evolving capacity and the use of multipurpose data bases such as Medicaid's (1st Conference) or evolving methodology such as data and information linkage and its limitations (2nd Conference). The focus of this Conference is upon the enormous difference that pharmacoepidemiology has already made and is currently making—a difference that improves the quality of public policy decisionmaking regarding the safety of medicines, which has already contributed substantially to protecting, promoting, and assuring the health of the people who take them.

An essential attribute of maturity is insight, and a critical component of insight is recognition of limitations as well as strengths. The limitations of the large automated data bases must be addressed. If a drug is not widely used or is restricted by formulary, populations large enough to provide power to answer important public policy questions soon enough may not be forthcoming. Or, if the outcome is important but subtle and is not likely to appear on a hospital discharge diagnosis list, then the data bases cannot pick it up. Refinement of existing resources is underway, but more efforts are needed. Considerable experience is needed to use data base technology appropriately. Certainly, the mere finding in the computer of an apparent association between an exposure and a set of outcomes is nothing more than the first step in proper epidemiologic analysis. Diagnostic verification and search for important potential confounders, especially through the use of the medical record, are minimum adjuncts in most such research.

Epidemiologists must be conversant in the vagaries of the applications of the new and powerful tools. A mindless meander through the data is likely to find chance associations that become dangerous to the public's health, because they are not properly understood, resulting in ill-advised or erroneous medical decisions. Standards for good research must be nurtured, including a sense of the best strategy and resource to address each problem. Large automated data bases enhance, but cannot replace, more traditional epidemiologic approaches. An enlightened and informed public—including the media, consumer advocates, and the courts—will also help improve the effectiveness of epidemiology.

To support all of these activities, we need to develop a careful system of checks and balances that includes *ad hoc* or project-specific funding among "users" and core support. Core support is critical to ensure that researchers themselves will continue to maintain capacity between demands to enable them to undertake publicly or academically important research for which an individual sponsor cannot be found (e.g., multisource drugs). These, then, represent the challenges that derive from the same limitations. The contributions reflected in this book provide more than ample justification for the efforts that will be involved, now that pharmacoepidemiology has clearly come of age, to be sure that it finds gainful employment!

Hugh H. Tilson, MD, DrPH

Contributors

ELIZABETH B. ANDREWS, MPH
Epidemiology, Information & Surveillance Division, Burroughs Wellcome Co., Research Triangle Park, North Carolina

SHARYN R. BATEY, PHARMD, MSPH
Hall Psychiatric Institute, University of South Carolina, Columbia, South Carolina

PAUL H. G. BEARDON, MSC, MPS
Research Coordinator, Medicines Evaluation and Monitoring Group, Department of Clinical Pharmacology, Ninewells Hospital and Medical School, Dundee, Scotland

PETER G. BERNAD, MD, MPH
Fairfax Medical Center, Fairfax City, Virginia

WAYNE BIGELOW, MS
Center for Health Systems Research and Analysis, Madison, Wisconsin

RUDOLF BRUPPACHER, MD
Pharmaco-Epidemiology and Central Drug Monitoring, CIBA-GEIGY LIMITED, Basel, Switzerland

GRAHAM H. BURTON, BSC, MRCP
Medicines Division, Department of Health and Social Security, London, England

JEFFREY L. CARSON, MD
Division of General Internal Medicine, UMDNJ-Robert Wood Johnson Medical School, New Brunswick, New Jersey

ELIZABETH A. CHRISCHILLES, PHD
Department of Preventive Medicine and Environmental Health, College of Medicine, University of Iowa, Iowa City, Iowa

WINANNE DOWNEY, BSP
Saskatchewan Prescription Drug Plan, Regina, Saskatchewan, Canada

JOHN M. EISENBERG, MD, MBA
Hospital of the University of Pennsylvania, Philadelphia, Pennsylvania

THADDEUS H. GRASELA, JR., PHARMD
The Pharmacoepidemiology Research Center, Millard Fillmore Hospital, Buffalo, New York

DAVID A. HENRY, MB, CHB
Senior Lecturer, Faculty of Medicine, Discipline of Clinical Pharmacology, University of Newcastle, New South Wales, Australia

MICHAEL C. JOSEPH, MD, MPH
Epidemiology, Information & Surveillance Division, Burroughs Wellcome Co., Research Triangle Park, North Carolina

DAVID H. LAWSON, MD
Professor and Consultant Physician, Royal Infirmary, Glasgow, Scotland; member, Committee on Safety of Medicines and chair, Committee on Review of Medicines, United Kingdom

JOHN R. LIVENGOOD, MD
Division of Immunization, Center for Prevention Services, Centers for Disease Control, Atlanta, Georgia

NEWELL E. MCELWEE, PHARMD
The Intermountain Regional Poison Control Center and the Colleges of Pharmacy and Medicine, University of Utah

ROBERT C. NELSON, PHD
Assistant Director, Office of Drug Evaluation II, Center for Drug Evaluation and Research, U.S. Food and Drug Administration, Rockville, Maryland

AUDREY SMITH ROGERS, PHD
Maryland State Health Department, AIDS Administration, Baltimore, Maryland

ROGER M. SACHS, MD, JD
Pfizer Pharmaceuticals, New York, New York

BARRY L. SHAPIRO, JD
Sills Beck Cummis Law Office, Newark, New Jersey

RONALD B. STEWART, MS
Professor and Chairman, Department of Pharmacy Practice, College of Pharmacy, University of Florida, Gainesville, Florida

BRIAN L. STROM, MD, MPH
Assistant Professor of Medicine and Pharmacology, and Co-Director, Clinical Epidemiology Unit, School of Medicine, University of Pennsylvania

Scott Stryker, MD, DrPH
Worldwide Regulatory Services, Product Safety and Surveillance, E. R. Squibb & Sons, New Brunswick, New Jersey

Patricia Tennis, PhD
Epidemiology, Information & Surveillance Division, Burroughs Wellcome Co., Research Triangle Park, North Carolina

Hugh H. Tilson, MD, DrPH
Director, Epidemiology, Information & Surveillance Division, Burroughs Wellcome Co., Research Triangle Park, North Carolina

Mari-Ann Wallander, BSc
Department of Drug Surveillance, AB Hässle, Mölndal, Sweden, and Department of Family Medicine, Akademiska sjukhuset, Uppsala, Sweden

Sidney H. Willig, JD, MA, BSPH, AB
Professor of Law and Director of Unit of Law and Health Sciences, Temple University, Philadelphia, Pennsylvania

Contents

SECTION FOUR–DRUGS, POPULATIONS, AND OUTCOMES: SPECIFIC STUDIES

Figures

Tables

Pharmacoepidemiology

SECTION ONE

Social Impact of Pharmacoepidemiology

Introduction

Professor David H. Lawson of Scotland reports on international progress in pharmacoepidemiology, but reminds us that the large automated data bases powerful enough to generate important signals or confirm signals from spontaneous voluntary monitoring exist primarily in North America. The Grahame-Smith Working Party in the United Kingdom has issued a clear call for structured postmarketing surveillance of new chemical entities, particularly those that will be widely used.

Dr. Robert C. Nelson from the U.S. Food and Drug Administration adds specific, powerful examples of current applications of data from multiple sources, including the spontaneous voluntary adverse reaction reporting system and its unique and powerful contribution as a signal generator.

Dr. Roger M. Sachs combines the skills and training of a physician and an attorney and directs them into the perspective of a user of the tools of pharmacoepidemiology. His report reflects his experience in public policy debate about the issue of the relative safety of various nonsteroidal antiinflammatory drugs. He does not debate the merits or legitimacy of the proposed policy; rather, his perspective is that such deliberations should consider the best information available and that pharmacoepidemiology has rendered such information accessible and affordable. Specifically, Dr. Sachs reports on the use of the large automated data bases linking automated prescription data with automated hospital diagnosis data and demonstrates that the spontaneous voluntary adverse reaction reports alone, fraught as they are with the vagaries of under- and overreporting and complexities of uncertain ascertainment of the denominator of exposed person, cannot and should not be expected to do the job.

1. *Pharmacoepidemiology and Public Policy*

DAVID H. LAWSON

It is a great honor to have given the Keynote Address at the 3rd International Conference on Pharmacoepidemiology to such a distinguished group of investigators. However, it is tempered by the realization that this puts me firmly in the position of being labeled an "elder statesman," whereas my self-image is of one who is still very much learning the skills of the trade. Perhaps these two apparently opposing views are not so incompatible as they appear to be at first sight. After all, the application of basic epidemiologic principles to the study of drug use is a relatively recent development—one which really began in earnest only a quarter of a century ago. I will not attempt to summarize the history of the subject at this time—others more qualified than I have done so elsewhere, and indeed at this very conference in 1986 your keynote speaker, Leighton Cluff, did just that. Who better to do it than the first major figure in the United States to address the problem in a systematic way?

In this chapter, I would like to bring to your attention several aspects of the subject that are of importance at the present time and then try the dangerous trick of looking ahead and seeing where we should be going in the 1990s. In doing so, I hasten to emphasize that my remarks should be seen as being purely personal and not in any way necessarily reflecting the views of any of the institutions with which I am now associated.

PUBLIC PERCEPTIONS OF DRUGS

I begin by reminding you that we live in a time when the public's perception of drugs and the pharmaceutical industry is far from a happy one. Increasingly both in the United States, in Europe and in Australasia drug abuse causes alarm and despondency amongst policymakers, who see no way of controlling the epidemic. The association between drug abuse and the AIDS complex increases concern, producing a general feeling of impotence as we fail to see any obvious way to stop the crisis getting quite out of hand. In parallel with this concern about drug abuse and its consequences, the public is increasingly exposed to reports of new suspected adverse drug reactions which are treated in a most irresponsible way by the media. If a drug is removed from sale because either its manufacturers or national regulators feel that the risk-benefit spectrum is no longer in its favor, there is a blaze of publicity about "bad drugs" and about the failure of government to protect us, the public, from them. We rarely, if ever, hear about bad prescribers, who may have given the drug in excessive dosage to inappropriate patients for longer than advised by the manufacturers or regulators. Nor do we hear about bad patients, who have found the drug to be helpful so have given it to friends/relatives, who have subsequently suffered in consequence. I do not mean to suggest that these latter are common causes of serious adverse drug reactions, but rather to emphasize that in virtually all instances when serious reactions lead to drug withdrawal, the issues are complex, incompletely elucidated, and rarely simply instances of otherwise healthy patients taking a prescribed drug in the correct dosage for the prescribed period and suffering quite unforeseen and unforeseeable consequences.

If the public perception of the pharmaceutical industry is indeed as bad as I suggest, and the media's view of drug toxicity quite as distorted as it appears to be, we have a major problem on our hands—one which will not go away on its own and one which will have to be carefully studied and defined if we are going to solve it in the near future. What then are the constituents of the problem posed by drug toxicity in the late 1980s? I suggest these are that

1. the public has become fixed in the idea that drugs can solve all ills physical and social (a "pill for every ill" mentality pervades our culture)
2. the public has naive faith in premarketing testing of new medicines ("you've tested these medicines in so many animals over many years, they must be safe")
3. the public by contrast has very great faith in our drug regulatory agencies' abilities to filter out all potentially toxic drugs while not preventing powerful new compounds gaining a license lest some might not receive their benefits

These are the concepts with which all who are interested in the provision of safe, effective, and high quality medicines are going to have to battle in the 1990s. How are we going to approach the challenge? Clearly it will require efforts on many fronts. However, it will be unsuccessful if we do not develop good information systems. Here is where the pharmacoepidemiologists come into their own.

PHARMACOEPIDEMIOLOGY

Drug Utilization Studies

Our first duty is to obtain good information on drug use patterns in the community. This is an area where most previous workers have feared to tread, claiming with considerable justification that their prime objective is to study the safety and efficacy of drug treatment rather than the prescribing patterns of doctors. I can understand this view, and indeed sympathize with the expressed feeling that we might alienate the very prescribers upon whom we

Table 1. Antidiabetic Drug Treatment: Variation by Region in Norway, Sweden, and N. Ireland

	Norway	Sweden	N. Ireland
Population (millions)	3.86	8.11	1.49
No. of regions	20	8	8
Insulin*			
range	1.4–4.7	6.2–8.0	3.2–4.3
mean	3.5	6.9	3.7
Oral agents			
range	4.9–12.8	11.1–19.5	3.6–5.4
mean	7.3	15.8	4.2

Source: Bergman et al.[1]
*Defined daily dose/1000 persons/day.

rely for our information by appearing to scrutinize their prescribing habits too closely. This in turn could jeopardize their cooperation with studies of greater interest to us as scientists. Nevertheless, several studies, including those by Wade and his colleagues in Northern Ireland in the 1970s have emphasized the impressive variability in drug use in that province. For example, he showed major variation in oral hypoglycemic drug prescribing in different Irish regions. This lead to a collaborative study with Norwegian and Swedish authors giving interesting overall pictures of the inter- and intracountry variations in antidiabetic therapy (Table 1). Studies such as these force us to view that more detailed enquiry in this area is justified and indeed indicated. We do not, however, need to look as far afield as Europe to notice major differences in prescribing habits. Look, for instance, at the data on IV fluid use accumulated by the medical monitoring wing of the Boston Collaborative Drug Surveillance Program (Table 2). Here major differences in IV fluid administration were noted between hospitals. Indeed even in my own city, two collaborating hospitals, which showed virtually identical drug use in all other respects, displayed a twofold difference in IV fluid use (Table 3). This in turn has considerable economic consequences which are often overlooked. Indeed when you compare the drug use patterns in apparently identical patients in medical wards in Glasgow and Boston, one sees major disparities in prescribing patterns (Table 4). We do not know whether the U.S. patients benefited more from the greater drug use; we certainly know that they experienced more

Table 2. Intravenous Fluid Use: Medical Wards, Boston Collaborative Drug Surveillance Program

Hospital		IV Fluids		Hospital		IV Fluids	
		No.	%			No.	%
U.S.	1	1871	53.7	N.Z.	1	260	22.7
U.S.	2	521	51.4	Scot	1	156	16.2
U.S.	3	364	37.5	N.Z.	2	30	14.0
U.S.	4	589	32.0	Isr	1	61	12.9
U.S.	5	754	28.1	Scot	2	71	7.8
U.S.	6	687	24.7	Isr	2	176	7.4

Source: Lawson.[2]

Table 3. Drug Use in Medical Wards, Scots Hospitals, Boston Collaborative Drug Surveillance Program

	Scots 1		Scots 2	
Drug	**No.**	**%**	**No.**	**%**
Nitrazepam	287	29.8	270	29.7
KCl	278	28.8	247	27.2
Furosemide	224	23.2	198	21.8
Ampicillin	164	17.0	170	18.7
Diazepam	147	15.3	146	16.1
Digoxin	179	18.6	138	15.2
Paracetamol	121	12.6	118	13.0
IV fluids	156	16.2	71	7.8**

**X^2 – 30.9, $p < 0.01$.

adverse effects during hospitalization (Table 5) and that the financial costs were greater than their Scots counterparts. It seems to me, therefore, that we pharmacoepidemiologists could, with profit, turn at least a small part of our attention to investigating these wide discrepancies in prescribing habits. The results obtained in these studies (which could be relatively inexpensive to conduct) would be most useful and interesting to many prescribers and also to those who pay for our health care systems.

The expertise developed in studies such as I have outlined could also be applied to scrutinizing the uptake of new medicines as they are introduced into a community, thus facilitating one of our major aims—to learn about the

Table 4. Drug Use in Medical Wards: International Comparison

	Scots		U.S.	
	No.	%	No.	%
Patients*	721		1442	
Drugs				
pre-hospital	1.2		2.0	
in hospital	4.5		9.4	
on discharge	1.3		2.1	
>4 drugs pre-hospital	52	7.7	283	21
>10 drugs in hospital	63	9	603	42

Source: Lawson and Jick.[3]
*Matched 1:2—age/sex/death/1st diagnosis/duration of stay.

Table 5. Adverse Drug Reactions in Medical Wards: International Comparison

	Scots		U.S.	
	No.	%	No.	%
Patients	721		1442	
ADRs				
patients	107	15.0	370	26.0
heparin	2/14	14.3	29/188	15.4
furosemide	19/155	12.3	34/280	12.2
digoxin	12/111	10.8	46/415	11.1
ampicillin	11/107	10.3	24/223	10.8
diazepam	1/91	1.1	22/420	5.2

effectiveness and safety of new medicines as rapidly as possible after their introduction to the marketplace. In turn, this would allow us to improve on the trend of the last decade whereby we have just about acquired sufficient information on several drugs to be able to use them wisely and relatively safely by the time that their useful life is past. Far from going away, this problem is going to get worse as our premarketing studies are prolonged and a drug's effective patent life is reduced. That is to say, we will have to improve our techniques just to stay still, and hopefully we can do better than that. My first major message today must therefore be:

> Pharmacoepidemiology will not prosper if it develops as an intellectual subject which plots the history of why drugs fell from favor. It must be a live and contemporary subject providing answers to current problems of drug use and drug safety in real time.

Adverse Reaction Studies

I should now like to consider the question of drug toxicity, a major problem for the pharmacoepidemiologist. It is clear that we have good information on the common acute toxicity expected from most drugs in widespread use today. Studies such as those conducted by the Boston Collaborative Drug Surveillance Program and others in the 1970s and early 1980s clearly covered this ground at least for hospitalized patients[4] and it seems to me that there is little need to repeat those general nontargeted in-hospital monitoring studies on any large scale. Personally, I would like to see routine in-hospital monitoring of some 20,000 medical inpatients undertaken in the United States or in Europe under the auspices of the Boston Collaborative Drug Surveillance Program or other similar groups with similar expertise on a regular basis once each decade or so. This would update the available information to include many newer drugs and possible interactions and would, I suspect, give much information of great value, particularly if undertaken in Europe where there has been a tendency for new drugs to be licensed earlier than here in the United States!

For a few drugs which have been around for a long time, we have reasonably good information about their long-term safety derived from formal studies of large cohorts. I am thinking of oral contraceptives, cholesterol-lowering agents, oral hypoglycemics, some beta-receptor blocking agents and some H_2-receptor antagonists. Almost invariably these studies have been slow to start and have proven very costly to conduct. They have also not been free of controversy as regards their interpretation. This is an area which requires more attention and education of the public and of physicians alike. Let me give you an example from a study I conducted recently with some colleagues. It was a nonexperimental postmarketing surveillance cohort study of some 10,000 cimetidine recipients and a similar number of age/sex-matched controls.[5] We recorded all events occurring in such patients in the year after entry (and continue to follow up takers on a long-term basis) (Table 6). Analysis of the resulting information revealed, among many other associations, a twofold

Table 6. Cimetidine Postmarketing Surveillance Study: First Year, Significant Events

	Takers	Controls
Number	9,928	9351
Follow-up (%)	98.8	97.7
Diagnoses	15,325	5002
Deaths (%)	3.8	2.1
Inpatients (%)	18	8
Outpatients (%)	39	21

excess of lung cancer in the takers (Table 7). This seems predictable and due to confounding by cigarette smoking, cimetidine tending to identify peptic ulcer patients who have a high prevalence of smokers and are thereby at a high risk of developing lung cancer. In presenting these results, my colleagues and I are often accused of "explaining away" this association. We are asked, "How can you be sure that the drug alone or in association with cigarette consumption did not play a significant role in the onset of the cancer?" This is one problem that will face us all as our studies get better and more sophisticated. We will therefore be required to put more effort into educating our readers well into the coming decades! This educational effort will need to run parallel to the development of more formal and economic systems for assessing effectiveness and, more important, safety of drugs used long-term in reasonably healthy subjects.

What does the public and the profession need from us in the 1990s? There are several areas of importance which need a mention. I make no apology for starting by commenting on spontaneous reporting schemes as these still give us very valuable information about new drugs.

Spontaneous Reporting Schemes for Suspected ADRs

Most major Western nations have such schemes in operation at the present time. They are generally accepted to be very valuable alerting systems, signalling possible drug-related events in the early years after marketing of a new chemical entity. Their great strength lies in the vast populations kept under observation by potential reporters. They have proven of greatest benefit when signalling rare events, usually occurring relatively soon after exposure to the suspect agent. They do, however, provide only incomplete (partial) numerators. Skillful attempts can be made to estimate an appropriate denominator

Table 7. Cimetidine Postmarketing Surveillance Study: First Year, Incidence of Cancer

Patients with Cancer	Takers	Controls	Ratio
Lung	50	27	1.7
Lymphoma	40	12	3.1
Rectum	21	15	1.3
Colon	20	9	2.1
Pancreas	11	5	2.1

Table 8. Adverse Reaction Reporting Rates: International Comparison

Country	Population	Annual Reports	Reports/ million/yr	Reports 1000 MDs/yr	% Hospital MDs
Denmark	5.12	2,087	407.6	187.2	50
N.Z.	3.03	1,160	383.2	141.4	38
Sweden	8.32	2,785	334.7	167.3	75
U.K.	56.10	14,701	262.5	163.3	19
Australia	14.93	3,715	248.8	83.6	48
Finland	4.81	726	150.9	80.0	49
U.S.	226.54	33,314	147.0	57.6	7
France	54.09	4,198	77.6	29.4	71

Source: Griffin.[6]

and suggest a rate of ADRs with the suspected drug. These, however, usually fail to emphasize that the derived rate is based on a variety of assumptions which have some validity, but which give a result with, at best, extremely wide confidence intervals!

In the United Kingdom, we now have over 200,000 suspected ADRs on file, in the United States you have well over a quarter of a million, and other countries also have large data bases—notably, the Scandinavian countries and Australasia. A comparison of national reporting rates expressed by population and by physician recently published by Griffin[6] makes interesting reading, showing as it does substantial differences in these factors between countries (Table 8). As the data bases enlarge, they are usually computerized to ease handling and facilitate analysis. We all know there to be a tendency to place greater weight on printout from a computer than the handwritten word. Therefore, we must always remember that the quality of the final data (the printout) is not better than, and indeed may occasionally be poorer than, that of the original source. It is important, therefore, to keep in mind that these spontaneous reports are often brief and may well require to be amplified by more detailed study to prevent erroneous conclusions arising from their uninformed or noncritical use. Ideally, before any major regulatory action is considered, detailed follow-up of individual reactions should have been undertaken by qualified personnel. Sadly, this is not always feasible at present. The spontaneous report, which was orginally viewed as an "alerting signal," stands the risk of gaining too much credibility and becoming regarded by some as indicating a definite causal link. In situations where the adverse event experienced by a drug recipient is known to be associated both with the disease under treatment and the class of drug given, we have real problems. The best example of this is upper GI bleeding and NSAIDs. Here, in my view, no amount of massaging of spontaneous reports is going to be helpful in *understanding* the problem. In particular, from spontaneous reports no valid comparisons can now be made between different NSAIDs as regards their potential gastrointestinal toxicity because we usually have no idea of the previous medical history of the affected patient and the biases of the prescriber in choosing one particular drug over another.

Think for a moment of the situation which would arise were a new antiinflammatory agent to be discovered that was free of GI tract toxicity, both in animals and in clinical trials. As soon as it is licensed, it would be given to all those who needed analgesia and had known peptic ulcers with previous perforations or bleeding or severe rheumatoid disease or were anticoagulated—all patients at high risk of developing GI bleeding. Soon spontaneous reports of this suspected ADR would arrive at the Food and Drug Administration, Committee on the Safety of Medicines, and other regulatory authorities. Within months, this drug would probably look distinctly less "clean" than many NSAIDs, purely as a result of selection bias, a bias that would be exceedingly difficult, if not impossible, to control from within the spontaneous reports themselves. Indeed, the only way to solve this problem would be from other outside sources.

Despite all the problems of spontaneous reporting systems, they are clearly here to stay and justifiably so. What can we do to improve them? One of the interesting findings of Griffin and Weber[7] was the relatively low frequency of reports from hospital physicians in the United Kingdom. As most major diseases lead to hospitalization (or at least hospital contact), one would expect a big contribution to the system by such doctors—not so, however. We have therefore been encouraging dermatologists, hematologists, nephrologists, neurologists, hepatologists, and ophthalmologists in particular to be aware of possible drug hazards and report to the system any suspicions they might have. I think if we are seen to use the resulting information responsibly, we will encourage better compliance.

> It is therefore up to us as pharmacoepidemiologists to ensure that spontaneous reports of suspected ADRs are used wisely in the full knowledge of their substantial limitations.

There are three main areas which particularly concern me in our current use of spontaneous reports of suspected ADRs.

The first we have already touched upon: the inappropriateness of comparing estimated rates of reports of common suspected adverse events between different drugs of the same class, a problem most commonly seen with GI bleeding and NSAIDs.

The second regards our use of reports of new suspected reactions in drugs which have been in widespread use for many years. I shall give an example of this with the nontricyclic antidepressant nomifensine and its association with autoimmune hemolytic anemia in a moment. But many here can think of other examples of this problem.

The third regards data for new drugs during their first two to three years after marketing—their so-called vulnerable period. It is at this time that scattered reports may occur with sufficient frequency to sound an alarm bell. Regulatory authorities become alert to the possible problem, and if the numerator appears to be large in relation to the apparent use of the medicine, action may be taken. This may be justified, but often what is needed at this stage is

Table 9. Large Data Sources for Postmarketing Surveillance

	No. (millions)	Year
1. Group Health Cooperative, Puget Sound	0.3	1976
2. Medicaid		
COMPASS	6.0	1980
Tennessee	0.4	
3. Minneapolis	0.5	1982
4. Kaiser-Permanente		
Los Angeles	1.6	1983
Portland	0.2	
5. Saskatchewan	1.0	1986

Source: Tilson.[8]

time—time to arrange follow-up of suspected cases and to seek information from other data bases.

> It is therefore our duty as pharmacoepidemiologists to ensure that other sources of information are available and can be interrogated in a reasonably rapid time frame. (Good data in six years is no substitute for usable data in six months.)

Large Automated Information Retrieval and Record Linkage Schemes

What, then, are these alternative sources of information? In my view, in the long-term, we must rely on large automated information systems. These are developed to the highest degree here in North America. They depend upon others to collect information on drug use and on hospitalization occurrences for their own purposes. No one would go to the expense of setting such systems up purely for the delectation of pharmacoepidemiologists. However, if we are lucky, we will be able to gain access to them for our purposes at relatively low cost. Given that most such programs serve a defined population, we are in perfect shape not only to undertake long-term cohort studies of recipients of new or old drugs, but also to undertake case-control studies or even in-depth case history reviews. Knowing the population base, we can derive age- and sex-specific rates for common events and we can look for attributable risks as well as the more ubiquitous relative risks of nonpopulation-based case-control studies. To be of greatest assistance, these systems must derive from large populations, at least of the order of 0.5 million persons and possibly even 5 million or more in due course. Ideally, they must have data accumulated over several years and available in an accessible format. They should include patient-specific drug histories, all hospital discharge diagnoses, and death certificate information.

There are several examples of this working well in the United States, notably with Group Health Cooperative of Puget Sound and its link with the Boston Collaborative Drug Surveillance Program and with some Medicaid data sets (Table 9). There is also great potential with new HMOs developing in the United States and in the Province of Saskatchewan in Canada, if only these can be realized. Unfortunately, we in the United Kingdom have so far failed to get such a system off the ground. It is to be hoped that the group originally developed in Scotland by the late James Crooks will expand in the near future and become the first U.K. record-linkage scheme in operation. In developing these schemes several important points must be considered.

First, in all cases it is necessary to be able to refer to the original case notes of selected patients to verify diagnoses and details of current and previous drug treatments.

Second, it is highly desirable to be able to follow patients from birth to death. We should, for example, be able to link records of drug exposure during a person's working life with disease outcome, both before and after retirement. We must also include pregnant patients and be able to link maternal drug exposure to fetal outcome. Absence of either of these criteria can seriously impair the usefulness of these new systems.

Third, it is with analysis of these large data bases that we must face up to a major difficulty. If we accept the concept that, on balance, given their widespread use and abuse, drugs are remarkably safe, we must also accept that many of our studies will be "negative" studies. The question in many people's minds then will be, Is your negative study "negative" because nothing is happening or because you cannot detect that which is happening because of inherent faults or defects in the system? In order to be sure of their reliability and utility, I would like to see published several analyses defining and quantitating well-known drug hazards such as hemorrhage after oral anticoagulant therapy. These analyses would be expensive in working hours at the outset, but in the long-term the money would be well spent. It is not reinventing the wheel. Rather it is assuring ourselves and, more important, others of the potential of our systems. Having assured ourselves that a negative study means what it appears to mean, what other pieces of information can we obtain from these large data sources? There are three areas worth emphasizing.

First, they could be of great use in helping regulators and members of the pharmaceutical industry in understanding the meaning of early spontaneous reports of ADRs after marketing of a new chemical entity. To do so, the new drug will clearly have to be used in the monitored population, and the analyses of data within the system will have to be rapid, efficient, and accurate. This means final reports must be possible within months of an alert being sounded and that, in turn, means dedicated full-time staff and adequate computer backup. This is not the place for the part-time amateur.

Second, they provide one of the only ways open to us to evaluate drug hazards in pregnancy. This is a particularly difficult area to research nowadays. Analysis of routinely prerecorded exposure information could give us the ideal answer to this vexed problem. We badly need this type of information if we are to prevent another Debendox/Bendectin saga, although perhaps you will forgive me if, as a European, I beg leave to doubt whether any good data will ever prevent the sort of consequences we have seen here in the United

Table 10. Spontaneous Reports of Hemolysis: Nomifensine

	Year								
	1977	1978	1979	1980	1981	1982	1983	1984	1985
Prescriptions (× 10^3)	18	227	190	188	165	202	245	251	191
Reactions									
hemolysis	0	1	1	0	0	2	5	16	23
hepatotoxicity	0	3	3	4	4	2	8	10	17
others	2	3	4	6	6	2	2	18	12
Total	2	7	8	10	10	6	15	44	52

Source: U.K. data.

States surrounding emotive areas such as potentially drug-induced fetal damage.

Third, such systems also give us a unique ability to investigate the consequencies of regulatory action. I have yet to see them used in this way; however, the opportunity is there and could be used. Let us consider, by way of an example, the antidepressant nomifensine to which I have already referred. This nontricyclic antidepressant was first marketed in the United Kingdom in 1977 and was withdrawn worldwide for safety reasons in January 1986. The reasons for this decision were many and varied. Spontaneous reports of acute hemolytic anemia (AHA) thought to be due to nomifensine were a major factor in the final decision of the company.[9] U.K. spontaneous reports are shown in Table 10. You will see a major increase in reports in 1984 and 1985, despite usage patterns in the form of prescriptions remaining fairly constant. Why was this so? Was this a new event arising only in long-term users, or in those exposed on more than one occasion to the drug? Was it the result of publicity in medical or lay press? Did it reflect a general concern about all antidepressants after withdrawal of one (zimeldine, causing Guillain-Barré syndrome)? Who can tell? The association between nomifensine and AHA was reported in a case study from France in *Lancet*,[10] and the same workers subsequently documented an antinomifensine antibody present in serum of their patient.[11] By April 1985, a detailed review of the subject showing metabolite-specific antibodies in patients with nomifensine-dependent immune hemolytic anemia was published in the *New England Journal of Medicine*.[12] Publication of these and other articles around 1984–85 almost certainly gave rise to at least part of the observed surge in reports. That is to say, the increased number of reports could have reflected but did not necessarily reflect *more* actual cases. How could large information systems help us here? They could have allowed us to review details of therapy among all nomifensive recipients in a large population, paying particular attention to the presence of AHA and other blood problems, and thus permit estimation of the risk in that population—a retrospective study, if you will. This would have been most helpful if the analyses came rapidly to the company or the regulators. It was not, however, available to the company: the drug was not used here in the United States for any length of time, and as yet no others have on-line sophisticated large record linkage systems. At the time of its withdrawal by the company, nomifensine appeared to be an effective antidepressant drug which had been used extensively for nine years. It was known to cause two types of hemolytic anemia: one a mild, gradual onset hemolysis, the other an acute, severe condition which may be fatal. The likely frequency of these reactions appeared to be low (1:10,000 prescriptions). On the basis of these data, to withdraw the drug is easy and should lead to cessation of reported adverse effects. However, what happens to recipients following withdrawal? We do not know. No one seems to have done a postwithdrawal surveillance study: an audit, if you will, of the company decision to withdraw. In this case, I would be interested in the proportion of former recipients who discontinued all antidepressant medication (and hence presumably did not need long-term therapy). What proportion converted on to older medications (e.g., amitriptyline/imipramine) for which we have more clinical experience and so a better overall feel for their risk/benefit status. What proportion converted to newer antidepressants for which we have no or insufficient experience on their safety? What proportion committed suicide as a result of inadequately treated depression? And so on. In other words, what were the risks experienced by this cohort of former recipients after withdrawal of the drug? The only practical way of obtaining this knowledge would be in large information systems.

Linked Multipurpose Data Schemes

Although several large data sources are in existence at present and more are in the offing, as far as I know, there has been little effort expended on arranging links between the systems. This is understandable but regrettable, and I think this is an area that deserves more concern. Given that any one HMO will at best have access to perhaps a million patients, it will on its own be insufficiently large to address important issues of rare adverse events. For example, a recent analysis of the Puget Sound data showed some 391 blood dyscrasias in 250,000 patients over 10 years (Figure 1). Of these, only 26 (6.6%) were probably drug-induced (ignoring for the moment dyscrasias linked to antitumor chemotherapy).

Thus, this major program with a very high reputation in the field is unable, by virtue of limited size, to mount a case-control study of agranulocytosis or aplastic anemia in a meaningful time frame. From the data presented, however, it seems that several HMOs acting in concert could address the issue. Were this possible, it would be much less expensive than conducting formal patient interviews as part of an ongoing case-control surveillance program such as that undertaken by the Slone Drug Epidemiology Unit in Boston. This is not to criticize that program in any way; indeed, I have had close personal links with late Denis Slone and with Syd Shapiro for many years and have been impressed with their progress in this difficult area. Nonetheless, it seems likely that the expense and problems of data acquisition by patient interview could

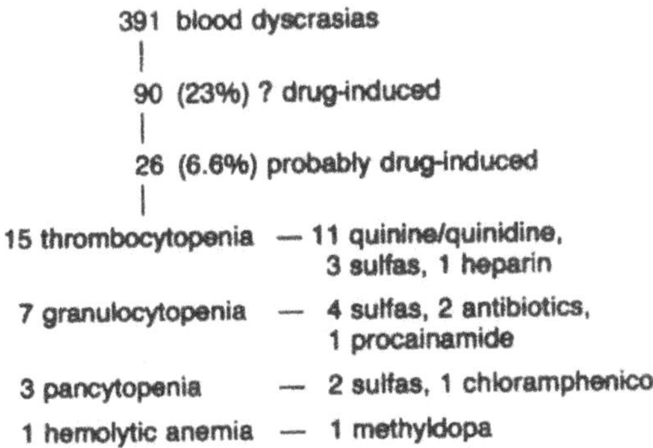

Figure 1. Blood disorders in HMO of 300,000, 1972–1981. From Danielson et al.[13]

be avoided by automated retrieval from several HMOs were they to be linked even in an informal way.

Linkage between large information systems will give us another urgently needed benefit, the ability to rapidly test hypotheses generated in one system with information from another. This ability will obviate at least partially one of my major concerns as a pharmacoepidemiologist: the problems arising if we get our studies wrong. At present, the consequences of error in this type of study are often much greater than would be the case were an animal experiment to go wrong. This is simply because of the ease of repeating animal experiments compared with the difficulties in validating nonexperimental data in different data sets. Let us hope that such developments become feasible in the future.

Over the years, we have seen many large expensive programs set up to study one area in great detail. Examples would include the University Group Diabetes Project, The Metoprolol Secondary Prevention (MI) Study, and The International Agranulocytosis & Aplastic Anemia Study. All share several features in common: long gestation periods, difficulty in data acquisition, variability in outcome between centers, large expense, and substantial controversy generated by their final conclusions. It seems likely that we will see more such studies in the future. I feel, however, that in this last decade of the 20th century, with costs of health care spiraling everywhere, it is up to us as a relatively new specialty to set a good example to the others. Should we not be exercising our influence toward achieving attainable goals at economic costs? Giant, single-drug or single-event studies costing several million dollars or pounds or yen or whatever seem to me often to be a waste of resources. Better by far surely to direct adequate funds into several multipurpose schemes than to carry on as at present. We have the technology to answer many of our problems at low cost through observational studies. Perhaps these do not give as perfect an answer as the randomized, controlled double-blind trials (RCCT) of our more experimentally minded colleagues. Nevertheless, once several good controlled trials have been undertaken and have demonstrated efficacy of a medication in a closely defined population, it is the duty of the pharmacoepidemiologist to observe populations of users and determine by observational means whether the results of the RCCT in the idealized type of population studied actually apply to other different subsets of recipients. Our large data bases either on their own or working in loose federations should be capable of answering these questions at relatively low cost.

The Pharmacoepidemiologist in Industry and Regulatory Affairs

From the remarks I have already made, it will be obvious to you that I feel the time has arrived for pharmacoepidemiologists to leave their ivory towers, where they can conduct "interesting" studies at a relatively leisurely pace in congenial surroundings, and infiltrate two areas where their expertise is urgently required: the pharmaceutical industry and the regulatory authorities. Some have made the move already and have been instrumental in demonstrating the usefulness and relevance of their training in these new environments. We need more to make this move in the coming years.

Speaking as one who advises our regulatory agency on new and old drug license applications, I am continually amazed by the poor quality of many submissions even from first-class firms. We hear continually of the increasing delays in processing new drug applications through Food and Drug Administration or Committee on the Safety of Medicines. The implications are that the delays are all due to faults in the regulatory agencies. Certainly, these agencies are not without fault! Nevertheless, there is ample evidence that a substantial proportion of the delays arises from poor applications. Trained pharmacoepidemiologists have much to teach industry and could benefit it by helping to minimize the delays at this stage in license applications.

At the same time, pharmacoepidemiologists could, by exercising their expertise, save industry substantial amounts of time and money by advising reduction in the number of methodologically flawed studies currently undertaken. These flawed studies are particularly prevalent in the field of adverse reactions. It is my view that most large national or international pharmaceutical houses should now employ one or more trained pharmacoepidemiologists. This will be one of their more cost-effective appointments!

Similarly, regulatory authorities also urgently need access on a full-time basis to the expertise of the pharmacoepidemiologist if they are to avoid the pitfalls of overinterpretation of their spontaneous reports of suspected adverse drug reactions and also to avoid making too rigid demands for postmarketing surveillance studies on too many compounds for too long periods of follow-up. In my judgment, a trained pharmacoepidemiologist would be a very valuable addition to the permanent staff of any large regulatory authority in the 1990s.

Table 11. Road Traffic Accidents, Western Europe, 1984

Country	Deaths per 100 million km	Total Deaths
U.K.	1.0	5,633
Denmark	1.2	706
W. Germany	1.6	8,942
Italy	1.8	6,928
France	3.1	10,961
Spain	6.3	9,419
Greece	12.0	1,511

Source: Toomey C: Spotlight on deaths on European roads. *Sunday Times*, July 12, 1987.

RISK PERCEPTION AND THE PHARMACOEPIDEMIOLOGIST

Having covered a large area rather patchily, I would like briefly to broaden the discussion somewhat. The size of this conference alone attests to the interest in our subject and gives me at least great hope for the future. With much ingenuity and moderate effort, we should be in a position in the near future to capitalize on existing information systems set up for other purposes to give a fairly precise quantitation of the variations in drug usage in different parts of our countries and also of adverse drug effects, both of old drugs and, perhaps, more important, of new drugs, these hopefully being accomplished within a meaningful time scale after release of a new chemical entity to the marketplace. What will we do with the resulting information, particularly the adverse reaction data? Clearly, we will disseminate it to prescribers, to regulators, and (possibly) to patients. It is in this area that we meet what I see as the biggest problem of the decade to come: the relative inability of patients and near total unwillingness of the media to relate risks of drug therapy to the possible benefits sought and to the risks of everyday living—risks such as those of smoking, alcohol consumption, car driving, or crossing the road. This entire area of risk perception has been relatively neglected until recently and, in my view, it is one in which pharmacoepidemiologists must play an increasing role in the years to come.

We live in a period where there are increasing concerns over risks and hazards arising from technological advances. People seem to accept certain risks, e.g., those of car driving, if the risk taker appears to be in charge of the situation. By contrast, they abreact violently if placed at risk by unknown forces. Consider the United Kingdom, for example. In 1984, some 5633 people died on our roads, a rate of 1.0 per 100 million km traveled by car drivers. Comparable data for other Western European countries were 1.2 (Denmark), 1.6 (W. Germany), 1.8 (Italy), 3.1 (France), 6.3 (Spain), and 12.0 (Greece). Total deaths seen in these countries are as shown in Table 11. The average member of the U.K. population seems to accept these 5633 deaths with equanimity. By contrast, what an uproar there was when 180-odd people died in a car ferry disaster in winter 1986, the first to hit that company in its entire existence, during which time it had carried many millions of passengers safely.

Now, of course, that was a disaster and a tragedy. My concern, however, is that we get the entire issue out of perspective.

As evidence to show our lack of perspective in this area of risk perception, let me remind you that recent best estimates suggest that we spend 2500 times as much money on assessing safety in the pharmaceutical industry as is spent on safety in the agricultural industry. I am not suggesting that we reduce our expenditure on drug safety, merely wondering if an odds ratio of 2500 is an appropriate one.

Perhaps I should conclude now by making a plea to the pharmacoepidemiologists of the 1990s: Pursue your studies enthusiastically yet always be mindful of their costs in relation to the possible benefit to accrue to patients from the results. Be reluctant to find yourselves conducting vastly expensive studies to try to save some medicine whose time to be laid to rest has clearly arrived! Keep your minds clearly on our main objectives which have been so well summarized by Hugh Tilson in the past. These are to learn as much as we can as accurately as we can and as quickly as we can about new drugs so that we can use them appropriately in the best interests of our patients. At the same time we must be in the vanguard of attempts to educate ourselves and our patients on the true magnitude of the hazards which will face them if they take our medicines, either appropriately or inappropriately, relating these risks to the benefits to be obtained from treatment and to the risks inherent in everyday living.

REFERENCES

1. Bergman U, Elmes P, Halse M, et al: The management of drug consumption: Drugs for diabetes in Northern Ireland, Norway & Sweden. *Europ J Clin Pharmacol* 1975;8:83–89.
2. Lawson DH: Intravenous fluids in medical inpatients. *Brit J Clin Pharmac* 1977;4:299–303.
3. Lawson DH, Jick H: Drug prescribing in hospitals: An international comparison. *Amer J Pub Health* 1976;66:644–648.
4. Cohen MR: A compilation of abstracts and index published by the Boston Collaborative Drug Surveillance Program – 1966–85. *Hospital Pharmacy* 1986;21:497–559.
5. Colin-Jones DG, Langman MJS, Lawson DH, et al: Postmarketing surveillance of the safety of cimetidine: twelve-month morbidity report. *Q J Med* 1985;215:253–268.
6. Griffin JP: Survey of the spontaneous drug reaction reporting schemes in fifteen countries. *Brit J Clin Pharmac* 1986;22:83s-100s.
7. Griffin JP: Weber JCP: Voluntary systems of adverse reaction reporting. Part II. *Adv Drug React & Ac Pois Rev* 1986;1:23–55.
8. Tilson, HH: *Post-Marketing Surveillance: The Way Forward, Center for Medicines Research Annual Lecture, 1986*. London, Center for Medicines Research, 1986, p. 14.

9. Committee on Safety of Medicines. Update: Withdrawal of nomifensine. *Brit Med J* 1986;293:41.
10. Bournerias F, Habibi B. Nomifensine-induced immune hemolytic anaemia and impaired renal function. *Lancet* 1979;2:95–96.
11. Habibi B, Cartron JP, Bretagne M, et al: Anti-nomifensine antibody causing immune hemolytic and renal failure. *Vox Sanguinis* 1981;40:79–84.
12. Salama A, Mueller-Eckhardt C. The role of metabolite-specific antibodies in nomifensine-dependent immune hemolytic anaemias. *N Engl J Med* 1985;313:469–474.
13. Danielson DA, Douglas SW, Herzog P, et al: Drug induced blood disorders. *JAMA* 1984;252:3257–3260.

2. *Risk Assessment of New Drugs, Pharmacoepidemiology, and Regulatory Decisionmaking*

ROBERT C. NELSON

INTRODUCTION

The safety or risk assessment of a pharmacotherapeutic agent begins early in its development, matures during its premarketing clinical evaluation, and continues throughout its use cycle. The practice of pharmacoepidemiology is the art of using the sciences and the tools of science to generate information about pharmaceutical outcomes, including associated risks, in the postmarketing environment. A pharmacoepidemiologist must be capable of functioning with a matrix constructed of three components: a knowledge base, a conceptual framework, and an interpretive framework. From this perspective one can establish surveillance schemes, or understand a posed research question, select strategies, apply methodologies, and interpret the results of purposeful investigations. The appropriately interpreted results of a properly conducted risk assessment when conveyed to the risk manager can be used in regulatory decisionmaking. Risk assessors should strive to provide a best estimate and the range of uncertainty. From the regulator's perspective decisionmakers must choose the proper amount of conservatism in setting the standard.

The existing U.S. statutes and regulations provide the basic requirements for determining the safety and efficacy of new drug products. The process includes the development of safety and efficacy data during the investigational or IND phase, and the submission of these data in support of a marketing application—the new drug application (NDA). As a basic principle, the sponsor of a new drug or biologic bears the responsibility for identifying and characterizing actual and potential safety issues associated with the use of the product that is proposed for market approval.

The evaluation of a new drug during its development and throughout the regulatory review process involves a continual risk analysis, which is later coupled with a benefit analysis. These culminate with the ultimate risk/benefit

Phase IV studies, postmarketing surveillance and drug use experience

Phase II and III human clinical trials

Phase I human clinical trials

In vitro and preclinical toxicity testing

Initial evaluation

Figure 1. New drug development and review of growth of drug knowledge.

determination, which takes the form of a decision to allow or not allow marketing of the drug product. If marketed, the basis for that decision appears in the labeling that is approved for the product.

Simplistically, these risk analyses flow along a continuum, from *in vitro* testing (e.g., mutagenicity), to preclinical animal testing (e.g., toxicity and carcinogenicity), through the three phases of premarketing clinical testing (in humans), to Phase IV studies and postmarketing surveillance efforts. In actuality there is a coordinated interaction between specific sets of preclinical tests and each phase of clinical testing. In the ideal, there should be coordinated interaction between premarket testing and postmarket observation.

Figure 1 depicts an inverse pyramid. When read from the bottom, it pertains to a process which can be termed either new drug development and review *or* the growth of drug knowledge. Each step up is considered possible only when the preceeding is fully explored and a sense of understanding is obtained. A risk analysis occurs at each level.

Thus far, I have used the words *safety* and *risk* interchangeably and that may lead to misunderstanding. Safety is the reciprocal of risk. In order to judge a drug's safety one must identify, characterize, and assess (quantitatively and qualitatively) its risk. Then a conceptual conversion to safety needs to be made.

To further clarify terms, I use *risk analysis* as a bi-compartment concept that includes risk assessment and risk management. *Risk assessment* includes the identification and characterization of the hazards (risks). *Risk management* involves a decision based upon the risk assessment. A benefit analysis is similar in structure. The risk-to-benefit decisionmaking requires the judgmental balancing of the results from both forms of analyses.

Drugs make up the only group of chemicals that are deliberately used or are administered at doses intended to have an effect on the body. By definition, a drug is biologically active and can therefore be expected to be toxic at some dose. Ideally, a drug's wanted effects are separable by dose-range from its unwanted effects.

Before a new potential drug can be administered to humans, reasonable assurance of its safety must be developed. A brief overview of the drug development process will provide a basis for understanding the role of pharmacoepidemiology in that process.

PREMARKETING RISK ANALYSIS

To begin, we draw a distinction between the evaluation and the testing of a new drug. A proper initial evaluation will aid in directing the preclinical testing efforts. An initial evaluation should take into account the known structural, biochemical, and pharmacologic properties as well as all information, experimental or epidemiologic, domestic or foreign, which can be obtained from similar or related compounds. Any special *in vitro* or preclinical testing requirements should be guided by what was learned.

The preclinical evaluation includes a standard battery of *in vitro* and *in vivo* tests plus those judged necessary for that type of chemical, specific dosage form, route of administration, and anticipated duration of human exposure. The reasons for performing preclinical testing are:

- to detect overt toxicity
- to establish dose-response estimation of pharmacologic and toxic effects
- to assess drug distribution to organ systems
- to identify metabolic, kinetic, and elimination pathways
- to assess carcinogenic potential
- to assess reproductive toxicity and teratogenic potential
- to direct clinical safety assessments

Acceptable toxicity for drugs is not based on a mathematically derived upper limit of acceptable exposure, but rather on an acceptable separation of toxic and beneficial doses that vary according to the particular disorder being treated, the therapeutic benefit sought, and the extent to which the particular type of toxicity can be detected early and reversed in humans.

In drug development, toxicology and other types of preclinical studies precede and then interdigitate with the clinical investigation. These toxicology data are not intended to assure or establish safe human use, nor are they typically used for de facto prediction of probably human risk. Instead, the primary purpose of the preclinical toxicity studies is to provoke and maximize the drug's effects in two or more species of animals and to determine the dose and time relationship of these effects under various experimental conditions. This characterization of the drug action may identify certain toxic effects or narrow margins of safety which pose an unacceptable risk for the proposed patient population or for humans in general. More commonly, however, the toxicology information serves to direct attention to potential adverse effects that may warrant particularly rigorous clinical monitoring or patient selection until the drug effects in humans are known.

The purpose of the FDA investigational new drug regulations is to assure that no compound is tested as a human drug without appropriate safeguards. To rephrase, the major function of preclinical toxicology data is to provide an

Table 1. General Outline for Animal Toxicity Studies for New Drugs

Category	Duration of Human Administration	Phase	Subacute or Chronic Toxicity
Oral or parenteral	Several days	I,II,III,NDA	2 species; 2 weeks
	Up to 2 weeks	I	2 species; 2 weeks
		II	2 species; up to 4 weeks
		III,NDA	2 species; up to 3 months
	Up to 3 months	I,II	2 species; 4 weeks
		III	2 species; 3 months
		NDA	2 species; up to 6 months
	6 months to unlimited	I,II	2 species; 3 months
		III	2 species; 6 months or longer
		NDA	2 species 12 months (nonrodent) 18 months (rodent)

integrated background of basic information about the drug to support and guide the clinical investigations.

Specific requirements for animal toxicology studies for INDs and NDAs generally depend upon the extent and duration of intended or actual human use, the dosage form to be used, the severity of the illness being treated and the availability of acceptable therapeutic alternatives. The sequence of these tests proceeds in lock-step with the successive phases of clinical investigation.

In brief, the three phases of premarketing clinical investigations are as follows:

> *Phase I*—clinical pharmacology usually in normal volunteers with attention to pharmacokinetics, metabolism, and both single dose and dose-range safety.
> *Phase II*—limited size, closely monitored investigations designed to assess efficacy and relative safety.
> *Phase III*—full-scale clinical investigations designed to provide an assessment of safety, efficacy, optimum dose, and more precise definition of drug-related adverse effects in a given disease or condition.

Toxicity testing is based upon anticipated human exposure in the developmental phases and the ultimate projected human exposure. The guiding principle behind the preclinical testing is to have exposure durations exceed the anticipated duration of human exposure in the clinical trials (Table 1). The durations of preclinical testing in each developmental phase are also a function of the anticipated use; thus, the closer one is to the anticipation of multiple dose exposures in large numbers of patients (Phase III), the longer the toxicity studies would be to support the relative safety of that duration of human exposure. Further relative assurances of safety are built into the toxicity trials by using multiple doses, the highest dose generally producing measurable toxicity. The data generated from toxicity tests are compared to those that produce the desired pharmacologic effect. This can be done by comparing acute and, if possible, subacute ratios of ED_{50} to LD_{50} doses. Of course, it is also possible to learn about the problems of toxicity by comparing the slopes of the dose-effect curves for pharmacologic and toxic effects, their steepness, and degree of overlap.

An assessment of the risk profile derived from the preclinical workup is performed. Decisions are made about whether to proceed. The composition of the ADR monitoring techniques in the clinical trials is guided by knowledge gained from the initial evaluation and the animal test results.

Upon reasonable assurance of relative safety from the preclinical testing, Phase I investigations can commence. These studies involve a small number of persons (normal volunteers and/or patients) and are conducted under carefully controlled circumstances by clinical investigators qualified to determine pharmacologic effects, toxicity, metabolism, absorption, elimination, and safe dosage ranges. At the end of Phase I the sponsor should have preliminary information on the drug's pharmacologic effects in humans and sufficient information on the short-term toxicity of the drug and its pharmacokinetics in humans to design Phase II trials. This second phase of clinical trials consists of well-controlled studies conducted on a limited number of patients to determine the drug's effectiveness for treatment, prevention, or diagnosis of a specific disease and to obtain additional data on short-term toxicity. Additional and/or longer duration toxicologic studies performed concurrently on animals may be necessary to provide further support of safety. For example, reproduction studies would now be carried out for drugs to be used in women of childbearing potential. At the end of Phase II the sponsor should have sufficient information to determine whether the drug should be developed to the new drug application (NDA) stage. An end-of-Phase II conference may be held between the FDA and the sponsor to discuss the results to date and to identify the need for further studies. Phase III studies, involving more extensive clinical trials, are undertaken if the information obtained in the preceding phases demonstrates reasonable assurance of effectiveness for the intended use and if the drug has potential benefits that outweigh the potential risks discovered up to that point. These studies are intended to assess the drug's safety on the basis of exposure to a reasonably large population group, to appraise effectiveness for the intended use in broader patient populations than those studied in Phase II, and to obtain the additional information needed to write a comprehensive package insert, i.e., to provide adequate directions for use. Phase III studies may include both controlled and open studies and may more closely approximate the use of the drug in medical practice than do Phase II studies. The NDA is prepared following successful completion of the Phase III studies. The clinical safety section of the NDA describes the extent of exposure to the drug, and contains listings of adverse drug reactions with their incidence and comparison to that found in the placebo group, a summary of clinical laboratory data highlighting abnormal values, any evidence concerning the consequences of acute overdosage, and a description of any reason for dropouts.

An assessment regarding the need from a regulatory perspective for formal

Phase IV studies is made prior to NDA approval. This decision is based on the assessments made of the scope of knowledge of the risks and benefits developed to this point.

While acknowledging that the data base for safety produced by this development process is incomplete, it is usually complete enough to make a regulatory decision as to adequacy of information to permit initiation of marketing.

Only a minority of Phase IV studies are conducted primarily to assess residual safety concerns. Furthermore, only a minority of Phase IV safety studies utilize epidemiologic techniques. In fact, only 6 of 46 studies required as conditions for approval in 1985 and 1986 were observational safety studies. Most Phase IV studies are requested to test the drug in specific patient subpopulations, i.e., elderly, children, women of childbearing age, thereby increasing the generalizability of the preapproval clinical trails (in a *post hoc* fashion).

THE PRACTICE OF PHARMACOEPIDEMIOLOGY IN A REGULATORY ENVIRONMENT

The FDA monitors a newly approved drug in the marketplace by a variety of mechanisms: Phase IV studies requested as conditions for approval; NDA periodic reporting requirements, compliance inspections and good manufacturing practices (GMP) requirements; and regulations and pharmacoepidemiologic surveillance and study for adverse outcomes. The remainder of this chapter deals with the last of these mechanisms.

The Division of Epidemiology and Surveillance (DES) within the Center for Drug Evaluation and Research (CDER) is FDA's functional pharmacoepidemiology unit, i.e., the *risk assessors*. This division houses the Spontaneous Reporting System (SRS), manages the cooperative agreements with extramural sources for epidemiologic data, and employs epidemiologists and other health professionals to assess drug safety in the postmarketing arena. Interaction with the regulatory components of the Center is vital. The new drug product review divisions within the Office of Drug Evaluation I (ODE I) and the Office of Drug Evaluation II (ODE II) are the functional regulatory decisionmakers and, therefore, the *risk managers*.

The three general areas for interaction are (1) important new adverse event signals received through the SRS; (2) consultations from or areas of regulatory concern to the reviewing divisions; and (3) recent literature reports and relevant epidemiologic studies.

The data which support a new signal are presented to the regulatory divisions either for their information or as an action item, depending on the strength of the case. The DES staff, as advisors and consultants to these new drug evaluation divisions, prepare epidemiologic reports on areas of regulatory concern and present these results at meetings referred to as safety conferences. The goal is, whenever possible, to narrow the regulatory decision gap with a well-conducted and comprehensive safety assessment. While it is generally recognized that the most concentrated postmarketing effort should be placed on the detection and verification of new, unexpected, and serious reactions, they constitute only a small portion of the total amount of safety and relative safety issues which arise.

The actual research questions that must be dealt with are varied in their nature and their importance. The operative word in the last sentence is *must*. The FDA must address all the safety issues brought to its attention and make a decision as to action. High-quality, accessible data sources used by well-skilled risk assessors increase the likelihood of a valid and timely risk assessment. This promotes rational decisionmaking.

When a new drug (hereafter referred to as a drug product) enters the FDA review process, it receives a priority designation based on its chemical uniqueness and a prediction of its eventual medical utility. In an ideal situation, the epidemiology staff from DES monitors the in-house progress of the new drug application (NDA). They obtain advanced information (usually a draft of the summary basis of approval, the SBA) on the new molecular entities (NME) and other designated drug products of special concern from the reviewing divisions before they are marketed so that an efficient and effective postmarketing surveillance effort can be set in place. If residual concerns about safety remain at the potential approval point, a formal Phase IV study can be negotiated with the manufacturer. In either case, full knowledge of the new drug product which includes the adverse-event profile seen in the Phase III clinical trials, data from foreign marketing experience, and knowledge of the adverse-event profile of pharmacologically-similar marketed drugs is mandatory. The goal here is to increase the probability of predicting and detecting the problems that may occur in the marketplace. The ideal goal of postmarketing surveillance is to bring the time of discovery of a major proportion of new information as close to the time of marketing of the new drug as possible.[1]

FUNCTIONAL FRAMEWORKS

Pharmacoepidemiology, an epidemiologic specialty, requires a synthesis of multidisciplinary information. The practice of pharmacoepidemiology is the art of using the sciences and the tools of science to generate information about pharmaceutical outcomes. In an extension of this theme, the practice of pharmacoepidemiology in a regulatory environment is the art of using the sciences and the tools of science to generate information which is then used as part of the basis for regulatory decisionmaking. That, in turn, by affecting drug therapy, affects the public health.

A pharmacoepidemiologist must be capable of functioning with a matrix constructed of three distinct frameworks. These are a *knowledge* framework made up of the accumulated information on drugs and disease states as well as clinical and general medical care principles; a *conceptual* framework for understanding, orientation, and direction which includes the epidemiologic

Table 2. Pharmacoepidemiologic Conceptual Framework (Part A): Ascertainment by Drug

Method	Detection or Signalling	Hypothesis Generation	Description	Strength of Association	Hypothesis Testing
A: Monitoring (without controls)	A–1 yes	A–2 yes	A–3 no	A–4 no	A–5 no
B: Numerator analysis across events (without controls)	B–1 yes	B–2 yes	B–3 yes	B–4 no	B–5 no
C: Cohort study (with controls)	C–1 no	C–2 no	C–3 no	C–4 yes	C–5 yes

principles and methodologies; and an *interpretive* framework which relies heavily on logic and the elimination of alternative explanations. A knowledge and understanding of the availability and the validity of the sources of data are required across all the parts of the matrix. These frameworks will be discussed next in more detail.

The *knowledge* framework is firmly based when the pharmacoepidemiologist has obtained a sense of understanding of the research question from the relevant medical and scientific disciplines involved. An epidemiologist should not begin any form of information synthesis until this sense of understanding is obtained. One must know when, why, and under what circumstances a drug is actually used. A full understanding of the pharmacology, the pharmacodynamics, and the pharmacokinetics of both the drug of concern and the other members of its pharmacologic and/or therapeutic class is required. A full understanding of the pathologic process for which the drug was indicated is also required.

It is the *conceptual* framework which will be discussed most extensively in this section. When referring to adverse consequences of drug use, one can envision a five-segment continuum in the pharmacoepidemiologic approach. These are (1) the detection of an event (which is often referred to as a signal or signalling), (2) the generation of a hypothesis, (3) description, (4) assessment of the strength of an association, and (5) the testing of a hypothesis. These endpoints appear as column titles on Tables 2 and 3. The last two columns are distinguished by the validity of underlying statistical assumptions. The conceptual framework for pharmacoepidemiologic techniques as presented in Tables 2 and 3 has been modified from the frameworks developed by Jones.[1,2] It allows one to organize the many approaches and the even more data sources available for the study of drug effects. The two main conceptual categories, ascertainment by *drug* and ascertainment by *event*, were originally described by Finney,[3] but are presented here in a revised and modified form. The strategies in each category are those in current use and are not exhaustive listings.

These two conceptual categories differ in directionality, in the time lapse until functional, and in their utilization. Each category contains a number of

Table 3. Pharmacoepidemiologic Conceptual Framework (Part B): Ascertainment by Event

Method	Detection or Signalling	Hypothesis Generation	Description	Strength of Association	Hypothesis Testing
D: Numerator analysis, event-specific (without controls)	D–1 yes	D–2 yes	D–3 yes	D–4 no	D–5 no
E: Single drug-event analysis (with denominator) (without controls)	E–1 no	E–2 yes	E–3 yes	E–4 no	E–5 yes*
F: Comparative proportional analyses (with internal controls)	F–1 no	F–2 yes	F–3 no	F–4 yes	F–5 no
G: Case-control study design (with controls)	G–1 no	G–2 yes	G–3 no	G–4 yes	G–5 yes

*With external or historical controls.

strategies or methods employed either in a surveillance mode or when addressing a specific research question. The ascertainment by drug category begins with the drug, then addresses the question, What adverse outcomes are associated with this drug? In a larger sense, this is not limited just to adverse outcomes but includes new beneficial ones. This concept is similar to that which underlies the practice of clinical epidemiology: the evaluation of the consequences of therapeutic interventions. The ascertainment by drug category has three components which are varied in function: (A) monitoring, (B) numerator analysis across events, and (C) cohort study design. The first two do not have the advantage of controls (see Table 2).

The primary surveillance mode, i.e., monitoring, is practiced through the utilization of the FDA-SRS and the medical literature. In general this large scale operation is used for the detection of new events, or signals. When the signal is an unexpected one from the perspective of biological plausibility, or one for which the interpretation is controversial, additional confirmation is necessary, and a hypothesis is generated. A numerator analysis (across events without denominators and without controls) can present a qualitative and a quasi-quantitative description of a drug's safety profile. For example, reported adverse events can be plotted across physiologic body systems, then at a finer level across diagnostic terms within a body system. The comparison of these profiles among drugs within a pharmacologic class is often informative and may lead to new signals and/or new hypotheses. The formally designed prospective cohort study with a control group can be used to assess the strength of an association or for a formal test of a hypothesis.

A reversal of directionality yields ascertainment by event (see Table 3). This addresses the question, What are the pharmaceutical risk factors for this adverse outcome? The four methods in this conceptual category are (D) numerator analysis (event-specific, without denominators and without controls); (E) single drug-event analysis (with denominators, without controls); (F) comparative proportional analyses (with denominators, and internal control); and (G) case-control study design. The event-specific numerator analysis can be used to examine which drugs are reported to be associated with a specific adverse event, e.g., hepatotoxicity. The single drug-event analysis can examine the context in which the events occur through a content analysis of the data. Comparative proportional analyses assess the strength of associations relative to other members of a comparable drug group. The formally designed case-control study can be used to generate hypotheses, but is most valuable when used to test a hypothesis. The integration of existing data sources into this conceptual framework is illustrated in the next section.

The *interpretive* framework concerns interpretation, utilization, and decisionmaking. An axiom of empirical research states that the more well controlled and internally valid the study design, the more straightforward, statistically valid, and less judgmental the interpretation of the results. At best, a properly designed analytical epidemiologic study, which is based on observational data that did not have the benefit of random allocation and other design features of prospective controlled trials, is difficult to interpret. The open research methods often used to address pharmacoepidemiologic questions contain most (if not all) of the threats to internal validity listed by Campbell and Stanley.[4] Interpretation of such results usually requires the use of additional outside sources of information, including the utilization of multiple data bases, to eliminate or assess the relative likelihood of alternative explanations. The most important source of information used in the interpretation of pharmacoepidemiologic findings is the previously described knowledge framework, the core of which is the knowledge gained from the new drug development process.

Utilization of the results of epidemiologic research requires information dissemination. The DES staff submits in-house reports on its risk assessment efforts to the reviewing divisions for regulatory decisionmaking and elective dissemination in regulatory media. For selected issues, publication in the medical literature is also sought.

Regulatory decisionmaking often occurs in the environment of uncertainty. In the postmarketing arena the decision gaps—that is, the difference between the amount of information one has and the amount required for a comfortable determination—regarding drug safety may be quite large. The interpreted pharmacoepidemiologic results are of regulatory value to the extent that they serve to narrow this gap for the risk component of the benefit-to-risk decision, a decision which must be made in a timely manner to protect the public's health.

In order to establish an effective postmarketing system for the evaluation of drug safety, a network of data sources must be supported and maintained. Selection of the appropriate types of sources is contingent upon a clear under-

Table 4. Relation of Current Data Bases and Methods to the Conceptual Framework

Data Base or Method	Primary Function	Secondary Functions
"Alerting"	A–1	A–2
Automated surveillance	A–1	B–3, A–2
SRS "safety profile"	B–3	B–1, B–2
SER-type analyses	F–4	F–2
Registries	D–3	D–1
Medical literature	A–1	C–5, G–5
Medicaid	C–4	B–2, G–4
Puget Sound (BCDSP)	G–5	C–5, E–3
DAWN	A–1	B–3, F–4
DEU	G–2	G–5

standing of needs and goals. Early detection and reliable and valid assessment are the general goals. The assessment goal, however, is often elusive due to the many forms a drug safety research question can take.

APPLICATION OF PHARMACOEPIDEMIOLOGY STRATEGIES

The first line of "defense" is ascertained, by drug, through the active use of the passive case report monitoring system: the FDA-SRS and published reports in the literature. Use of spontaneously submitted case reports can be considered both an inherently limited and an abundantly useful endeavor. Proper use of the submitted reports is somewhat like panning for gold. Valuable nuggets can be found among the massive quantities of common matter. Diligent "panning" by the DES staff is required to actualize the potential of the SRS. Recent changes (August 1985) in the adverse drug experience reporting regulations have made this mining process more efficient.[5] Also, the receipt of well-documented reports from health professionals can increase the potential. It remains to be seen whether these changes have a positive or negative impact of the effectiveness of the system.

The next challenge to the pharmacoepidemiologist is to find strategies that maximize the quality and value of a risk assessment, given a signal and/or a specific research question. Tables 2 and 3 display a conceptual framework, which will now be used to integrate the presented strategies with the available methods and data sources. Some of those, as they represent specific research methods, and a variety of research methods used with the FDA-SRS data base are listed in Table 4. The annotations in the primary and secondary function columns on Table 4 refer to the cells in Tables 2 and 3. It is readily apparent from the tables that the primary function of many of these methods is detection of events, or signalling (cell A-1). Fortunately, often their value is not limited to these indicated functions.

Alerting implies the hands-on review of a 15-day (i.e., serious and unlabeled) or a direct (from a health care provider) SRS report by an in-house health professional. Algorithms for causality assessment are used in this review. *Automated surveillance* refers to the computer-controlled screening of all received reports. Programmed output reports are used to screen for large changes in type or frequency of labeled reactions and those unlabeled reactions that fall short of the serious outcome criteria, as outlined in the revised regulations (CFR 314.8).

An SRS *safety profile* refers to the numerator analysis of all events, clustered by a meaningful unit of examination, e.g., a body system, reported for a specific drug. These profiles are informative in the absolute and more so when compared to those of the other drugs in a pharmacologic or therapeutic class. A standardized event rate (SER) type of analysis is a form of a comparative proportional analysis. Essentially, this type of analysis examines whether the observed reporting rate for a specific drug-event pairing is greater than would be expected in a set of comparable drugs, given that it is an event that has been reported with use of the compared drugs. No causality assessment is conducted here. SER is used to examine the relative strength of an association using the reporting event rates for the comparable drugs as an internal control. The reader is referred to the citation for the upcoming case example of maprotilene for details of this methodology.

Registries, such as the FDA-supported ophthalmology and dermatology registries, are ascertainment-by-event vehicles used to describe the spectra of drugs reported to be associated with the outcome events of emphasis. On occasion, a new drug-event pairing is detected from these sources.

The medical literature is a rich but often underutilized source of data and information. The information available in the medical literature ranges from single case reports of adverse events (usually in the form of letters to the editor), through the formal reporting of the results of an epidemiologic or randomized investigation, to relevant research results from other disciplines and sciences, especially those that shed light on the pharmacokinetics or pharmacodynamics of a drug of interest or the pathogenesis of the disease under treatment as well as the one being characterized as the event.

Medicaid records form the largest but probably the most complex and confounded source of pharmacoepidemiologic data and much of it developed as part of the extramural program of the FDA. The most common use of these data is for formal cohort studies; however, case-control studies have been conducted using these data. Broad-based screening by drug has also been tried in these data bases. Components of the medical data base at the Puget Sound health maintenance organization are under the management of the Boston Collaborative Drug Surveillance Program (BCDSP). This arrangement provides data linkage suitable for a variety of study methodologies, especially the case-control design. The Drug Abuse Warning Network (DAWN), currently managed by the National Institute on Drug Abuse (NIDA), is one of a few useful drug abuse indicator systems. These data have been used to describe the abuse situations associated with specific psychotropic drugs and to perform a variety of comparative proportional analyses. The Drug Epidemiology Unit

(DEU) in Boston maintains a case-control surveillance program to generate hypotheses about drug-event associations and to test specific research questions.

Monitoring through ascertainment by drug is an effective means of detection or signalling; however, the nature of the research question, the nature of the drugs of interest, the availability of data sources, and the working time frame determine the optimal research methods used for risk assessment. Lack of full understanding of any of these factors can lead to a flawed and misleading evaluation.

CASE EXAMPLES

The dual intent of this Section is to illustrate the varied nature of drug safety research questions and to demonstrate what impact some recent epidemiologic risk assessments have had on regulatory decisionmaking. The case example format was chosen to provide a pragmatic approach. Full details of the methods used are contained in the cited unpublished documents (available through a Freedom of Information Act request).

CASE 1—AMOXAPINE TOXICITY UPON OVERDOSE

Signal: A literature report based on poison control center data that observed a greater likelihood of lethality from an amoxapine overdose relative to the tricyclic antidepressants. This paper also reported more seizure involvement.[6]

Purpose: Support or refute the conclusions of the literature report. Assess the relative toxicity and seizure profile of the marketed antidepressants upon overdose.

Data bases used: FDA-Spontaneous Reporting System (SRS), Drug Abuse Warning Network (DAWN), FDA-Poison Control Center Data (PCC), National Disease and Therapeutic Index (NDTI), National Prescription Audit (NPA), and the medical literature.

Methods: Relative case fatality rates were calculated for each antidepressant from a number of the above data bases. For example, a DAWN case fatality rate was estimated as DAWN Medical Examiner (DAWN-ME) mentions per 1000 DAWN Emergency Room (DAWN-ER) mentions. They then were rank ordered and compared. Consistent support was obtained from similar calculations performed independently on data from the PCC and FDA-SRS data bases. Therapeutic ratios were also calculated and compared after a content analysis of the SRS reports.

Results: No substantial difference in lethality on overdose was found between amoxapine and the standard tricyclic antidepressants. Amoxapine was found to differ in the clinical manifestations present on overdose. Most notable was the presence of intense seizure activity. A potential selection bias was alleged for the poison control center data used in the original literature report.[7]

Action: No regulatory action was considered necessary regarding the relative lethality issue. The overdose section of the label was revised as to the presence of seizures as a major symptom and a recommendation was added for an aggressive course of treatment. Physicians were encouraged to contact their local poison control center for the latest overdose treatment advice.

Follow-up: Monitor and reassess annually.

Comment: Strategies from Table 3 used in this case include cells D-3, E-2, E-3, and F-4. The consistency in results on multiple measures across multiple data bases provided a sufficient level of certainty for decisionmaking. However, all the event measures were from unvalidated data sources; therefore, continual reassessment and external validation is needed.

CASE 2—TRAZODONE: OVERDOSE TOXICITY VS PRIAPISM

Signal: Continuing concern over a previous signal regarding priapism and the contrasting allegations that the recently marketed (1984) trazodone was less toxic on overdose than other drugs used to treat depression.

Purpose: The regulatory division was weighing the need to recommend, via the labeling, that trazodone use be considered second-line due to the occurrence of priapism. The DES was asked to provide an assessment of the risks associated with trazodone overdose relative to its class and contrast that to the risk of the unique reaction of priapism.

Data bases used: SRS, PCC, DAWN, NDTI, NPA, literature.

Methods: Similar to that used in example 1, but on a more recent time frame.

Results: Overdoses with trazodone appeared less likely to be lethal in this initial analysis. Seventy percent of the overdose episodes were in females. Priapism in males is estimated to occur once per 7000 trazodone exposures.[8]

Action: Labeling was modified with new information. A second-line drug status was not conferred upon trazodone, although labeling recommended that use in males should be only with a clear understanding of the risk for priapism.

Follow-up: Monitor and reassess the overdose profile annually.

Comment: When this analysis was conducted, trazodone was only marketed for a brief time. Confirmation is needed. However, the suggestion that it may be less likely to be lethal on overdose was sufficient to retain its full indication.

CASE 3—MAPROTILINE AND SEIZURES

Signal: British Committee on the Safety of Medicines (CSM), FDA-SRS, and the medical literature.

Purpose: Seizures have been reported with the use of almost all of the antidepressants. However, the signal suggested a higher frequency with maprotiline exposure. The DES was asked to assess whether seizures that occur while on therapy (not on overdose as in the amoxapine case) are more strongly associated with maprotiline than with comparable antidepressants.

Data bases used: SRS, NPA, NDTI, literature.

Methods: Standardized event rates (SER) were calculated for a comparison of events for maprotiline, amoxapine, and trazodone. Seizures in overdose situations were excluded from the analysis.

Results: Seizure events were more strongly associated with maprotiline therapy than from therapy with comparable antidepressants.[9]

Action: Label was modified. A "Dear Doctor" letter was required.

Follow-up: Two hypothesis-testing studies utilizing Medicaid data were commissioned. Results are pending completion. In addition, external support for these findings appeared in a subsequent literature report.[10]

Comment: Strategies from Table 3 included cells D-3 and F-4. This innovative analysis was used to test for substantial differences in a specific event across a group of comparable drugs. It addresses a manufacturer's claim that all drugs in a class are associated with a specific event, and it is already in the labeling. Proper use requires the acceptance of a set of assumptions and adjustment for known biases in SRS data.

CASE 4 – PIROXICAM AND UPPER GI EVENTS (see also Dr. Sachs's accompanying paper)

Signal: Literature, CSM, SRS, Health Research Group's (HRG) Petition.
Purpose: To assess whether piroxicam was more strongly associated with upper GI events than the other drugs in the nonsteroidal antiinflammatory (NSAID) group. The signal was seen for the older age group.
Data bases used: FDA-SRS, NPA, NDTI, literature, Boston Collaborative Drug Surveillance Program (BCDSP), Vanderbilt University's Medicaid data base.
Methods: Standardized-event-rate calculation adjusted for a variable secular reporting trend over the past decade.
Results: When adjusted for known biases and trends in the SRS data based, then adjusted for drug use, a standardized-event-rate analysis showed that piroxicam was not substantially different from other NSAIDS for GI-associated morbidity and mortality. Findings from the other cited data bases were supportive of this finding.[11]
Action: The HRG petition was denied. At present, no labeling changes have been ordered.
Follow-up: Continual monitoring.
Comment: This was the most extensively researched drug safety question of the past few years. Some of the extramural data sources supported by the FDA were consulted with high priority due to the high visability of this issue. Their input supported the SER analysis performed by in-house staff.

CASE 5 – HUMAN GROWTH HORMONE (HGH) AND CJD

Signal: Three 1639 case reports of Creutzfeldt-Jakob disease were submitted to FDA in the NIH-sponsored treatment IND.
Purpose: To assess whether these three reports of this very rare neurological disorder were more than expected.
Data bases used: National Center for Health Statistics (NCHS) mortality data and exposure data from the IND.
Methods: The observed rate was compared to the expected rate to test the hypothesis of no difference.
Results: A rate of 3 in 10,000 exposed was significantly greater than could be expected in the population.[12]
Action: The production and distribution of pituitary-derived HGH was halted. A recombinant product received FDA priority, under orphan drug status, and was soon thereafter approved for use in HGH-deficient conditions. A departmental task force was created to identify and monitor the balance of the exposed individuals.
Follow-up: A Health and Human Services (HHS) task force will monitor and conduct a National Death Index (NDI) based study.
Comment: For the research question, a simple but innovative analysis was suffi-

cient to allow a confident decision. In reference to Table 3, this analysis is best described as a special case of strategy E-5, with a firm denominator and external control from the NCHS data.

CASE 6–IMPACT OF NALOXONE ON PENTAZOCINE ABUSE

Signal: An internal FDA request from our drug abuse staff.

Purpose: To assess the impact of a regulatory action taken about three years prior, when the narcotic antagonist naloxone was added to the oral tablet formulation of pentazocine.

Data bases used: DAWN, NPA, literature, FDA-SRS.

Methods: A hypothesis-testing trends analysis of DAWN emergency room and medical examiner data over NPA retail prescription mentions which compared data before and after the addition of naloxone to the oral tablet dosage form of pentazocine.

Results: There was a significant decrease in the number of drug abuse mentions per reporting quarter in each of the DAWN system parameters since the addition of naloxone.[13]

Action: No additional regulatory action was warranted. The intervention appeared successful to date.

Follow-up: Analysis to be repeated if a new signal requires another examination.

Comment: The strategy from Table 3 is a special case of cell E-5 using a historical control to test the hypothesis of no change in trend. This assessment of a prior regulatory action clearly demonstrated a public health impact. The original agreement to add naloxone illustrated a constructive spirit of cooperation between industry and government (FDA, DEA, & NIDA).

CASE 7–WITHDRAWAL SEIZURES WITH THE NEWER BENZODIAZEPINES

Signal: FDA-SRS.

Purpose: To describe the conditions under which seizures occur and to assess whether they are more strongly associated with any specific benzodiazepine anxiolytic.

Data bases used: FDA-SRS, literature, NPA, NDTI.

Methods: Content analysis of FDA-SRS reports.

Results: Seizures secondary to withdrawal from benzodiazepine anxiolytics are rare events. They are reported most frequently for the potent benzodiazepines, alprazolam and lorazepam. Data were plotted dose against duration of therapy. Risk appeared dependent upon sufficient exposure to produce a physical dependence state. Higher doses appear to decrease the time to risk. These data support the pharmacologic theory of cumulative exposure.[14] Further confirmation is needed.

Action: Awaits additional supportive data.

Follow-up: Continued SRS monitoring.

Comment: Strategies D-2 and D-3 from Table 3 were used. A comparative proportional analysis could not be conducted because the NDTI data demonstrated that alprazolam had a unique usage pattern. Therefore, there were no comparable drugs. Additionally, an appropriate denominator for this contingent event was not available. The generated hypothesis awaits testing. The conduct of confirmatory studies will be difficult, however, because these type of data are outside the scope of all the usual postmarketing data bases.

COMMENTARY ON THE CASE ANALYSES

Each of the above cases was, by necessity, presented in a very abbreviated format. The relationship with the three underlying frameworks, while present, may not be readily apparent due to this outline format. However, their importance in organizing and conducting inquiries in response to a drug safety research question cannot be overstated.

One last illustration of the use of epidemiologically derived information to form the basis for regulatory decisions involves the labeling of the combination oral contraceptive drug products. The April 21, 1987, issue of the *Federal Register* announced the availability of revised patient and professional class labeling. The main purpose of the revision was to update the risk sections, clarify the interaction with smoking, and the update the overall labeling in light of that the hormone content of these pills had been lowered. The unique aspect of this new labeling is that it contains information on noncontraceptive health benefits related to the use of oral contraceptives. They are supported by evidence from epidemiologic studies. They include various effects on menses, effects related to inhibition of ovulation, and effects from long-term use, including a decreased incidence of the following: fibrocystic disease of the breast, pelvic inflammatory disease, endometrial cancer, and ovarian cancer. I see this is a major example of the public health impact of epidemiologic data.

The regulatory actions cited in the case examples were not taken solely upon the results of these postmarketing risk assessments. The new findings are added to the existing knowledge data base, and the benefit/risk equation is recalculated or, more correctly, "rejudged" by the risk manager. Decisions are based upon consideration of the aggregate information available.

CONCLUSIONS

Risk (safety) assessment of a new drug is a continual process. Pharmacoepidemiology risk assessment is the postapproval stage of the continuum. Postmarketing risk assessment strategies should be guided by the cumulative experience with the new drug to that point. Phase IV studies should address specific residual concerns.

Responsibilities for assessing postmarketing risk and for the application of these to risk management and regulatory functions exist in different organized components of the FDA. The postmarketing decisionmakers are the same functional units who worked with the drug throughout its entire development process.

The practice of pharmacoepidemiology is not amenable to a standardized or cookbook approach. This chapter attempts to explain the concepts and foundations of the art in pharmacoepidemiology so that thinking, creative individuals can apply them as the research questions warrant. Each new research question requires a different individualized approach, and there are more exceptions than there are methodologic rules. The only valid rules in this field are those of research logic. The need for mastering a conceptual framework and a solid knowledge base cannot be stressed too strongly. Diverse data sources are required to address the breadth of potential questions that arise in this field. Due to the secondary and imprecise nature of most of the available data, multiple data sources should be examined for each research question in the expectancy that consistent, confirmatory findings are generated. Unfortunately, current extramural data bases are utilized only on a limited scale to address FDA-initiated research questions. Clearly, much room for improvement is present. Each question posed to the FDA must be addressed, and must be addressed in a timely manner. However, it is recognized within the agency that not all questions can currently be answered, and that is not a desirable situation. Additional data sources are needed.

Epidemiologic data on drug safety in the postmarketing arena have value in the regulatory environment when they can be used to form a risk assessment which is interpretable and capable of narrowing the often very large decision gaps, thereby facilitating rational regulatory decisionmaking. Regulatory adjustments made by the FDA still must be made through professional judgment. When made, they affect public health by affecting patient care through prevention and/or minimization of unsafe drug therapy.

Just as in the case prior to approval, it is also the sponsors who bear the responsibility for identifying and characterizing actual and potential safety issues associated with the use of *their* products in the postapproval environment. The new drug sponsors need to develop pharmacoepidemiologic capabilities so that they can carry out their responsibility. Solid, reliable, and valid data sources need to be funded and maintained. The FDA views pharmacoepidemiologic assessment of risk as a necessary component of its public health mission . . . a mission which does not end when an approval (to market) letter is issued.

The FDA will continue to refine its program and will assess risks using the best techniques and data sources possible. Better sources of epidemiologic data will increase the probability that the decisions FDA *has to make* on safety issues will be rational and correct.

REFERENCES

1. Jones JK: Broader uses of post-marketing surveillance, in Wardell WM, Velo G (eds): *Drug Development, Regulatory Assessment and Post-Marketing Surveillance*. New York, Plenum Press, 1981.
2. Jones JK: Regulatory use of adverse drug reactions. In *Skandia International Symposia. Detection and Prevention of Adverse Drug Reactions.* Stockholm, Almqvist & Wiksell International, 1984, pp 203–214.

3. Finney D: Statistical logic in the monitoring of reactions to therapeutic drugs. *Methods Inform Med* 1971;10:237–245. Revised & updated in Inman, WW (ed): *Monitoring for Drug Safety*. Lancaster, MTP Press, 1980, pp 383–400.
4. Campbell DT, Stanley JC: *Experimental and Quasi-Experimental Designs for Research*. Boston, Houghton Mifflin Company, 1963.
5. *U.S. Code of Federal Regulations*, Part 314.80.
6. Litovitz TL, Troutman WG: Amoxapine overdose: Seizures and fatalities. *JAMA* 1983:250:1069–1071.
7. Nelson RC: *Amoxapine Toxicity on Overdose* (unpublished report), Food and Drug Administration, Office of Epidemiology and Biostatistics, 1984.
8. Baum C, Nelson RC: *Trazodone Toxicity on Overdose* (unpublished report), Food and Drug Administration, Office of Epidemiology and Biostatistics, 1985.
9. Nelson RC: *Maprotiline and Seizures* (unpublished report), Food and Drug Administration, Office of Epidemiology and Biostatistics, 1984. Revised and presented at the APHA meeting, Washington, DC, November 1985.
10. Jabbari B, Bryan GE, March EE, Gundersen CH: Incidence of seizures with tricyclic and tetracyclic anti-depressants. *Arch Neurol* 1985;42: 480–481.
11. Rossi A, Hsu JP, Faich G: Ulcerogenicity of piroxicam: An analysis of spontaneously reported data. *Brit Med Journal* 1987;294:147–150.
12. Piper J: *HGH and CJD* (unpublished report), Food and Drug Administration, Office of Epidemiology and Biostatistics, 1984.
13. Baum C, Hsu JP, Nelson RC: Impact of the addition of naloxone on the abuse of pentazocine tablets. *Public Health Reports* 1987; 102(4): 426–429.
14. Nelson RC, Barash D, Graham D: *Intense Abstinence Syndromes and the Newer Benzodiazepine Anxiolytics* (unpublished report), Food and Drug Administration, Office of Epidemiology and Biostatistics, 1985. Revised and presented at the USPHS Professional Association meeting, June 1986.

3. *Industry Perspectives and the Contributions of Pharmacoepidemiology to Public Health*

ROGER M. SACHS
GRETCHEN S. DIECK

INTRODUCTION

This discussion is based upon the belief that the interests of public health and those of the pharmaceutical industry have many common threads despite their obvious differences. It further offers the hypothesis that pharmacoepidemiology can and should be a major force in the achievement of these common goals.

INDUSTRY GOALS

Pharmaceutical companies have been a major factor in improving public health through their development and distribution of pharmaceutical products. To continue to do this, however, the industry must remain economically viable, and this is achieved through the selling of its products for profit. Thus, the substantial expenditures devoted to research and development as well as to drug safety evaluation must be supported by a profitably conducted business.

A second goal of the pharmaceutical industry is to operate in a rational regulatory climate. *Rational* from the industry point of view implies that regulatory requirements are based upon scientific principles and are applied in a consistent manner.

A third issue of importance is relative freedom from irresponsible attacks from such sources as litigation, government (Congress as well as regulatory agencies), media, and special interest groups. This is not meant to imply that all actions against pharmaceutical manufacturers are unwarranted or to deprive injured parties of their rights. Rather, *irresponsible* refers to challenges that are not based on substance, but instead are motivated by secondary issues such as financial or political gain, or publicity. These attacks are particularly difficult to refute because they are not based in fact.

ACHIEVEMENT OF INDUSTRY GOALS

Many factors affect the sales of pharmaceuticals, but the most important of these are the safety and efficacy of the products themselves. However, since virtually nothing is absolutely safe and/or effective, these are terms of art which must be determined within a rational scientific framework.

Understanding of patient needs and population demographics is critical both in the premarketing and postmarketing periods. Assessment of these factors aids in determining who needs the products, where the products should be marketed, and how they should be sold.

A final consideration with respect to drug sales is public confidence—a recurrent theme when discussing pharmacoepidemiology and public health. If the public lacks confidence in a drug company or in a particular product, it will be difficult to sell the drug regardless of its actual safety and efficacy.

A number of issues are directly related to the goal of operating in an environment of rational regulation. An essential need is for a logical basis for drug approval. Related to this issue is the need to develop a rational approach to pre- and postmarketing drug safety and a proper balance between efforts to address the two. Some safety issues can be assessed in the premarketing phases whereas others, particularly the identification and quantification of rare events, can only be determined through postapproval drug surveillance. Finally, there is a pressing need for a regulatory bureaucracy relatively free from nonscientific pressures.

The third concern of the pharmaceutical industry is relative freedom from attack. From the industry's standpoint, there is a need for rapid and scientifically sound methods of evaluating drug safety. It is only through rapid and accurate studies that the industry can adequately address safety questions raised by the government, special interest groups, the media, physicians, patients, or other pharmaceutical companies, not to mention those which it feels itself stimulated to undertake as part of its ongoing commitment to rational drug development.

Therefore, in order to achieve industry's goals of selling pharmaceutical products, operating in a reasonable regulatory environment, and having relative freedom from attack, several important criteria must be met. These include the development of safe and effective drugs, the rapid assessment of health needs, and public confidence in the actions of industry and government. Within the context of pharmaceuticals, these represent basic public health needs and issues. Therefore, from the pharmaceutical industry standpoint, good public health is good business. And resulting from this assumption is the proposition that pharmacoepidemiology (as good science) leads to good public health which, in turn, promotes good business.

PHARMACOEPIDEMIOLOGY AND DRUG SAFETY

Pharmacoepidemiology can address the needs of both the industry and public health. What follows are some examples of how pharmacoepidemiology has been used recently in addressing drug safety.

The International Agranulocytosis and Aplastic Anemia Study (IAAAS) was carried out to quantify the risks of agranulocytosis and aplastic anemia with NSAID use. This major epidemiologic study determined that, although higher relative risk estimates were associated with some drugs compared to others, the absolute risks of both these conditions with the use of NSAIDS were extremely low.[1] The results were reassuring, and labeling changes were not made as a result of the study. In addition, it is unlikely that physicians would change their prescribing habits in light of these findings.

A similar conclusion was reached in a study of zomepirac sodium in relation to anaphylactic shock. A preliminary case-control study carried out using Florida Medicaid data estimated that users of zomepirac had a slightly greater than twofold increase in risk of allergic reaction or anaphylactic shock, but that the risk was extremely small in magnitude,[2] although in this case the manufacturer opted voluntarily to withdraw the product.

Epidemiology has also played an important role in the study of the relation between oral contraceptive use and myocardial infarction,[3] breast disease,[4,5] ovarian cancer,[6] and thromboembolism.[5] Another recent example is a study carried out to assess the risks of clinical bleeding with the use of certain antibiotics.[7] This information serves both industry and public health needs, since quantification of risk leads to appropriate use of therapeutic agents.

PHARMACOEPIDEMIOLOGY AND DRUG EFFICACY

Pharmacoepidemiology has also served, albeit less frequently, to assess drug efficacy (or, at least, importance) within the obvious limitations imposed by the biases introduced by observational methodology. Quality-of-life studies that examine patients' perspectives of how they feel on prescribed medications are often carried out using a cohort design. These studies are useful because they evaluate important subjective information that can be used both for positioning drugs for marketing and determining whether treatment truly benefits the patient. In addition to quality-of-life studies, some pharmacoepidemiologic studies have been carried out to formally examine unanticipated beneficial effects of drugs. Studies showing a lower risk of myocardial infarction with daily aspirin consumption,[8] or a lowering of the risk of ovarian cancer with oral contraceptive usage[6] are two examples.

EPIDEMIOLOGY AND DETERMINING HEALTH NEEDS

Epidemiologic methods can also be used to evaluate health needs. One example is in defining markets where there is no established therapy. The various treatment modalities for a particular disease can be examined along with the constellation of symptoms and other diagnostic factors, and then statistical modeling applied to assess which factors predict which treatment regimen will be used over another.

An example of how traditional epidemiologic methods are of value to industry is in determining the incidence or prevalence of a disease. Knowledge of whether a disease frequency is increasing or decreasing with time helps the pharmaceutical company in positioning its drug in the marketplace. The determination of whether the frequency of a condition increases after a drug has been put on the market can alert a company to a potential safety problem that should be examined further using more rigorous methods.

Traditional epidemiologic methods can also be used in identifying high risk groups. An example of this is the identification of flank pain in users of suprofen. Young males were found to be at higher risk for flank pain than other demographic subgroups.[9] Had the drug remained on the market, this information could have been of great value when weighing risks and benefits of therapy.

In summary, therefore, pharmacoepidemiology is well suited to evaluating precisely the types of public health issues which allow the pharmaceutical industry to successfully conduct its business. That is to say, good (i.e., scientifically sound) pharmacoepidemiology promotes good public health, which, in turn, is good for business.

PIROXICAM—A CASE STUDY

A related proposition, however, is that bad (i.e., scientifically unsound) pharmacoepidemiology is bad for both public health and for business. A recent example of this was the Imminent Hazard Petition filed against the nonsteroidal antiinflammatory agent piroxicam* by the Health Research Group (HRG), already outlined in the accompanying paper by Dr. Nelson.

Although carefully carried out epidemiologic studies have been effectively used to identify and quantify safety risks and to assess health needs, poorly executed studies have resulted in misinformation, confusion, and unnecessary concern on the part of the public. The piroxicam experience illustrates how damaging this can be to industry and to the public.

Piroxicam was approved for marketing in the United States in 1982, when the total number of ADR reports to the FDA had increased dramatically (almost doubled from 1981 to 1982).[10] Some of the observed increase in ADRs

*Piroxicam is manufactured by Pfizer Pharmaceuticals, New York, New York.

may have been prompted by problems with other drugs such as benoxaprofen and zomepirac.

In a January 8, 1986, letter to Secretary Bowen, Sidney Wolfe of HRG petitioned the Department of Health and Human Services (HHS) to have piroxicam declared an "imminent hazard" and to restrict its use in the elderly. The HRG petition relied in large part on spontaneous reporting data that had been previously reviewed by the FDA's Arthritis Advisory Committee and declared to be unacceptable as a basis for regulatory action.[11] In addition to comparing the number of reports for piroxicam (a new drug) to those of older NSAIDs, which had entered the market when reporting rates to the FDA were considerably lower, HRG's interpretation of spontaneous reporting data failed to account for such biases as differences in patient age and duration of therapy. The HRG petition was further supported by anecdotal case reports and case series, but contained no formal epidemiologic studies designed to control for biases and confounding factors.[10]

In spite of these limitations, when the HRG petition was submitted, an enormous effort was required by the manufacturer to defend the safety of the drug. Evidence supporting piroxicam's safety was derived from comparative clinical trials and observational epidemiological studies. Formal epidemiological studies using different methodologies and study populations confirmed the drug's comparative safety.[12] This was supported by data from 68 controlled clinical trials representing over 5000 patients.[13]

Although the HRG petition was denied six months after it was filed, it required an enormous expenditure of manpower and money by both the manufacturer and the FDA to address the issue. The FDA spent nearly one man-year of staff time and at least $50,000 on outside contractors addressing the petition (*The Pink Sheet*, March 2, 1987). Although HRG initiated the controversy with approximately 20 pages of documentation, the manufacturer responded with 10 volumes and over 600 pages. HHS denied the petition with a two-page letter (to Sidney Wolfe from Secretary Bowen, July 7, 1986) based on a seven-page memo (to Secretary Bowen from FDA Commissioner Frank E. Young, May 27, 1986), which, in turn, was based on a 60-page analysis by the FDA.[14]

The most persuasive data and over half of the FDA's analysis involved pharmacoepidemiology. If the resources that produced these data and analyses had not been in place when the petition was filed, the outcome could have been very different despite the fact that a problem did not truly exist.

In denying the HRG petition, the FDA stated "that in citing spontaneous reports the HRG ignored rudimentary precautions needed to evaluate such data . . . [and] instead ignored all the well known limitations."[14] The agency concluded that because "properly analyzed epidemiologic and spontaneous report data fail to provide evidence of an excess of GI toxicity with piroxicam . . . data from controlled clinical trials . . . is not critical to a decision" (memorandum to Secretary Bowen from Frank E. Young, May 27, 1986, p. 5).

Unfortunately, despite the denial of the petition, the fears of physicians and patients were aroused by the unfavorable publicity. Approximately 33% of patients surveyed had become aware of the petition, and about one-third of those stopped or changed medications because of concerns it raised about the drug. In addition, nearly 25% of the physicians surveyed had at least one patient ask to be taken off the drug because of the publicity (Pfizer Inc, unpublished data). Since drugs within a therapeutic class are often not interchangeable in a given patient, switching from one drug to another on the basis of scientifically unfounded concern creates the risk of either adverse reactions or loss of efficacy. The overall outcome, then, is a negative impact on public health as well as business.

OTHER ISSUES

There is a need to improve the quantity and quality of pharmacoepidemiology's resources and to promote greater understanding of its strengths and weaknesses. With respect to the quantity of resources, the industry should take an active role in supporting and expanding existing resources and in forming new data base linkages. In addition, the development of new, early postmarketing surveillance methodologies should be encouraged. No one resource or method is perfect, and no regulatory decision should be based on just one study. Supporting information from many sources using different study designs minimizes the risks of reporting erroneous or misleading conclusions.

As to the quality of epidemiologic studies, industry should promote the setting of standards for investigations as well as the setting of standards for publication. Implicit in this statement is the need for peer review. Critical review of study proposals and of findings presented for publication should minimize the quantity of poorly carried out studies obtaining widespread attention. The purpose of such review is not to eliminate studies that reach negative conclusions about drugs, but rather to eliminate the promulgation of poorly or irresponsibly executed research. It is the quality of the research that should be important to both the industry and the public health irrespective of the direction of the findings.

Finally, the quality and quantity of available resources has little meaning unless there is an understanding of the value of the research. It is in industry's best interests to promote a greater understanding of pharmacoepidemiology by the public, the press, government, and within industry itself. Along these same lines, greater cooperation between industry, government, and academia will aid in focusing support, assessing study quality, and advancing better understanding.

CONCLUSIONS

Valid pharmacoepidemiology plays a major role in furthering good public health practices. This, in turn, serves the industry's interests. Scientifically questionable pharmacoepidemiology, no matter how well-intentioned, may adversely affect public health and the pharmaceutical industry. It is therefore in industry's best interests to support the discipline of pharmacoepidemiology, to insist upon rigorous scientific standards for the field, and to increase awareness and understanding of its value.

REFERENCES

1. The International Agranulocytosis and Aplastic Anemia Study: Risks of agranulocytosis and aplastic anemia: A first report of their relation to drug use with special reference to analgesics. *JAMA* 1986;256:1749–1757.
2. Strom BL, Carson JL, Morse ML, et al: Anaphylactoid reactions from zomepirac and other non-steroidal anti-inflammatory drugs. *Clin Res* 1984;32:229A.
3. Jick H, Dinan B, Herman R, et al: Myocardial infarction and other vascular diseases in young women: Role of estrogens and other factors. *JAMA* 1979;240:2548–2552.
4. Vessey MP, McPherson K, Doll R: Breast cancer and oral contraceptives: Findings in Oxford-Family Planning Association contraceptive study. *Br Med J* 1981;282:2093–2094.
5. Boston Collaborative Drug Surveillance Program: Oral contraceptives and venous thromboembolic disease, surgically confirmed gallbladder disease, and breast tumours. *Lancet* 1973;1:1399–1404.
6. Vessey M, Metcalfe A, Wells C, et al: Ovarian neoplasms, functional ovarian cysts, and oral contraceptives. *Br Med J* 1987;294:1518–1519.
7. Brown RB, Klar J, Lemeshow S, et al: Enhanced bleeding with cefoxitin or moxalactam: Statistical analysis within a defined population of 1493 patients. *Arch Intern Med* 1986;146:2159–2164.
8. Jick H, Miettinen OS: Regular aspirin use and myocardial infarction. *Br Med J* 1976;1:1057.
9. *Minutes of the Arthritis Advisory Committee meeting*. Food and Drug Administration, Center for Drugs and Biologics, Bethesda, MD, December 1–2, 1986.
10. Sachs RM, Bortnichak EA: An evaluation of spontaneous adverse drug reaction monitoring systems. *Am J Med* 1986;81(suppl 5B):49–55.
11. *Minutes of the Arthritis Advisory Committee meeting*. Food and Drug Administration, Center for Drugs and Biologics, Bethesda, MD, April 29–30, 1985.
12. Bortnichak EA, Sachs RM: Piroxicam in recent epidemiologic studies. *Am J Med* 1986;81(suppl 5B):44–48.
13. Meisel AD: Clinical benefits and comparative safety of piroxicam: Analysis of worldwide clinical trials data. *Am J Med* 1986;81(suppl 5B):15–21.
14. *Recommendation in Piroxicam Imminent Hazard Proceeding*. Food and Drug Administration, Center for Drugs and Biologics, May 14, 1986, pp 16, 56.

SECTION TWO

Drug Epidemiology and the Law

Introduction

Professor Sidney H. Willig brings to the debate years of counsel to individual companies and to the public policy apparatus. His chapter provides insights into the extent and basis for much of the liability dilemma that currently faces America and presents examples in which bad information irredeemably damaged an otherwise good defense and good pharmacoepidemiologic information promoted better, more equitable settlements.

Barry L. Shapiro and Marc S. Klein are attorneys who have represented the pharmaceutical industry for over a decade in a wide variety of drug and medical device litigations. In this chapter they illustrate the need for epidemiologists to agree on standards for the courts to use to qualify expert epidemiologic witnesses and to accept or reject arguments of causality made in expert testimony. They discuss legal and scientific interpretations of proof of causality and detail a case that exemplifies the embarrassing way some courts have ignored the qualifications of experts and soundness of expert testimony, relying instead on the personal demeanor and tone of the witnesses.

4. Impact of Drug Products Liability on Needs for Pharmacoepidemiologic Studies and Expertise

SIDNEY H. WILLIG

INTRODUCTION

Evidence consisting of analysis of pharmacoepidemiologic studies of drugs subject to drug products liability litigation are of prime importance to both plaintiff and defendant when the adequacy of the prescription drug package insert is at issue. Protagonists of their use say they may offer proof or disproof on important legal issues (such as failure to warn or properly instruct as to use or administration or even as to causation) more objectively than traditional expert testimony and diminish the number of expert witnesses required. Antagonists often find them legally unsound and would admit their use sparingly, if at all. Many lawsuit results have already been determined by experts using elementary principles of pharmacoepidemiology even though not identified as such.

Recent developments in FDA adverse drug reaction (ADR) reporting and documentation for drug sponsors before and after new drug application (NDA) approval are tailored to recognized pharmacoepidemiologic concepts and facilitate timely or episodic pharmacoepidemiologic analyses. These concepts and analyses are fundamental to a plaintiff's claim as well as to an answer to the claim based on the usual state-of-the-art defense.

The challenge to the pharmacoepidemiologist is to take the data available, plumb clinical experience, and determine whether an association manifest from the data is or differs from a causal connection. The more the technique is applied, and the more it proves itself, the greater will be the need for experts in pharmacoepidemiology to apply their skills.

Every pharmaceutical manufacturer who seeks to develop, research, produce, and distribute drugs and devices for the American public, must of necessity hew to the statutory mandate of the Federal Food, Drug and Cosmetic Act.[1] The exact terms of these statutory tasks are further implemented and detailed by the Federal Code of Regulations in regulatory material both substantive and interpretive, and administered by the Federal Food and Drug Administration.[2] Since both the law and the regulations are dynamic in nature, they serve established scientific and economic needs responsively and offer collaterally support or qualification not only to manufacturers, whom they govern, but also the many technical, professional, and associated specialty groups involved.

The epidemiologist has long been involved in assisting public and professional understanding of new and established public health concerns that can be approached from this special discipline.

THE FEDERAL STATUTE AND REGULATIONS

One of the purposes of this chapter is to acknowledge the renewed vigor with which, by redesign of methodology and by enlisting additional resources, the Food and Drug Administration has embraced pharmacoepidemiology to carry out the statutory mandate requiring drugs to be proven safe and effective for their intended uses.

Complementing this purpose is another that recognizes the realities of American life and acknowledges that the Federal Food, Drug and Cosmetic Act is a public safeguard, but not a route to public economic or legal redress for individual injury arising from defects in product design or product description.[3] In these instances, the role in litigation of pharmacoepidemiologic studies and derived testimony has become undeniably important and is increasing. (Pharmacoepidemiology encompasses the same public health interest and professional expertise as the parent study, epidemiology, but is directed to the narrower and more specialized areas of pharmaceutics and pharmacal and pharmacologic concerns.) Spokesmen for the FDA bureaucracy established in this epidemiologic mold point out frequently that postmarketing surveillance (PMS) of prescription drugs is a necessary element in determining the accuracy of the accompanying labeling. Thus, PMS is spelled out carefully in regulation[4] and seeks to provide routine ongoing information on the safety of prescription drugs, with reviews using statistical methodology as well as medical analysis and interpretation. The final purpose is public dissemination of such accumulated information. Since the FDA is short on medical officers trained in epidemiology, and since the package insert remains the best form of dissemination, it becomes obvious that the product's sponsor must be responsible for much of the process.

The act of gathering adverse reaction reports is itself salutary to the manufacturer as a public service and can provide early warnings of major design or labeling defects. In a cumulative sense, since many drugs are molecularly similar, relative safety profiles are created within certain classes of drugs on the basis of composition as well as therapeutic or diagnostic use. In the process, among subdivisions of the general public host population, special host susceptibility factors will be demonstrated.[5]

Faich[5] divides the commonly used epidemiologic studies into descriptive and analytic. While descriptive studies are nonanalytic and not controlled, they hold a fascination for attorneys because they lend themselves to interpretations that may suit their needs. Using them, the attorney may point to early signals of the safety problems that ultimately troubled his client.

Case control studies played a large role in determining the need to add and clarify warnings as to dangers associated with oral contraceptives, which of course developed into a fertile field of litigatory exploration. Faich also points out their historic application to studying carcinogenicity and teratogenicity where there was suspicion that they were drug-induced or contributed to by the delayed effects of the suspect chemicals. A recent case control study concerning the nebulous Reye's syndrome is another example. Before concluding on anything that might sound like causation in a case control study of a syndrome rather than a disease, good epidemiologic analysis, as in the swine flu studies, may need to rule out all factors of input except the most exactly defined and nonbiased selection of cases and controls, something difficult to accomplish under conditions of media fervor, regulatory panic, or "public research group" flagellation.[6] Analysis of a syndrome especially lends itself to use of Bayesian methodology, where the profile of the syndrome, as manifest in various highly diverse reports and patients (and observers), is constructed and used as the net to measure retrospectively encounters within the study.

Thus, the diagnostic criteria are very sensitive to the manner in which the patient to be reported is approached by the physician questioner. Faich uses the example of gastric cancer cases being studied by pharmacoepidemiologic methods. Since at least early symptoms of gastric cancer mimic gastric ulcer symptoms, the patients will show high use of aluminum and magnesium hydroxides and similar drugs, as will as potent anticholinergics, all of which would appear to pose a nexus between the disease and the drug, but in this case "observed association between the drug and the disease would be noncausal."

DEVELOPMENT OF EPIDEMIOLOGIC TECHNIQUES BY FDA

The Food and Drug Administration has gradually sophisticated its technique of implementing the statutory mandate of 21 USC 355 (j) since it came into being via the New Drug Amendments of 1962. Today at last, the epidemiologic approach is overt and in the hands of competent staff[7] capable of understanding and applying substantive elements comprising pre- and post-marketing surveillance of prescription drugs and devices. An evolutionary process must go on seeking improvement and practical achievement; however, good tools, good procedures, good motivation, and good people are in place.

Although the statutory changes that led to these reformative concepts and procedures were accomplished to require proof of *effectiveness* in addition to the older need for showing proof of *safety*, the thalidomide tragedy did much to promote seeking greater proof of the latter at every phase of drug development, including the pre-NDA phases (the so-called IND work) and postapproval surveillance. However, required reporting of unsafety in trials preceding the Phase III clinical trials could (1) modify or terminate further activity with the investigational drug, (2) require vast changes in the provisional investigational labeling, and (3) alter product design and composition.

Within the clinical trials, the need to report adverse reactions was continued and the method gradually formalized, so that introductory product labeling reflected experience with the new drug and/or similar or related compounds, to that date, give or take a few months. The controlled clinical trials that gave rise to the first labeling accompanying the approved marketing of the new drug often described almost all adverse reactions that had been reported. In their omission of some, they made obvious that such reports had not been clearly observed or validated and were perhaps illogical or aberrational.[8]

It has been said that scientific hearing procedures, seeking the establishment of fundamental principles and ideas, could learn much from application of the adversary system used in law.[9] Both deal in probabilities. Indeed the acceptance of probabilistic analysis by scientists appreciates such end results. However, while science uses deductive processes and probabilities for predictive purposes, law uses probabilities to determine economic liabilities.[10] Thus the scientist's approach to epidemiologic models, their study, and utility does not necessarily envision legal utility. Law still prefers reliance upon cause and effect and a deduction therefrom that can be used as an integer in a total sum.

Most medical curricula that teach either the epidemiologic approach, or epidemiology per se consider it a study of the relations of various factors determining the frequency and distribution of diseases and other undesirable conditions in the human body. It is sometimes described briefly as medical ecology.

Epidemiology, by use of scientific methods, use of statistical sampling techniques, and application of analyses that employ reasoned concepts of probabilities, charts out the *who*, the *where*, and the *how* of disease distribution. That is, within given parameters of interest, the epidemiologist offers an insightful prediction of disease dispersion and, to some extent, the causal factors that seemingly appear. The epidemiologist's knowledge of the frequency and dispersion of disease in populations has created a new ability to make and forecast comparative impact of disease entities upon mankind.

Traditionally, epidemiologic investigations consider information gathered among preestablished factors such as sex, age, prior conditions, concomitant health status, and so on. As a simple example, if among 100 whites living in a temperate climate, one incident of a given disease had occurred within a one-year period, then it would be anticipated the same fate would befall 1% of all whites living in an equivalent climate. If the rate, the likelihood, or the probability seems insufficiently qualified, you are probably thinking like a lawyer instead of an epidemiologist.

In fairness to the latter, however, he/she bases analysis and predictions on as many epidemiologic factors as is reasonable to a scientific outlook, which in turn is based upon prior training and experience. A major concern for the epidemiologist is that he/she must accrue and use factual information provided by a diverse group of fact gatherers, no matter what their skills, their biases, or their competencies.

SCOPE OF PHARMACOEPIDEMIOLOGIC INQUIRY

Pharmacoepidemiology is a special area of epidemiology that deals with one special source of disease or illness: that derived from ingestion, application, or administration of pharmaceuticals to humans or animals.

Pharmacoepidemiologic studies are either prospective or retrospective in purpose and approach. The Food and Drug Administration and the manufacturer utilize both in the new drug investigation and approval procedure, and in postmarketing analysis this plays a role in the FDA's determination as to acceptability of proffered new product labeling from the time of product introduction to research and to the market.[11] Change of any factor in the mix of epidemiologic conclusions can be devastating. For example, following years of careful study at a particular dosage level, age group, or indications for use, a change occurs in one such factor. Obviously, the rates of both safety and effectiveness may thereafter be at first unpredictable and later show complete disparity with prior rates. The chloroquine experience in the 1950s is a good example. Serendipitous augmentation of product use indications is a frequent cause of this kind of an event.

Thus, at the present time, no prescription drug that engenders ADRs is immune from epidemiologic analysis. However, in the most recent past, some particular drug entities have been studied closely for these purposes.

THE SWINE FLU EXPERIENCE

For example, when former President Gerald R. Ford initiated widespread swine flu immunization, there was some suspicion that this vaccine would suffer the mixed fate of other important vaccines such as the one for polio. That is, there would be good news and bad news: large numbers of the public freed from fear of the dreaded flu, and some persons suffering ill effects from the vaccine. The result was special preparation by the federal government to offer a degree of insulation against the "blockbuster" lawsuits that put many manufacturers out of the vaccine business. Nonetheless, even with the virtual removal of the opportunity for plaintiffs to use the favorable strict products liability route, there was extensive use of epidemiologic data to seek to prove causation in the negligence suits filed against the United States Government via the Federal Torts Claim Act (FTCA).

The villain of the piece was Guillain-Barré syndrome (GBS), described in the medical literature *(Taber's Cyclopedic Medical Dictionary)* as acute idiopathic polyneuritis or infectious neuronitis. This sometimes seemed to follow in the injected patients. Through the work of National Centers for Disease Control, the epidemiologic tag of causation was finally offered for those cases that evidenced at 10 weeks or less following inoculation with the vaccine.

There is considerable public acceptance of the value of pharmacoepidemiologic studies in reviewing classes of effects toward establishment of standards. In the handling of claims of GBS arising from the swine flu vaccination program, epidemiologic data having indicated vaccination could entail risk of GBS in the first 5 to 10 weeks, the government treated plaintiffs who claimed GBS developed after that period as improper claimants. Those who persisted in litigation usually failed to gain a verdict.[12] Only about 15% of the courts found for plaintiffs.

CAUSATION PROBLEMS

It is difficult, however, to establish cause-and-effect relationships through the use of epidemiologic techniques, as evidenced in the Agent Orange situation.[13] Often, unfortunately, the results of the study suffer from the "eyes of the beholder." Thus, the advocate for the defendant is more likely to hew to the belief that the plaintiff's seemingly favorable pharmacoepidemiologic analysis, of itself, cannot supply the causal link between a given product and a given plaintiff. Operating with statistics, how can it answer the bottom-line question of whether the defendant's product (or conduct in marketing, labeling, etc., the products) actually caused the damage to the plaintiff in the instance subject of the suit?[14] On the other hand, the plaintiff's advocate says the nexus between product and injury, if it can be shown inferentially by statistical analysis, is as good as any other relevant circumstantial evidence that would be used to prove the plaintiff's allegation.

Interest in this approach has been escalating. As Dore points out,[15] epidemiologic expert witnesses have been permitted to answer to hypothetical questions on causation, solely upon the basis of their own or other epidemiologic studies, declaring death was causally related to the employment in a uranium mine. Death of a plaintiff's decedent had been from cancer. Both plaintiffs and defendants have found journalistic interest in theories of liability predicated on epidemiologic studies. In a press release following an unfavorable verdict in a Bendectin case (*Philadelphia Inquirer,* Jan. 21, 1987, B-2), Merrell-Dow, one of the defendants, asserted: "The safety of Bendectin has been well supported by over 35 published epidemiologic studies or reports, [and] the evidence in this trial did not show that Bendectin causes birth defects specifically." Epidemiology as a determinant for causation must meet the qualifications that traditionally distinguish real evidence. Like statistical studies, they may offer bricks to build a theory of causation, but without the mortar of fact to maintain the cohesion and the edifice, they may fail the task.

The history of Dalkon Shield litigation is another well-known mass of cases where first knowledge of danger was developed through epidemiologic studies. Although the various problems associated with its use caused the proprietor, A. H. Robins, to withdraw it from the market in 1974, thousands of product liability suits in the United States and elsewhere have been filed. The results of the epidemiologic studies and the history of the product are well described.[16] The role that epidemiologic reports played in *Dalkon Shield* was to indicate that such analyses are fruitful to demonstrate an increased level of risk of which the supplier should be aware or should have been aware.

When Faich and others are discussing PMS of the prescription and diagnostic modalities in use today, they are describing systematic accrual of incident information concerning such drugs available in the marketplace.[17] Preferably, these reports deal with use of the product named as labeled. Therefore, although the primary components of PMS involve monitoring ADRs and feeding these into epidemiologic studies, qualification of the information tendered in the ADRs must be of great concern lest it develop or disturb hypotheses constructed therefrom.[18] Like all other data for analysis, the competency, the bias, and the interest of the source, apart from mere mechanical errors, must cause concern.

Much could be written concerning the epidemiology of the antibiotics involved in numerous class cases. Similarly, in those cases dealing with individual complaints, one finds cases similar to *Wooderson v. Ortho.*[19] In the *Feldman* tetracycline case, where eventually the New Jersey Supreme Court reasserted the importance of Comment k and the "state of the art" in defense, the FDA had earlier denied the manufacturer's offer to warn of risks of staining of the teeth of infants on the basis of insufficient evidence.[20] However, in some states, compliance with governmental regulations, and specifically with those of federal agencies of acknowledged expertise in implementing particular statutes, is seen as an affirmative defense. One such state is now Kansas, perhaps in reaction to *Wooderson.*[21]

THE VARIETY OF PURPOSES SERVED BY PHARMACOEPIDEMIOLOGIC REVIEW

The importance of ADRs and epidemiologic studies for the supplier of drugs and devices is that these afford a means of keeping the labeling at a state-of-the-art level. A supplementary new drug application to improve or add warning information to the package insert may be undertaken by the supplier unilaterally under certain conditions.[22] However, there is much concern that the practice, which protectively lists every suspicion aroused by every ADR, will make the package insert inaccurate and unreadable for the practitioner.

Another purpose of epidemiologic review by the FDA, facilitated by the recording and reporting requirements at 21 CFR 314.80 and 314.81, is to distinguish reported effects of the drug from other influences, such as spontaneous changes in the course of a disease; placebo effects; biased observations; or the confusion that can arise from concomitant pharmacologic entities and procedural accidents. This is also why the FDA requires adequate and well-controlled studies to create original labeling.[23] They will not allow lesser standards of validation to change labeling.

Traditionally, the FDA has stated that the 15-day reporting requirements in Para. (c)(i)(ii) of 21 CFR 314.80 apply to a significant increase in frequency of a serious, expected adverse drug experience as well as reports of adverse drug experiences that are both serious and unexpected. These may come from reports found in scientific and medical journals either as the result of a formal clinical trial, or from epidemiologic studies or analyses of experience in a monitored series of patients.

All communications between the FDA and holders of a new drug application are required to be emplaced in the NDA file,[24] and these are therefore available to counsel in their litigatory review of that file.

LEGAL THEORIES OF REDRESS: CIVIL LIABILITY

It is hornbook law that the manufacturer of a product can be liable to the user if the user is injured due to failure of the manufacturer to exercise reasonable care in warning potential users of product hazards—though the product is itself neither negligently designed, nor negligently researched prior to agency submission, nor negligently manufactured for either its research or commercial use.[25] To exercise reasonable care in warning potential users of prescription drugs, the innovator, manufacturer, or other supplier is to provide an accompanying product description that reflects state-of-the-art knowledge for the patient who uses the product or for the learned intermediary who directs use of the product in accordance with the labeling. Reasonable ways of maintaining such current state-of-the-art knowledge are for manufacturers (1) to share with the FDA the ADRs that are received, regardless of how they were obtained—bibliographically or otherwise; and (2) to be responsive to FDA's suggested changes in the package insert, especially to warnings, contraindications, and indications for use.

The exercise of reasonable care includes not only a willingness to add warnings, but also a willingness to exclude unscientific hypotheses, rumors, or unsubstantiated reports. It is much easier to just add the latter, but both the FDA and the drug labeler understand that they must encourage recourse to the package insert by discouraging haphazard additions and other clutter that may obscure important precautionary recommendations.[26] But not all manufacturers or lawyers will take the risk. Prescription drug suppliers are more likely to add even unverified reports that stand as aberrations in pharmacoepidemiologic studies when they associate a use of the product with an appreciable gravamen of injury. It may even make sense to consider additional warnings based upon the allegations of a legal complaint. While substantiation may not be proven, the claims of a similar nature likely to follow in some instances may thus be tempered.

Within the statutory scheme of adverse reaction reporting, recording, and monitorial activities, special attention is given the serious and unpredicted reactions, although quantitatively the major substance of report systems tends to be pharmacologically predictable based upon the composition of the drug, its labeling, and its track record in clinical use prior to general usage. It is the strange occurrences—whether idiosyncratic, bordering on the incredible, or unpredictable—that usually play a role in product liability considerations. However, what has distinguished some plaintiffs' attorneys is not their ability to convince a jury that the unpredictable should have been predictable, but rather that the package insert statements concerning the predictable were inadequate in the light of the frequency and the gravamen of the injury.

By a system based upon pharmacoepidemiology, the Food and Drug Administration has translated the statutory mandate (mainly as expressed in 21 USC 355) into a vast bureaucratic mechanism for accumulating notice and description of adverse drug reactions incidental to the use of modern potent therapeutic and diagnostic drug products. The objective of such programming, at least as it affects prescription drugs, seems to assure the contemporary character of the accompanying labeling. The belief is that, on notice of not heretofore noted adverse drug reactions, these will be added to the package insert in the appropriate category, or that increased frequency, or growth of gravamen of injury, will similarly cause changes to the package insert and update its usefulness to the physician intermediary in terms of safety considerations. All of this depends upon systematic scientific validation.

Subsequent to this mainly time-tethered accrual process, tally sheets are available which chronicle the number of reports received in the various categories, not all of which are mutually exclusive. Examination of the underlying reports often shows them to have substantial dissimilarities but be categorized together. Lawyers have found that there are ways of using these counts, following their discovery, (1) as a means of accomplishing early pressured settlement of incipient litigation; (2) as a means of remaining in the court despite a lack of facts to support such a right; and (3) as evidence where judicial unsophistication may gain admission for them despite their hearsay character or a legally insufficient show of relevance or materiality.

In federal courts, and under federal rules, certain species of data gleaned by the district agency so charged to do may come in as exceptions to the hearsay rule. The Census Bureau, the National Highway Traffic Administration, and the Federal Energy Regulatory Commission all contribute to use for such purpose. In the health care field, the Consumer Product Safety Commission, the Food and Drug Administration, the National Centers for Disease Control, and National Institutes of Health provide data and statistics that are widely used and often admitted for some purpose. If one examines the basis for these statistical summaries— for example, such as developed by the FDA from reports of incidents of adverse drug reactions—the medical scientist must be for the most part disappointed, while the lawyer (or at least the defense lawyer) is outraged at times.

FLAWS IN SUBSTANCE OR OBTENTION OF EPIDEMIOLOGIC "EVIDENCE"

First of all, the events are generally a hodgepodge of statements and information recorded by persons frequently not themselves positive of the actual happening. The data are often preliminary and not in sufficient detail, and sometimes follow-up, where possible, is contradictory. The data are neither initiated nor recorded by individuals in purely objective terms in most instances. There are insufficiencies as to patient history, manner of administration, concurrent procedures or medications, and so on. Often the reporters are persons concerned with the possibility of lawsuits against themselves, their professional associates, or the hospital that may be involved. In multiple cases where generic equivalents are used, the report is most likely to go, as does the inquiry, to the pioneer brand manufacturer, because the latter is likely to offer the most resources for the present and future. The reports are not at all likely to describe whether the product was itself changed, diluted, or admixed, or whether it was used in the manner recommended by the manufacturer. The subsequent result is a multiple-hearsay nightmare for the plaintiff and the defendant to sort out if the incident becomes the subject of litigation. Then there exists the possibility that somehow admissibility and relevance will extrude from the compost.

The FDA is quick to state that such reports, whether individual or tabular, are prepared and published without any assertion that they signify an observation as to cause and effect.[27] But there they are, and whether the fundamental complaint is for failure to design or failure in warning or instructions for use, a handhold is apparent that all too frequently enjoys far more respect and attention than it merits. "The fact that someone had made a claim is, applying established principles of evidence law, of questionable relevance."[28]

A plaintiff's attorneys seek to use the FDA's adverse drug reaction information either as a claim or as reports for proof that the manufacturer was "on notice" of the kind of effect his drug might have earlier than its acknowledgment in the package insert as a possible hazard of use. They are seeking to elevate a report riddled with hearsay to the status of notice of danger—even, notice of product defect and, sometimes, the loosely worded status of a claim—and all too frequently judges are failing to distinguish such documents (because they are couched in language of another discipline) from acceptable documents for purposes of notice. They are using these conjectural pieces to intone strict liability requirements. Worst of all, they are not getting discriminatory guidance from the scientific community, which has become caught up with the phenomenal potential of pharmacoepidemiology to bulwark the therapeutic and diagnostic selective processes. The interesting thing is that an ADR—or DER (drug experience report), as they may be alternatively called—does not rise to the level of a complaint or a claim. An adverse drug reaction is defined by the agency generally as "any unwanted occurrence experienced while on treatment with a specific drug, that is not part of the expected and intended pharmacologic action of the drug. A causal relationship is not necessarily implied."[29]

Complaints carry an allegation of causation, dealing with the complainant's adverse experience with the use of the product due to some kind of defect that is part of the allegation. Whether in the form of a letter, an oral report reduced to writing, information on a governmental form or within legal proceedings, the writer is identifiable and signifies a belief on his own knowledge or from the knowledge of one he represents privately or publicly that the product is defective in some manner, causing the injury or loss subject of the complaint.

With respect to adverse reaction reporting, manufacturers usually initiate changes in the package insert when the reports, by increased number, kind, or seriousness, need to be reflected to the prescribers. But regardless, the FDA is constantly reviewing adverse reaction reports and will initiate package insert changes on their own.

Many ADRs are based solely upon allegations in the legal complaint served upon the drug or device manufacturer and may even prove entirely fictitious at the time of litigation two, three, or more years later.[30] In such cases, the adverse reaction may have already become permanently entrenched within the official product description (package insert).

Because the complaints are then part of a litigation process that generally involves the various treating or diagnosing practitioners, the hospitals, and the manufacturer, all at some point in time will have been instructed to provide no further information on the claimed incident until the later trial, thus frustrating any attempt by either the FDA or the reporters, in seeking further information toward details that are essential, or following that, may aid validation or invalidation.

ADRs that have been filed by many manufacturers concerning dependency and dermatotoxicity with regard to strong analgesics rarely consider drug abuse. Thus some reports that come in are predicated on acceptance of the often unreliable word of drug abusers as to the identity, the form, and the dosage of the product used, to say nothing of frequency, materials, or mode of ingestion or injection that may have been used.[31] These ADRs too appear in the files of the FDA and on the charts.

Evidence of prior instances of defect effect is generally admitted on the issue of existence of the design defect and perhaps also defendant's notice of same, but only where the plaintiff shows they occurred under circumstances substantially similar to those at issue in his case. Even then, it is within judicial discretion, considering Federal Rule of Evidence (FER) #403 and similar state rules, to exclude such evidence on the ground that their prejudicial effect, likelihood of confusion, or undue delay outstrips their probative value for the jury's determination.[32] Thus trial judges similarly have the power to exclude reports from the Food and Drug Administration, including tabular summaries and other exhibits that fall into the area of epidemiologic analysis.

Failure to warn of hazards associated with foreseeable uses of a product is of itself negligent conduct, so that where such an omission proximately results in a plaintiff's injuries, damages may be recovered. In the same vein, the inadequacy of the package insert is a defect in the product, providing the vehicle for the strict liability claim. However, many ADRs are surely the hearsay tales of disguised misuse. Thus the report may be issued "defensively" and even with inaccuracies as to dosage, procedure, concomitant medication, and so on. It is not too farfetched to speculate that some physician and some institutional reports are predicated on a fear of being sued, and the report is intended to potentially deflect the onslaught of those who represent the patient. I know of one instance where the drug named was not used, but another drug used in error caused the paralytic injury. Despite the original ADR and the follow-ups, it was not until plaintiff's attorneys discovered the error, and an attempted cover-up in their wholesale gathering of hospital documents, that this came to be noted. On the tables prepared by the FDA, this is still shown as an ADR involving paralysis following "use" of the not-used drug.

Accrual of incident reports that show various risks will no doubt be seen by many (including firms) as creating a duty to warn where there was no warning prior. Here, however, agency purposes, scientific thinking, and legal thinking may become separables. Despite occasional statements otherwise, the agency is perceived to want every report, no matter how remotely associated the reported incident may be, no matter how incomplete or uncorroborated, and no matter the degree of hearsay that figures in the communication. And that's what they often get! Scientific usage of the reports from any source requires an acceptable degree of hearsay, because the report is scientifically valueless unless subject to corroboration. They need complete information, including a usual medical history, the stated observations of those immediately in attendance, accurate time intervals where involved, test findings when and where taken, concurrently and concomitantly used drugs, devices, and even foods. They need follow-up, that is, past reaction history, operations, and testing. It is only rarely that the initial report of the adverse reaction incident has any follow-up and still more rare that it has the kind of follow-up required for the medical scientist to validate, that is, credit or discredit the report.

For legal thinking, the plaintiff notes that the reports categorically deny they can establish causation, as a matter of the formal language on the FDA's individual or cumulative incident reports. Yet he/she also notes that this language does not of itself deny causation. In fact, frequently the unadorned formal language and the captions on the forms cloak the product subject of the report with suspicion of malfeasance and draw history that infers a line of occurrence from use of the product to the patient's final injury.[33]

It is true, strictly speaking, that if the injured individual is not the author of the complaint, in its ultimate form it too is hearsay. But if there are degrees of hearsay, and there are, it is likely of a lesser degree than the ADR and FDA's accrual of statistics of ADRs.

USE OF ADRs BY PLAINTIFFS

In either case, where an adversary seeks to use either complaints or ADRs in an affirmative manner to rebut motions for dismissal, or to establish an evidentiary basis for proof of notice prior, or for similar purpose, the other party can and should be expected to claim hearsay disqualification. Whether that will be granted becomes a matter for contrasting judicial philosophies and traditions to determine, often leading to inconsistency.[34]

While business records are frequently hearsay, most attorneys quickly sweep all company adverse reaction reports and correspondence concerning their products into that category by citing regulatory and statutory requirements for such record keeping. But if put strictly to the test of admissibility as a business record, in either a state or federal court it might fall short of meeting the requirements of the rules governing admissibility as such. Adversaries should put each such grouping of material to whatever test the rule calls for in the court of trial. Their flaw is apt to be that they are made without recourse to direct knowledge of the circumstances recorded. Thus in testing admissibility on hearsay objection, surprising results may occur, differentiating a legal approach from a regulatory or bureaucratic approach.[35]

In *Paul v. Winthrop*, N.Y. State Supreme Court (Westchester County), Sept. 1981, the plaintiff attempted to have his expert witness, a physician who ran a drug abuse clinic for the Veterans' Administration, read into the record drug experience reports that the manufacturer had filed with the FDA following the doctor's telephoned reports to them.[36] Judge Sifken would not admit the reports either as evidence of truth that the subject drug caused dermatotoxic reactions or that they were notice of same. The doctor had not used injections of the drug in these patients. The drug abusers and addicts presented themselves to him with various complaints, which they attributed to injections of the drug they had given to themselves following illicit procurement of same. In short, the expert was accepting this hearsay as gospel from persons who were known to be unreliable, and he was seeking to present it as evidence. The same is often accomplished by an expert describing a bibliographic reference he has selected which on examination, in many instances, is the author's hearsay recounting of events not personally known to him.

Of course at the very least, the attorneys should demand a limiting instruction which will advise the jury that what is being said is no evidence of truth of the substance of the statement, but at best is evidence that the manufacturer was put on notice as to an allegation.[37] In short, "we don't know if it really happened, or happened the way they said, but this shows when they told defendant it happened, and how they let him know." Thus since "notice" voids the hearsay objection, the hearsay comes into the record for that limited purpose.

In rejecting evidence of consumer complaints on hearsay grounds for any useful purpose, the Fourth Circuit in *Ellis* emphasized judicial economy and the danger such materials pose in prolongation of the time of trial. This is eminently true, and any lawyer who has suffered through the discovery procedure when such economy is discouraged by the wide latitude afforded discovery procedures sees more than mere judicial economy here. Discovery, where adverse reaction reports, prior complaints, claims, and so on are examined in detail, pile on legal fees for the litigants mercilessly.

For the defendant's legal representatives, as might be expected, they consider the incident reports of the FDA, individual or accumulative, to be hearsay of the worst order, unreliable as to causation, and mischievous if in any way communicated to the court and jury.

IMPACT OF ADRs ON EVIDENTIARY PRODUCTION

The existence of these reports, dated as they are for time of occurrence, is often utilized to defeat the defendant's motions for aborting a lawsuit in which, up to the time of trial, the plaintiff has shown no credible grounds on which to remain suited.

Further, the reports, unless redacted, carry the names of patients, physicians, and treating institutions, and the two latter are especially sensitive to the need that any suspicion of difficulty suffered by the patient be attributed to someone else. Thus the plaintiff's attorneys will examine ADRs filed by a defendant drug manufacturer with their FDA history brought forward. They will then approach physicians, preferably located in the jurisdictions in which they operate, and query them about each report that bears their name. By inference, by persuasion, and by other means, they seek to induce the physician to speculate for them as to causation, and even to testify.

Thus it should be obvious that epidemiologic data and testimony may provide a twofold bonanza to a plaintiff. It is very valuable in the discovery phase, the preparation of the case. It may also have great value in developing proof of "failure to warn" or "failure to redesign" as related to product defect and defendant's conduct.

As for the defendant, during discovery, the rules are so liberal and the preponderant majority of trial judges so unwilling to restrict a plaintiff's access to any information that may lead to useful evidence, that they can make very little objection to epidemiologic exploration in the defendant's files. There are a few exceptions to this unfettered plaintiff privilege. Defendants need only access epidemiologic data that applies to the kind of injury or occurrence claimed, and only up to the date of the plaintiff's alleged incident of injury. Further, insofar as the FDA by regulation requires strict maintenance of confidentiality as to reporters of adverse reactions, their names may be redacted from the ADRs.

Needless to say, there are jurisdictions, judges, attorneys' competence and personalities, and particular plaintiff or defendant circumstances admixed into the handling of epidemiologic discovery that may influence breadth and degree of the exceptions noted.

EXPERT WITNESSES, EPIDEMIOLOGISTS, AND OTHERS

Another dimension in the problem of epidemiologic testimony and evidence which is often rather vividly shown is that, as in other branches of medicine, while peer consistency and consensuality is cherished, it need not exist.[38] Epidemiologists may find the study, the analysis, and the conclusions of other epidemiologists flawed. Taking that even further in the matter of prescription drugs, national impressions as to competency, resources, and sometimes merely national self-esteem may bias epidemiologic evaluations made in particular countries. For easy example, in *Wooderson,* it was the FDA's distrust of the validity of British epidemiologic conclusions as to a connection between certain generally formulated contraceptive tablets and hemolytic uremia syndrome (HUS) that delayed adoption of the warning in Ortho's package insert. Similarly, many other nations with sophisticated systems for drug approval (i.e., Japan, Canada, and France) will not accept the U.S. FDA's approval of a product here for safety and efficacy as labeled, but will require independent proof in their own country and to their own standards. This speaks of epidemiologic distrust, since the new drug approval process, no less than postmarketing surveillance programs, is heavily dependent upon epidemiologic systemization and accrual of first experimental, then clinical case report forms that are carefully evaluated as a primary step in drug approval.

In establishing the swine flu immunization program at the urging of then President Ford, the Congress provided that the United States would serve as a substituted defendant for actions brought to redress personal injury or death evolving from the program.[39] Thus, the standard for determining liability is the same as under the FTCA. Liability, further, should be determined according to the law of the jurisdiction wherein the tort occurred.[40] In almost all instances, this will require the application of state law. Those laws, in turn, create the need to prove that a defendant's conduct actually and proximately caused plaintiff's injury and damages. In the often-quoted language of Cardozo at the turn of the century, the court must be satisfied of more than a mere possibility of causation, because reasonable foreseeability depends upon probabilities.

In his opinion in *Francis Szczepaniak v. U.S.A.,* District Judge Mazzone heard the testimony of six medical expert witnesses, including the plaintiff's treating physician who was a board-certified neurologist, Martin Goldfield, an epidemiologist, Charles Poser, a neurologist, as well as three other board-certified neurologists: David Dawson, H. Royden Jones, and James Coatsworth. Judge Mazzone analyzed the initial and dispositive issue as to whether this plaintiff had suffered a transverse myelitis as a result of his swine flu injection. The opinion clearly indicates that it was the plaintiff's burden to prove medical causation by a fair preponderance of the evidence and that the mere possibility of a partial Guillain-Barré syndrome might be inadequate to trigger the probability of an epidemiologic trail leading from the flu vaccination. The district judge, having heard especially the testimony of Goldfield, who had spent 20 years with the New Jersey State Department of Health and was an old hand at swine flu virus, was not of a mind to accept the doctor's techniques of statistical extrapolation, commonly used in epidemiology. Epidemiologic evidence all too often becomes the handmaiden for possibilities rather than probabilities, unless they can fairly establish through preponderance of the evidence that there has been proximate cause.[41]

Thus, as in *Szczepaniak*, epidemiologic evidence of association between the product and an injury is likely to be by itself insufficient without additional means to establish causation. This is certainly in keeping with the FDA's admonition on its ADRs that such a reported association is not deemed proof of cause and effect.

Incidentally, another problem with the use of testimony by accredited epidemiologists such as Gold is the likelihood that they have spent the great majority of their careers in administration, academic, and research posts rather than as practicing physicians who have examined patients and taken medical history from patients. When, as in this case, such an expert is set against a prominent practitioner, the academician suffers from the comparison in court.

Many legal writers find pharmacoepidemiologic studies for regulatory ends extremely desirable and effective, even though they are much less enthusiastic about using such studies in litigation. For example, none will quarrel with the value of postmarketing surveillance as epidemiologic oversight as to use patterns of drugs made available through the NDA procedure. Not only does this provide information on the safety and effectiveness of the product in the hands of the larger and less expert body of practitioners than those who carried out the Phase III work prior to NDA approval, it also informs on the effectiveness of the labeling in terms of product use, and it does provide the denominator for select numerators that reflect particular factors of interest. For the attorney, a denominator figure can also be achieved by calculating the volume of the product used from either sales figures or FDA records. There may also be danger in how each advocate views what sometimes appears to be egregious abuse of judicial discretion exercised by the trial judge.

But the major differential is that in regulatory efforts, epidemiologic data are collected and addressed as a prelude to evaluation, while in the courtroom such data are all too frequently sought to be introduced as truth or fact for evidence or evaluation of causation. And in the courtroom, when and if counsel has not been able to bar its admission to the jury, it can create unavoidable prejudice. For even where the admission is conditioned upon restrictive purpose and judicial instruction, the attorney must despair. "It is true that lawyers rightly mistrust instructions that tell juries to disregard what they have just heard; our memories are independent of our wills."[42]

We have previously noted that whether called DERs (drug experience reports) or ADRs (adverse drug reactions) for the plaintiff's attorney in discovery proceedings for drug or device products liability litigation, these records and reports represent a great resource. He/she can usually gain access to those in possession of the defendant(s), but with a little foresight he/she can increase his/her survey or improve it with refinement and particularity via use of the Freedom of Information Act (FOIA). Except through the use of FOIA requests, no manufacturer can ever have the complete file of such reporting to the same extent as the Food and Drug Administration. To the FDA come the reports of independent reporters as well as those of the manufacturer. Frequently, reports go to them from sources around the world—practitioners, hospitals, domestic organizations, and even competitors—who do not inform the product proprietor. In addition, one can particularize the interest in the reports to those that deal with one style of injury that has been reported, whether or not described in the current product package insert.

While judges should not admit ADRs into evidence individually as such except in the rarest of circumstances and for the narrowest of purposes, these reports can play a role in the testimony of expert witnesses and often do despite their quintessential hearsay nature. When they are allowed into evidence as such, despite their nature their prejudicial effect is apt to be so dangerous that the adversary would have to run a mini-trial for each one. But experts can and do opine on the basis of their study of ADRs.

EVIDENCE OF PRIOR COMPLAINTS

There is some similarity here to the ordinary practice of seeking to discover and later introduce evidence of complaints against the product. So, for example, in a suit to show a french fryer of potatoes supplied by General Electric was defective in design, the plaintiff sought information as to all other instances where persons, beyond employees of fast-food establishments, were burnt using the fryer. The defendant objected in that the plaintiff's burns arose because, as he bent over the fryer, his aerosolized antiasthmatic device fell into the hot oil and exploded, causing the burns. General Electric said this was a one-of-a-kind occurrence.[43] (I am surprised the plaintiff's attorney did not go after the manufacturer of the antiasthmatic device for failure to warn about its danger when dropped into french fryers full of combustible oil at high temperature. That would not be reportable as an ADR under current FDA guidelines.)

Circuit Judge Mikva differed with District Court Judge Green, who had directed a verdict for the defendant and refused to sanction GE for refusing to comply with the plaintiff's discovery demand. Following Judge Mikva's review, the court on retrial would have to allow the "epidemiologic" history of the french fryer into evidence for some purpose and in some form, and the defendant would need to rebut or qualify each incident, even though none such involved dropping a pressurized aerosol antiasthmatic device into the cauldron of oil. Judge Mivka nonetheless argued that the other incidents were admissible as relevant to show both dangerousness and notice, no matter that they were substantially dissimilar to the plaintiff's episode.

Defense attorneys are more likely to emphasize the legal deficiencies of postulations dependent heavily on pharmacoepidemiologic or chemoepidemiologic studies, because they are seeking to nonsuit claimants for failure in causation connection between product and plaintiff, and plaintiff and injury. Judges who likewise concern themselves with jury instruction that requires findings of causation and proximate cause of injury based on some facts are seen by plaintiffs' attorneys as obstacles. For easy examples, in *Robinson,* the federal judge cited vast differences between experts in the field of epidemiology that translated into an unreliable basis. He also explicitly stated that epidemiologic evidence could no more establish cause and effect than bare statistical evidence. The probability-of-causation connection calls for a greater than 50% possibility that defendant's product caused damage.[44] In a southwestern federal court[45] a year earlier, the trial judge would not admit epidemiologic evidence to show causation, to a class of persons, for purposes of showing increased risk to the class. Yet one purpose of FDA epidemiologic studies is to ascertain whether patients are at greater risk from the product than the package insert indicates.

Szczepaniak v. U.S. (see earlier discussion) in the northeastern part of the United States about a year later indicates the same wholesome skepticism of the use of epidemiologic studies in litigation, but there the plaintiff had to overcome a subtle reluctance to find the sovereign liable in the swine flu vaccine–Guillain-Barré controversy. ". . . The broad-based statistical conclusions that are its product (epidemiology) do not alone establish the legal causation necessary for demonstrating liability in a court of law." When the swine flu vaccination program was terminated December 16, 1976, after about 42 million doses had been administered, it was because of the epidemiologic notice of large numbers of Guillain-Barré syndrome among recipients. What made the role of epidemiologic studies more tenuous in GBS was that it was a syndrome rather than a specific disease. Thus epidemiologic factoring in the class of users was as difficult as medical diagnosis in the individual. And, if medicine can lay no claim to exactitude, how can epidemiology?

A so-called tag-along case, *Baker v. U.S.,*[46] which was filed just as Judge Gesell ended his judicial panel on multidistrict litigation in regard to the swine flu inoculation cases, was finally decided April 30, 1987. Significantly, the only liability issue for the court was causation, and while the court found for the plaintiff, the battle was fought on medical diagnosis and countered on that basis rather than on mere epidemiologic evidence. In fact, as in *Manko v.*

U.S.[47] a year earlier, it was the expert testimony of qualified neurologists that carried the plaintiff to an award. However, here also the fact finder's role was to carefully weigh the medical and scientific evidence and their sources to reach finding of legally acceptable causation.[48]

Earlier cases involving diethylstilbestrol (DES) have also lent themselves to epidemiologic guidelines for the product's federally uniform labeling. The history of DES litigation and the theories of finding or rejecting liability are too well known to repeat here, but both the Food and Drug Administration and epidemiologic studies continue to play a role in these proceedings. In one case that served many plaintiff's causes, the California appellate court did affirm a jury decision for the plaintiff without proof of causation for her condition. They relied on epidemiologic studies fortified by medical expert opinion.[49]

In the swine flu cases as in *Baker,* plaintiffs were found to have offered proof in their cases that met the preponderance of evidence test by offering medical proof that they contracted GBS in a reasonable period, epidemiologically constructed, following their vaccination. Thus, using epidemiologic studies to establish growth of awareness of risk and actual risk may be sounder than using it to prove causation, no matter the judicial orientation in the particular court.

In *O'Gilvie v. International Playtex Inc.,*[50] the court found sufficient evidence, mainly in the form of epidemiologic testimony, to support the trial court's finding that the Playtex tampon package inserts did not keep pace with the development of association with toxic shock syndrome. The evidence further supported a $10 million punitive damages award for the conduct of the manufacturer in not keeping abreast of its competitors' labeling and design changes. The catch-22 in this situation is that defendants argued their warning was adequate since there was no legal proof that a causal link existed between toxic shock and their superabsorbent tampon. But, under Kansas law, an inadequate warning causes a presumption of causation, bridging the gap between article and injury.[51] Since the causation issue here was placed in the hands of a Kansas jury for determination, inadequacy of warning was the key to their positive finding.

In recalling *Wooderson v. Ortho,* a case which elicited *amicus curiae* on behalf of the contraceptive manufacturer whose labeling comported with FDA requirements contemporary with use of the product by the plaintiff, it was distrust of other than U.S. epidemiologic evidence which dissuaded both the FDA and the suppliers from warning of hemolytic uremia syndrome (HUS).

On the other hand, it was copious epidemiologic data gathered by the FDA which had induced it to create "direct to patient" labeling for products prescribed by a learned intermediary.[52] It was that same epidemiologic data that described all the inherent risks in the use of the oral contraceptives and required uniform warning language. *Wooderson* therefore, among other things, stands for the concern that suppliers should have when information on additional or greater risks of injury are communicated to them, even when the

FDA is content with the product package insert they have in use. For in retrospect, the fears created by the English studies, if they were proven true, were creating a change in the legal status of that package insert. Comment k of the Restatement of Torts 2nd 402A,[53] in dealing with potent therapeutic and diagnostic drugs and devices, offers an exemption from strict liability theory if the package insert is not misbranded. But that is a simplification of how state liability theory touches on federal law and vice versa. State courts accept misbranding as a sign of product defect. But they accept all admissible evidence that, federal law and agency regulation notwithstanding, the package insert is actually misbranding the product by not including a warning that should have been the knowledge of the manufacturer when the product was issued. If within his knowledge, it should have been in the package insert accompanying the product. The bottom line here is that a jury, as fact finders, can second-guess the FDA with its experts and consultants, and such a second guess, as in *Wooderson,* can uphold punitive damages.

PROOF AND PHARMACOEPIDEMIOLOGIC REPORTS

The defendant argued: "I have properly reported all adverse reactions that have come to my notice to the Food and Drug Administration in accordance with the regulatory system that implements the FFDC statute; I have done so in a timely and appropriate manner. The FDA has never suggested a change or augmentation of the warnings, the contraindications, the precautions, the recitation of adverse reactions, as we have stated that in our product labeling. Does not this compliance with the regulations and this absence of criticism or recommended change from the FDA betoken that our labeling is epidemiologically sound?"

While state courts deem compliance with law or administrative agency regulations as merely a sign of meeting the minimal standards, that is certainly untrue in terms of standards imposed by the FDA. Yet, the Tenth Circuit, reading Kansas law, said compliance with FDA standards is not of itself dispositive of the charge the manufacturer has been negligent or indifferent. The real issue, they said, is whether "a reasonable manufacturer would have done more." Thus, in *O'Gilvie,* not only did Playtex's supposed labeling compliance fail to prove nonnegligent labeling or a nondefective product, but it also failed to preclude punitive damages (of $10 million in this case).

CAUSATION AND PROXIMATE CAUSE

Proximate cause is that cause which in natural or probable sequence produced the stated injury. While it need not be the only cause or the one closest in time to the occurrence of injury, it must be clearly and distinctly causal. It can concur with another causal element acting at the same time, the combination causing the injury, but concurrent or contributory cause is not to be confused with alternative cause.[54]

In products liability, whether on theories of strict liability or traditional negligence, proximate cause must be shown for liability. That is, either the product defect in strict liability or the defective conduct in tort liability must have proximately caused the injury of which the plaintiff complains. Therefore, epidemiologic analysis, however useful in characterizing the growth of notice as to product defect or failure of design or warning, is not meaningful legally unless the product or labeling defect has caused the damage in the particular instance.

In considering the necessity for pharmacoepidemiology, one need only hark back to the advent of the two styles of polio cases that arose following vaccination with first the "killed" vaccine of Salk and then the "live" vaccine of Sabin. The former gave rise to numerous lawsuits, based actually on "adulterated" vaccine, so that the children vaccinated developed polio in some small numbers *(Gottsdanker v. Cutter Laboratories).* In the case of the Sabin vaccine, certain narrow population groups of adults, again in small numbers, developed polio through contact with vaccinated children. These were "misbranding" cases in legal parlance, since the plaintiffs argued failure to effectively warn of the risk *(Givens v. Lederle Labs).*[55] Here were two distinct kinds of drug-induced clusters of reports.

The earlier thalidomide disaster that served to change the Federal Food, Drug and Cosmetic Act was literally a universal occurrence of phocomelia in the newborns of a class of female patients who used the drug as a nonbarbiturate sedative during pregnancy. Although I do not know much of the history of thalidomide subsequent to the epidemiologic analysis that eventuated in its withdrawal, it would seem the same data would have established it as a useful nonbarbiturate sedative for males and women past childbearing age.

In the Agent Orange cases,[56] "the weakness of the evidence of causation as to all plaintiffs," as well as the strength of the military contractor defense, moved the court to develop a settlement figure and fashion an appropriate distribution scheme. In the appellate court 818 F.2d 145 (1987), the opinion of Justice Winter made clear that Chief Judge Weinstein's press to settle appreciated the fact that a ragtag assembly approach to evidentiary proof was epidemiologically unsound. The effort of media pundits, who seized upon the sympathetic tale of dioxin damage and tried to create a web of unfortunate occurrences in a quantity and of quality to simulate chemoepidemiologic evidence, was transparently inadequate. Epidemiologic studies of Vietnam veterans, many of which were undertaken by the United States, Australian, and various state governments, demonstrate no greater incidence of relevant ailments among these veterans than among any other group. To an individual plaintiff, a serious ailment will seem highly unusual. For example, the very existence of a birth defect persuade grieving parents as to Agent Orange's guilt. However, a trier of fact must confront the statistical probability that thousands of birth defects in children born to a group the size of the plaintiff class might not be unusual without exposure to Agent Orange. A trier of fact must also confront the fact that there is almost no evidence, even in studies involving animals, that exposure of males to dioxin causes birth defects in their children.

In the Agent Orange case, one would say chemoepidemiologic studies provided defense against the legally defective proofs sought to be mustered by a well-orchestrated plaintiffs' barrage of horror and sympathy journalism.

But it was only by the exertion of judicial prerogative that this had any influence, and the substantial settlement fund established in the process exhibits concession to the lack of certainty that the defendants' epidemiologic studies offered. So while the Agent Orange saga illustrates the defensive value of chemoepidemiologic studies, to be used as evidence, no less than where sought for plaintiff purposes, it may remain suspect as legal proof.[57]

Defendants argue in the usual prescription drug products liability case that bibliographic references to undesired reactions in human or animal use are to be considered like drug experience reports, as undocumented coincidences, unless a process of scientific validation, contemporary or retrospective, offers certain proof to the contrary. Plaintiffs, on the other hand, enlist the use of pharmacoepidemiologic studies to prove that a failure in the design of the product was manifest at a time previous to the occasion of the plaintiff's injury.

When there are design shortcomings, the supplier is expected to correct the design if that is feasible, given the usefulness for which the product is intended. If these changes are not possible without sacrifice to the benefit and the utility of the product, the supplier has a duty to warn the user. In the case of prescription drugs and devices, that means warning the learned intermediary who is directing use of the product, directing its administration, or administering it. Thus if a state-of-the-art warning accompanies the product to the learned intermediary, if *ab initio* contemplated benefits outweigh known deficits providing a rationale for introduction to the learned intermediary, then principles of strict liability do not apply. At best, an injured plaintiff must undertake the burden of providing a case in negligence or professional malpractice.

Therefore to a plaintiff seeking to establish a case against a supplier on a bottom-line failure to warn, although strict liability via 402A, 402B, or breach of warranty is desired, proof of defective labeling may require more than mere epidemiologic statistics.

REACTING TO ADRs: THE TAMPON EXAMPLE

For defensive purposes however, as in *O'Gilvie v. International Playtex,* reaction time of warning accretion becomes very important. Epidemiologic studies purporting to show failure to warn despite reasonable gathering of adverse reaction notice attain greater credibility where a defendant can be shown to have demonstrated a posture of ignoring such notices. The ignorance may be manifested by failure to report as well as by failure to follow up. Failure to follow up, in turn, may be deduced from lack of internal procedures and instructions, unwillingness to attempt contact with reporters, or even failure to respond to FDA Drug Surveillance inquiries. Lagging behind competitors' labeling changes is also condemnatory.

In the case of prescription drug products, strict liability applies when a product is dangerous to an extent beyond which would be contemplated by the average intended user of the product (the average learned intermediary), on the basis of either knowledge commonly held by his professional peers, or information provided in the labeling and promotional materials accompanying the product to its ultimate prescriber. While, conceptually, the product defect necessary for a strict products liability claim might be found by imperfection in the product or defective design, more often the defect is in the warning or instructions for use, stated or implied by the manufacturer.

For strict liability actions, design defect is better for the plaintiff, since it is easier to show that the defect was there when it left the manufacturer's control, and thus incorrect or abnormal postdistributive handling cannot be intervening. However, since the design of prescription drug compounds, their development, composition, testing and release are closely regulated by objective hands (the FDA), plaintiffs frequently rely upon the defect as one of inadequate, fraudulent, incorrect product information, and the product deficiency is derived from the insufficient, untimely, or missing warning to be read with the product information by the person prescribing or administering the product.

Thus, to recover for his/her plaintiff in the rather simplified circumstances of drug product strict liability, the plaintiff's counsel needs to prove that the product was defective on use, having left the supplier as such, and that the defective product caused the plaintiff's injury, resulting in the damages claimed. But the legal inference of defection in the product may not be drawn for strict liability purposes solely on evidence the injury happened.[58]

Injuries ordinarily are not compensable under strict liability theory where they arise from inherent properties of a product, obvious or known to all who come into contact with such product or a similar or related product with the same properties. For that reason the supplier's package insert, having described the adverse reaction later encountered, can only be defective if it minimized the possibility of the adverse reaction quantitatively or qualitatively. Epidemiologic study and analysis can be utilized to address such an issue by either a plaintiff or a defendant.

While the issue of whether a product is defective so as to justify imposition of strict liability usually becomes a question of fact for the jury to determine, the court may move that question from them if, as a matter of law, a plaintiff has not adequately set forth such an issue.[59]

The reason for counsel seeking ADR information directly from the FDA under FOIA is that almost one-third of the ADRs the agency accrues come from sources other than the manufacturer. This is true also where a plaintiff seeks ADR information that developed in the course of controlled clinical trials. In these, the drug has been in the hands of especially expert clinicians and reporters, and ADRs are more carefully evaluated and explained because of their impact on the approvability of the drug and its initial labeling. As Faich put it: "Contrast this with the usual postmarketing situation where confounding, noncausal associations and biased data must be dealt with."[60] As further purpose to the agency's epidemiologic approach, he suggests that "epidemiology provides a scientific approach to interpretation and collection of such PMS [postmarketing surveillance] data. When applied to observational situations, epidemiology deals with confounding and biases by stratifying, matching and other analytic means."

What excites plaintiffs especially about the pharmacoepidemiologic approach is that one can probe the existence of a prescription drug or device product defect inferentially by either direct or circumstantial evidence, and epidemiologic testimony, minus judicial discipline, may be described to a jury as use to the latter.

A problem surfacing in recent cases has been the willingness of sympathetic or apathetic judges to allow jurors to determine not only whether the warning was adequate for the plaintiff, but also to determine whether a duty to warn the plaintiff existed. The latter is clearly a question of law, not fact.

Proximate cause of the injury to the plaintiff, like existence of defect, is ordinarily a question for the jury.[61] Therefore both parties in the suit will look to epidemiologic studies to bolster their theory of the absence or existence of proximate causation from product defect to injury. Since as a practical matter juries may be majoritatively favorable to plaintiffs in drug and device products liability litigation, epidemiologic testimony may be impressive enough, in the absence of analytic guidelines from the judge, to sway them in the affirmation of proximate cause.

BENDECTIN

In *Will v. Richardson-Merrell Inc.,*[62] the U.S. District Court for the Southern District of Georgia held plaintiff parents to the usual legal burden of proof to support their allegation that the mother's ingestion of Bendectin during the early part of her pregnancy was direct cause of the child's birth defect.

The plaintiff, as in other cases involving this product and these allegations, relied upon pharmacoepidemiologic studies to show the drug had teratogenic properties. "Because the parties reached an agreement among themselves on the issue of the FDA Advisory Committee Hearings," the Court had no need to accept or challenge their admission or the FDA correspondence involved. The pharmacoepidemiologic studies relied upon by these plaintiffs were taken from animal toxicity data available both in the NDA for the product and literature in the field. The liberal Federal Rule of Evidence #702, on which various state rules are patterned, permits experts to testify in the form of an opinion or otherwise. Of course, the court must recognize them as experts first. In Rule 703, the base upon which they may opine is described. An expert may base his opinion or inference on facts or data supplied to him in a particular case, or those made known to him at or before a hearing. If these facts or data are, to the view of the court, such as would be reasonably relied upon by experts in the field to base such an opinion or inference, the facts or data could be hearsay material that need not be admissible in evidence. In short, without credible support, the expert's opinion feeds no litigable "issue of fact" for a jury. For the reasons qualified by these rules, the plaintiff's expert opinion on the Bendectin injury premise was not admissible. He admitted in an earlier deposition that he had not reviewed the epidemiologic studies published on Bendectin. Under Federal Rule of Evidence #403 the trial judge has broad discretion to exclude evidence in order to prevent needless accumulation of evidence.[63]

When there is extensive and conflicting testimony regarding the validity of studies performed and when human—as opposed to animal—studies have not borne demonstrable evidence of the defect claimed, this court felt that the plaintiff had not settled the significant issue as to causation in humans.

The key point is that epidemiologic data, whether pre- or postmarketing in nature, may be insufficient to successfully create an issue of fact for the jury as to injury causation by product defect, unless it is truly overwhelming in quality or quantity, and opinions are available from bona fide experts in the particular physiologic and pharmacologic area at issue. Defendants do not have the burden of showing the product did not cause the injury; rather, plaintiffs have the burden of showing the product defect did cause the injury.

In *Warner Lambert v. Heckler,*[64] the Third Circuit recognized that the FDA does not err, as a legal matter, when they take the position that each study could be evaluated "to determine that the results were therapeutically significant rather than merely statistically significant." Granted that this case contemplated most closely another subsection of 21 USC 355 than that which fathers FDA epidemiologic analysis involved in postmarketing surveillance, but the same reservation is appropriate here as well. In that case, the FDA refused to consider a body of expert opinion and clinical study analysis purporting to substantiate the efficacy of oral proteolytic enzymes sought to be marketed by four pharmaceutical companies. In addition to the fact that the FDA hearing did not have an opportunity to cross-examine some of these experts, Judge Sloviter noted judicial deference to FDA expertise in the evaluation process and conclusions to be derived therefrom. Despite the adverse results in cases such as *Wooderson,* there is every reason to respect the FDA's similar authority in evaluating ADRs as to the need to add or alter precautionary and warning advice within a current package insert.

SUMMARY

1. Clearly, the FDA considers their renewed adverse reaction reporting scheme as better constructed epidemiologically than ever before. If so, this will have some bearing on whether product manufacturers should see a need to redesign, relabel, or withdraw the product. And indeed, that is part of the theory of implementation by the agency of the statutory objective established at 21 USC 355 (j).

   Even more obviously, the receipt of epidemiologically evaluable reports concerning adverse reactions observed within some period of the drug's ingestion, application, or administration will construct a more complete and accurate safety profile of the drug for its continued use.

2. As previously stated by the agency in this context (44 Fed. Reg. 37434, 37453, 37455, June 26, 1979), mere association of an adverse result with use of a drug is not of itself a call to change labeling. Such "effects coincidental to the use of a drug are not necessarily synonymous with adverse reactions . . . [to] be included in prescription drug labeling." Important product information concluding warnings ought not be diluted with incidental descriptions of unsubstantiated risks.

3. From *Will v. Richardson-Merrell* (supra), we conclude that epidemiologic findings to support causation should select quality observations of association between the product and injury which are consistently observed in different settings and by different observers.

   In *Ferebee v. Chevron* (supra), we learn that sound scientific methodology and judgment, including quality observation confirmed through careful technique, design, and cautious analyses and interpretation of results, must be applied for useful epidemiologic assessment of causation.

4. From the "Report of the Tort Policy Working Group . . ." (62–63 Feb 1986, Attorney General's Office), it is clear that "courts must be more aggressive in determining the credibility of scientific and medical evidence and opinions before trial "and not allow parties to present unique, non-peer scrutinized statistics and theories to juries."

5. Pharmacoepidemologic studies and principles are used by plaintiff or defense counsel via expert witnesses, in advocacy of their cause in particular litigation where injury is alleged from drug or device use. (This includes of course, vaccines and contraceptive devices, whether with or without physician intermediaries in the scheme of availability.)

6. The use of ADRs or DERs, as they have been submitted to the FDA and recorded, is of assistance to the FDA in their pharmacoepidemiologic

analysis, even though to the legal system they appear to be cumulative hearsay. It is therefore when private advocates in drug products liability litigation seek to use them to prove product defect that judges and attorneys should and do grow wary. To the extent these are sought to be in trial, their purpose must be narrowed and the jury carefully instructed, because the bare materials are prone to bias in favor of either participant.

7. One means to seek to utilize or to overcome the bias of introducing information from ADRs or DERs is by expert witnesses, who may on one hand seek to fortify their significance, or on the other hand to ridicule, rebut, or diminish their significance. Thus the credibility of such expert witness becomes a matter of great impact. While credentials and experience play a great role in this weighing process, all the usual factors that apply to the acceptability and credibility of witnesses generally, do apply here additionally. Battles between quantity and quality of such witnesses are mediated in the main by evaluation and restrictions within the discretionary imposition of the trial judge. Much of this depends on court rules and individual application of their broad discretionary guidelines (see FRE 403, 702, 703).

   The district court was willing to grant a summary judgment in the Agent Orange litigation, where it found there was no genuine factual dispute and where expert opinions could be characterized as unreliable so "that the danger of prejudice substantially outweighed their probative value" under the rules of evidence (FRE 403).

   The next decade may tell us that FDA's use of pharmacoepidemiology is one of the most valuable applications of epidemiology from a medical and scientific view. From a legal point of view, the source material for such FDA study may become a major source of seeding for litigation. That is obviously not the FDA purpose. Postmarketing surveillance is pointed toward prospective use of the information in improvement of product design and product labeling for the public and the professions generally, not to retrospective use as to cause of injury in an individual. In the language of the FDA, no ADR can stand for a definitive statement with reference to individual causation, and no accumulation of ADRs can do so either. Experts who argue or hypothesize contrarily are suspect. If a case depends solely upon their testimony for causation, it can lead to a judicial exercise for dismissal on failure to establish cause in fact.

8. The misuse of ADRs or DERs has various manifestations. Admitting them and/or giving them evidentiary weight of any kind is fraught with danger and unfairness unless meticulously qualified and restricted. So is permitting them to provide the basis for granting or refusal of motions

that seek dismissal or summary judgment because attorneys have shown no other basis for suit. Use of them in the discovery process may invade privacy of physicians, patients, or others who have submitted such reports believing their names and institutions would not be disclosed. The exact language of the regulations states an intent not to disclose for fear of inhibiting reporting (21 CFR 314.81 (h)).

Using ADRs or DERs to stand for an approximate causation, despite the admonition on the ADR form, violates scientific as well as epidemiologic considerations of the FDA (21 CFR 314.80).

9. Government agencies in all nations undertaking governance of a distribution system involving safe and effective drugs, vaccines, devices, and so on require epidemiologic scientists. Their personnel needs are really not met by the number of those so credentialed, educated, and otherwise prepared by our medical and scientific educational institutions.

   Industry has similar needs in order to comply with the statutes and regulatory agenda implemented by many federal and state agencies (e.g., Occupational Safety and Health Administration, Food and Drug Administration, Consumer Product Safety Commission, and Environmental Protection Agency). They, too, have insufficient opportunities for recruitment. In fact, when the practitioners in the subspecialty in pharmacoepidemiology are sought, those small numbers become minuscule.

   The legal community has the same special need for epidemiologists and pharmacoepidemiologists that they have for any species of expert witnesses, but the pool is probably much smaller for these specialists than they have been accustomed to noting. A quick review of several major plaintiff and defense journals reflects the shortage of persons available. However, lawyers are inventive, and as with other medically related specialties they will innovate in selecting experts, arguing to a court if challenged that every physician has had some variety of epidemiologic training from which his education and experience can qualify him/her in the situation at hand. In addition, a jury as well as a judge is much more likely to find credible a physician with clinical experience rather than one who has had no hands-on experience with patients. For this reason, academic title and degree may also play a part in choice of expert.

10. The types of expertise and the needs of the epidemiologist's, (or pharmacoepidemiologist's) three major constituencies probably cannot be met by the product of unitary training. However, the transfer of skills between the three areas is certainly feasible.

    For the candidate's education at the university, where he/she seeks to gain academic recognition of special skill, certain suggestions are in order from my own perspective gained from years of practice in law, the teaching of law, and earlier experience as a pharmaceutical industry executive.

CONCLUDING RECOMMENDATION

I would suggest that each university program arrange for a legal course at the university or another affiliated law school. The 28-hour course should explore the legal burden borne by governmental agencies in implementing their statutory mandates. It should also provide a brief excursus into medicolegal and pharmacolegal principles associated with litigation involving both health professionals and suppliers of health care products. The design, as I envision it, would evolve to be credited as a 28-hour (14 weeks at two hours) course.

I would also suggest that within the university curriculum an internship be offered, placing candidates for certification as epidemiologists in an industrial habitat of their election among numerous eligible companies that would file with the university, indicating their needs, their resources, and their capacity for affording the intern with the additional training to which he/she aspires.

REFERENCES

1. Crout, R., "The Drug Regulatory System: Reflections and Predictions," 36 Food Drug Cosmetic Law Journal 106, 113 (1981).
2. 21 USC 355 statutorily outlines the needs to make a new drug available to clinical researchers 21 USC 355 (i); to make a new drug publicly available 21 USC 355 (a) et seq.; to make reports and keep records concerning the new drug, postmarketing surveillance 21 USC 355 (j). 21 CFR 314 et seq. are regulations drawn to effectuate the foregoing statutory mandate, which promulgations are used by FDA for their implementation procedures; 21 CFR 314.80, 314.81 is the mainstay of the FDA's epidemiologic review process.
3. Drug products liability suits are brought on various theories of redress. (Citations available from the author.)
4. 21 USC 355 (e); 21 CFR 314.80, 314.81.
5. Faich, Gerald A., "Post Marketing Surveillance of Prescription Drugs: Current Status," Washington, DC, Clinical Medicine Research Institute, October 1986.
6. Hurwitz, E. S., 313 New England Journal of Medicine 849–857 (1985). PHS study on Reye's syndrome and salicylates.
7. Data from the Office of Epidemiology and Biostatistics, Center for Drugs and Biologics, Gerald A. Faich, MD, MPH, Director).
8. 21 CFR 314.80, 314.81.
9. Kantrowitz, "Controlling Technology Democratically," 63 American Scientist 505–509 (1975).
10. Iacocca, L., Address to Opening Assembly of American Bar Association, San Francisco, August 10, 1987, as reported, litigation based on mere

possibility rather than probability as inflationary and adverse to America's capability to compete, innovate.

11. Statutory mandate provided by 21 USC 355.
12. Baker v. U.S., 660 F. Supp. 204 (1987).
13. 818 F.2d 145.
14. See 3 supra.
15. Dore, M., "A Proposed Standard for Evaluating the Use of Epidemiological Evidence in Toxic Tort and Personal Injury Cases," 28 Howard Law Journal 677 (1985).
16. In re A. H. Robins Co. Inc. . . . 406 F. Supp. 540, Judicial Panel Multiparty Litigation 1975, id 419 F. Supp. 710 (1976); id 438 F. Supp. 942 (1977); id 453 F. Supp. 108 (1978); id 505 F. Supp. 211 (1981); id 570 F. Supp. 1480 (1983). See also 745 F.2d 312 for attempt by foreign citizens to sue in U.S.
17. See 5 supra.
18. 41 Food Drug Cosmetic Law Journal 444 (1986).
19. 235 Kan. 387, 681, P.2d 1038 (1984), cert. denied 105 S. Ct. 365 (1984).
20. Feldman v. Lederle Labs, 97 N.J. 429, 479 A.2d 374 (1984).
21. See, for example, a proposed bill by the New Jersey Senate, No. 2805, introduced at the end of the 1986 sessions.
22. 21 CFR 314.8.
23. 21 CFR 314.126.
24. 21 CFR 314.102.
25. Laaperi v. Sears, Roebuck & Co. Inc., 787 F.2d 726 (1st Cir. 1986). Adequacy, failure of warning.
26. Cooper, "Drug and Labeling and Product Liability: The Role of the Food and Drug Administration," 41 Food Drug Cosmetic Law Journal 233 (1986).
27. Paul v. Baschenstein, 105 App. Div 2nd 248 482 N.Y.S.2d 870 (1984).
28. Patterson, Donald, "Design Defect Cases: The True Cost of Settling for the Defense," 27 For the Defense 20 (May 1985).
29. "A Primer on Post Marketing Surveillance," 21 Drug Information Journal 99 (1987).
30. Karns v. Emerson, 817 F.2d 1452 (1987).
31. Perez v. Ford 497, F.2d 82 (5th Cir. 1974). Misuse. Steinmetz v. Bradbury, 618 F.2d 21 (8th Cir. 1980).
32. Brooks v. Chrysler, 786 F.2d 1197.
33. See FD1639.
34. See Rexrode Amer. Laundry Press 674 F.2d 826, 10th Circuit 1982 and similar cases; Ellis v. International Playtex Inc. 745 F.2d 292, 4th Circuit 1984; McKinnon v. Skil Corp. 638 F.2d 270 First Circuit 1981.
35. Wolf v. Proctor & Gamble Co., 555 F. Supp. 613, 2.I. 1982; Ellis International Playtex Inc. supra; McKinnon v. Skil Corp., supra.
36. In *Paul,* plaintiff's counsel recruited this "expert witness" from the adverse reaction files he examined at the defendant's offices.
37. Soden v. Freightliner Corp, 714 F.2d 498, 5th Circuit (1983).
38. Richardson v. Richardson-Merrell Inc., 649 F. Supp. 799 (D.D.C. 1986).
39. 42 USC 247b(k)(2)(A).
40. 28 USC 1346(b).

41. Neustadt, Richard E., and Fineberg, Harvey V., "The Swine Flu Affair: Decision-making on a Slippery Disease," 37 Journal of the Neurologic Sciences 136 (1978); see also McDonald v. U.S. 555 F. Supp. 935 (1983).
42. U.S. v. Wolf, 787 F.2d 1094, 1100.
43. EXUM v. GE 819 F.2d 1158. See also 818 F.2d 1161 (1987). Also Ferebee v. Chevron Chem., 736 F.2d 1529 (D.C. Cir. 1984).
44. Robinson v. U.S., 533 F. Supp. 320 (1982).
45. Hardy v. Johns-Manville Sales Corp., 681 F.2d 334 (1982), reversing 509 F. Supp. 1353.
46. 660 F. Supp. 205.
47. 636 F. Supp. 1419.
48. Abraham and Merrill, "Scientific Uncertainty in the Courts," Issues in Science and Technology 93, 104 (Winter 1986).
49. Grinnell v. Pfizer, 274 Cal. App. 2d 424 79 California Reporter (1969). See also 190 California Reporter 349, Mertan v. Squibb (1983). Also 196 Colo. 56, 581 P.2d 734 (1978).
50. (CA-10), CCH Products Liability Reporter No. 628, 7/21/87, 11428.
51. Wooderson v. Ortho 235 Kan. 387, 681 P.2d 1038 (1984).
52. This labeling was published after promulgation as a regulation in 21 CFR.
53. See 4 supra. Also Brown v. Superior Court (CAL 3/31/88).
54. Webb v. Angell, 508 N.E.2d 508 (1987).
55. Givens v. Lederle, 556 F.2d 1341 (5th Cir. 1977). Reyes v. Wyeth, 498 F.2d 1264 (5th Cir. 1974). Gottsdanker v. Cutter Labs, 182 Cal. App. 2d 602, 6 California Reporter 320 (1960).
56. In re "Agent Orange" Product Liability Litigation, 818 F.2d 145; 818 F.2d 179; 818 F.2d 187; 818 F.2d 204, 216, 226: 2d Arant, 1987. In re "Agent Orange," 506 F. Supp. 737 (1979); 500 F. Supp. 762, 795 (1980); 565 F. Supp. 1263 (1983); 597 F. Supp. 740 (1984); 611 F. Supp. 1396 (1985); 611 F. Supp. 1452 (1985).
57. In Re "Agent Orange" Product Liability Litigation, 611 F. Supp. 1223 (E.D. N.Y. 1985).
58. Renfro v. Allied, 507 N.E.2d 1213 (1987).
59. Marder v. G. D. Searle & Co., 630 F. Supp. 1087 (D. Md. 1986, aff'd 814 F.2d 655 (4th Cir. 1987).
60. Faich, Gerald A., "Post Marketing Surveillance of Prescription Drugs: Current Status," Washington, DC, Clinical Medicine Research Institute, October 1986.
61. See 54 supra.
62. 647 F. Supp. 544 (Ga. 1987).
63. Hopkins v. Britton, 742 F.2d 1308, 1311.
64. 787 F.2d 147 (1987).

5. *Epidemiology in the Courtroom: Anatomy of an Intellectual Embarrassment*

BARRY L. SHAPIRO
MARC S. KLEIN

INTRODUCTION

In *Wells v. Ortho Pharmaceutical Corp.*,[1] a federal district judge found that a child's exposure *in utero* to spermicide caused her serious limb anomalies. In so finding, the judge disregarded the clear consensus of the scientific community based on the great weight of the epidemiological data[2] because that data could not "rule out all possibility that spermicides can cause birth defects." He then focused on the experts' oral testimony and found in the plaintiffs' favor "primarily because the Court found plaintiffs' expert testimony to be far more credible than defendant's." In that regard, the judge stressed that he "paid close attention to each expert's demeanor and tone" and "perhaps most important, the Court did its best to ascertain the motives, biases, and interests that might have influenced each expert's opinion."

Rarely, if ever, has a "scientific factual finding" made by a court in a product liability action generated the type of controversy that followed. The Food and Drug Administration (FDA) took the highly unusual step of rejecting the *Wells* finding in a Talk Paper.[3] Prominent researchers from the National Institutes of Health (NIH) condemned the decision as one indicating that "courts will not be bound by reasonable scientific standards of proof."[4] The head of the Birth Defects and Developmental Disabilities Branch of the Centers for Disease Control (CDC) concluded that *Wells* shatters "the assumption that causality in the legal sense is the same as in epidemiology."[5] The authors of the principal epidemiologic study used by the plaintiffs' experts in *Wells* fought publicly over the scientific integrity and validity of their work.[6] Indeed, the controversy swept beyond the scientific community. In a lead editorial ("Federal Judges v. Science"), *The New York Times* (December 27, 1986) characterized the *Wells* decision as "an intellectual embarrassment."

Bert Black and David E. Lilienfeld, in their seminal law review article entitled *Epidemiologic Proof in Toxic Tort Litigation*,[7] discussed a long line of "ill-reasoned and inconsistent" judicial decisions dealing with speculative theories of "traumatic cancer" causation. Black and Lilienfeld argued that a sound use of epidemiologic evidence would "enable courts to adhere to both tort law and scientific principles" because it "would provide courts with a rational and consistent means for evaluating evidence of a causal relationship." Finally, they stressed that "judicial reluctance to examine the substantive basis of the testimony can easily permit unfounded expressions of certainty to carry the day."

Subsequent developments in the law imbue Black and Lilienfeld's classic piece with the quality of prescience. Courts have since divided into two distinct camps on the correct legal approach for evaluating evidence of a causal relationship. The majority more or less follow the traditional approach outlined by Black and Lilienfeld. A minority, however, have fashioned unique rules based in large measure on the premise that courts cannot make sense of the scientific issues involved. These courts will permit physicians to express causal hypotheses based on their "clinical impressions" unsubstantiated by epidemiologic or animal studies.

Wells is a perfect example of how poorly courts will deal with scientific issues if guided by the minority view. An analysis of that intellectual embarrassment exposes the fatally flawed premises of the minority view. While Black and Lilienfeld dealt lucidly with the more technical issues "on how to mesh law and epidemiology in a consistent way," it now appears that courts have gone astray on more profound issues, those which entail the very nature of proof in law and science. In the context of law and epidemiology, this chapter seeks to contribute fresh insights on these questions.

Part II of this chapter discusses the traditional legal standards governing the use of epidemiologic evidence in legal proceedings and explores the question whether proof of causation is truly different in science and law. Part III focuses on the *Wells* decision as an example of the irrational outcomes that might result from the minority view. It lays bare the antiintellectual predicates of that decision and uses it as a teaching vehicle to identify legal methodologies for finding scientific facts. Finally, in Part IV we address the role epidemiologists can and should play in assisting the courts to make rational findings of scientific facts.

EPIDEMIOLOGY IN THE COURTROOM

The science of epidemiology has come to play a prominent role in the resolution of many legal actions, particularly those characterized as toxic torts.[8] In a wide variety of toxic tort actions, courts have found that epidemiologic evidence is critical in resolving the question of causation.[9]

While courts have recognized epidemiology as an important and powerful science—one frequently necessary to the resolution of toxic tort cases—most courts have taken care to insure that only sound epidemiologic analyses are utilized. To insure reliability, a majority of the courts have subjected expert epidemiologic testimony to the traditional standards generally governing the admission and interpretation of all scientific evidence. Under these standards, a court will consider and credit expert epidemiologic testimony only if it is (1) given by a qualified epidemiologist; (2) based on reliable data; and (3) consistent with a sound scientific methodology. These criteria insure that any epidemiologic testimony is consistent with the role of expert testimony.

Courts have traditionally utilized these screening devices to "insure . . . that the flow to the jury of expert information is not wholly bogus in nature."[10] Courts have long been concerned that lay triers of fact may be misled by unreliable expert or scientific testimony precisely because it is labeled "expert" or "scientific." Consequently, before an expert is permitted to testify, the trial judge must make preliminary determinations regarding that person's qualifications,[11] the reliability of the data base,[12] and the validity of his/her scientific methodology.[13]

If a witness passes these threshold tests, the court will *permit* him/her to express opinions as an expert. This does not mean that these views must be credited. In deciding that question, the trier of fact (most often a jury) must also then weigh the expert's qualifications, the reliability of the data base, and the validity of the scientific methodology. This is true because the premises underlying the screening devices (used to determine whether the trier of fact is even permitted to hear the expert's opinion) necessarily play a critical role in determining whether to credit that opinion.

Of course, in a courtroom many other factors may affect a trier of fact's decision. These include a witness's appearance, tone, demeanor, and possible biases. How should a court make sense of these factors together with the scientific aspects of an expert's testimony? In a bench trial, where the judge, instead of a jury, sits as the trier of fact, the fact-finding process must be articulated. Several bench decisions reconciling conflicts in scientific opinion identify key elements of a sound fact-finding methodology.

The Importance of Objective Evidence

The law has long favored objective evidence over subjective evidence. For example, parties who dispute the terms or meaning of a contractual document are required to produce it, if available, rather than testify to their recollections of its contents. In this way the law would have the issue resolved through objective evidence, which it has appropriately termed the "best evidence," rather than the parties' recollections.

The preference for objective evidence becomes a necessity in the context of expert testimony. For an expert's testimony to be admissible, "there must be a demonstrable, objective procedure for reaching the opinion and qualified persons who can either duplicate the result or criticize the means by which it was reached, drawing their own conclusions from the underlying facts."[14] Thus, an expert's testimony must first satisfy these objective criteria before it can win on the basis of subjective criteria.

While a trier of fact should arguably be free to consider the "demeanor and tone" of all witnesses, as well as the "motives, biases, and interests that might have influenced their testimony," the nature of their testimonies must control the degree of importance attached to those factors if rational fact finding is the objective. This proposition is made evident by contrasting the litigation of a scientific question with the litigation of a common two-car intersection collision.

In the litigation of an intersection collision, witnesses may testify concerning which of the two litigants ran the red light. In that case, subjective credibility criteria may be decisive if there is no objective or tangible evidence to contradict their stories. On the other hand, expert witnesses called to address scientific issues are required to evaluate empirical data in light of scientific premises. Their credibility is primarily "a function of logical analysis, credentials, data base, and other [objective] factors"[15] and should be rooted in elements of science, not showmanship. Consequently, courts and legal scholars have recognized that "reliance on an expert's demeanor to determine credibility is dangerous"[16] and that "scientific questions . . . will not be decided upon the basis of the witnesses' behavior while testifying."[17]

The Consensible Knowledge of the Scientific Community

In dealing with scientific issues, courts do not make *de novo* determinations of scientific propositions. Rather, they look to what has been established in the relevant scientific community. In a medical malpractice case, for example, a jury does not study the human body and then independently determine what the physician should have done under the circumstances. Instead, it measures his/her action against an established reference point—what competent physicians do under similar circumstances.[18]

Thus, in determining whether epidemiologic data tend to support or negate a hypothesis, courts do not independently study the ramifications of epidemiologic data and reach their own conclusions regarding the methodology. Instead, courts consider whether the expert has utilized a scientifically sound methodology. In making that determination, courts use as their point of reference what other competent epidemiologists actually do in the pursuit of their science.

This information typically derives from three sources with special elements of trustworthiness. First, courts have accorded special weight to epidemiologic studies performed by the CDC, NIH, and other governmental agencies. In *Kehm v. Procter & Gamble Manufacturing Co.*,[19] a wrongful death action against the manufacturer of tampons, the district court admitted into evidence "reports of epidemiological studies conducted by the CDC and various state health departments. . . . Each of the studies analyzed the statistical relationship between tampon use and the incidence of [toxic shock syndrome]." In sustaining the district court's decision to admit these studies, the court of appeals reasoned:

> In the case at hand, the district court found the CDC and state case studies employed procedures and methods widely accepted in the field of epidemiology. Procter & Gamble does not dispute this finding. Dr. Dan, as well as Procter & Gamble's own expert, Dr. Feinstein, testified that *epidemiologists regularly rely on studies of this kind. Furthermore, we note the timeliness of the investigations, the special skill of the agencies conducting them, and their lack of any motive for conducting the studies other than to inform the public fairly and adequately.*[20]

Second, the law has long valued consensible knowledge reflected in scientific treatises. This is true because publication of a scientific treatise itself connotes trustworthiness:

> The writer of a learned treatise publishes primarily for his profession. He knows that every conclusion will be subjected to careful professional criticism, and is open ultimately to certain refutation if not well founded; that his reputation depends on the correctness of his data and the validity of his conclusions; and that he might better not have written than put forth statements in which may be detected a lack of sincerity of method and of accuracy of results. The motive [that insures trustworthiness], in other words, is . . . the unwelcome probability of a detection and exposure of errors.[21]

Third, the law has drawn from scientific studies themselves, particularly those published after suitable peer review. This emphasis on published data is highlighted by *Richardson v. Richardson-Merrell, Inc.*,[22] a recent Bendectin litigation. Noting the role of published scientific studies in the resolution of scientific questions, the court concluded that the most important evidence in the litigation resided

> in the presentation of the totality of the published literature on the subject of Bendectin exposure and the incidence of congenital malformations, which collectively represents the sum of all that can be said to be scientifically "known" of the matter at present. . . . [T]he "literature" is to scientists both the ultimate authority as to and the most respected repository of scientific knowledge.

Proof of Causation in Science and in Law

Three appellate courts have now expressed the view that, in toxic tort cases, proof of causation in law can precede proof of causation in science. Several legal commentators have endorsed this view.[23] In the main, it derives from a profound ignorance of basic scientific principles. Before examining the intellectual underpinnings of this view, it is helpful to discuss the principal cases that have adopted it.

The Ferebee Phenomenon

The leading authority for the proposition that, in toxic tort cases, proof of causation in law can precede proof of causation in science is *Ferebee v. Chevron Chemical Corp.*[24] In *Ferebee*, an agricultural worker alleged that he suffered from a lung condition akin to pulmonary fibrosis as the result of his long-term exposure to diluted solutions of paraquat. The parties conceded that "paraquat is known to be toxic and to cause acute injury if directly absorbed into the body." The scientific question presented was whether long-term dermal exposure to paraquat also causes chronic injury akin to pulmonary fibrosis.

In support of their causal hypothesis, the plaintiffs' experts relied on "the medical tests performed on [Ferebee]" as well as "medical studies which . . . suggested that dermal absorption of paraquat can lead to chronic lung abnormalities of the sort characterized as pulmonary fibrosis." Chevron's experts relied on a body of epidemiologic data in maintaining that "there has never been any evidence nor any suggestion that [dermal exposure to] paraquat can cause chronic injury of this sort."

The jury found in the plaintiffs' favor. On appeal, the court declined to analyze the bases of their experts' testimony. Instead, it fashioned a unique standard to govern the use of expert testimony in toxic tort litigations:

> Judges, both trial and appellate, have no special competence to resolve the complex and refractory causal issues raised by the attempt to link low-level exposure to toxic chemicals with human disease. *On questions such as these, which stand at the frontier of current medical and epidemiological inquiry, if experts are willing to testify that such a link exists, it is for the jury to decide whether to credit their testimony.*

The court then addressed Chevron's contention that the vast body of epidemiologic data, which detected no link between paraquat exposure and any chronic injury akin to pulmonary fibrosis, should have carried the day:

> *[A] cause-effect relationship need not be clearly established by animal or epidemiological studies before a doctor can testify that, in his opinion, such a relationship exists. . . . [P]roducts liability law does not preclude recovery until a "statistically significant" number of people have been injured or until science has had the time and resources to complete sophisticated laboratory studies of the chemical.* In a courtroom, the test for allowing a plaintiff to recover in a tort suit of this type is not scientific certainty but legal sufficiency; the fact . . . that science would require more evidence before conclusively considering the causation question resolved is irrelevant.

Thus, *Ferebee* stands for the proposition that causation may be established in a toxic tort action (1) so as long as "a doctor can testify that, in his opinion, such a relationship exists"; and (2) the law does not require "animal or epidemiological studies" to sustain that opinion.

With the exception of *Wells*, the only other published decision that has embraced *Ferebee's* logic is *Oxendine v. Merrell-Dow Pharmaceuticals, Inc.*,[25] the first to find that Bendectin is a teratogen.[26] In *Oxendine*, the plaintiff's expert based his opinion on four types of data. He testified that (1) structure-activity information "provided a clue about Bendectin's possible teratogenicity"; (2) one animal study "raised a *suspicion* of the teratogenicity of Bendectin"; (3) one *in vitro* study "indicates that the *potential* [for teratogenicity] is there"; and (4) an epidemiologic study supported a causal hypothesis even though it "did *not* show a statistically significant association between Bendectin and birth defects."

Following *Ferebee's* logic, the court in *Oxendine* left it to the jury to decide the "complex and refractory question" whether statistically significant data are necessary to establish a cause-and-effect relationship:

> Dr. Shanna Swan, an expert in biostatistics and epidemiology, testified that the mere fact that the number "1" falls within the confidence interval does not invalidate [sic] the study. She cited as an example an epidemiological study by a Dr. Smithells, in which the confidence interval was from 0.71 to 2.61, and the relative risk was 1.36. Dr. Swan testified that the relative risk calculation is the "best estimate of the true situation based on [these] data. . . ." A relative risk of 1.36 means that women who take Bendectin have a 36 percent higher risk of having a baby with a birth defect than those who do not. Confidence intervals, she said, are used to predict the range in which the relative risk would fall if the study were repeated several times. Thus, in the Smithells study, "the data [are] consistent with the relative risk being as high as 2.61," which means that women who took Bendectin would have a 161 percent higher risk of having a baby with a birth defect than those who did not take Bendectin. Dr. Swan's testimony thus contradicted that of Dr. MacMahon [Merrell-Dow's expert] on the question of whether many of the studies which he rejected could be relied upon as evidence that women exposed to Bendectin had a higher risk of giving birth to babies with birth defects. *That contradiction was properly left to the jury to resolve.*

Finally, the court justified the plaintiff's reliance on disparities in raw data that lacked statistical significance because "Dr. MacMahon *conceded* that statisticians must be careful to weigh other evidence and not to apply their rules rigidly and blindly." This "concession" came in response to a question that assumed its conclusion:

> Q. Doctor, one of the things you have to consider . . . when you come up with your statistics is what happens if you are wrong. You have to consider that risk, don't you, as a biostatistician?
> A. Yes.
> Q. And if the studies that show a relative risk as Smithells did at 36 percent greater chance of a defect, Mitchell, 50 percent, and the other ones that we referred to were right with that relative risk and you are wrong saying they are statistically insignificant, and Bendectin is in fact a teratogen, then the risk is that children are going to be born with limb defects of mothers who take Bendectin, isn't that right?
> A. That's very hypothetical, but yes.

In short, Bendectin was found to be a teratogen based on nonepidemiologic data showing a "clue," a "suspicion," and a "potential" for teratogenicity, together with epidemiologic data that could have been "wrong." Because the court felt that it could not understand "the complex and refractory causal issues" involved, it simply left them to the jury. Under the traditional approach to scientific testimony, the *Oxendine* analysis would not have passed muster.

The Traditional Approach

The traditional approach is well represented by two more recent Bendectin decisions. In *Richardson v. Richardson-Merrell, Inc.*,[27] "a virtual reprise" of *Oxendine*, the court stressed that epidemiologic studies could not be considered in isolation; rather, the fact finder had to consider "the significance of the literature in its entirety." The court cited the great weight of the epidemiologic data and the findings of an FDA advisory committee in concluding that "no reasonable jury could find . . . that this infant plaintiff's birth defects were more likely than not to have been caused by her intrauterine exposure to Bendectin." The court reasoned:

> It is unnecessary to revive debate upon the wisdom of that rule of law which, for purposes of awarding damages in personal injury cases, allows unschooled triers-of-fact, whether judges or juries, to resolve those "complex and refractory causal issues . . . at the frontier of medical and epidemiological inquiry," [citation to *Ferebee* omitted], for it is obvious that Bendectin's teratogenicity *vel non* is no longer such an issue. The ominous hypothesis of two decades ago, namely, that Bendectin might be another Thalidomide, has been reduced to the status of a perdurable superstition by the worldwide epidemiological investigations it provoked, surviving mainly by the *post hoc ergo propter hoc* logic which beckons whenever deformed babies are born to women who have taken any suspect substance.

What is perhaps most important in *Richardson* is how the court treated the contrary views offered by the plaintiffs' expert. The court wrote:

> *Though [the plaintiffs' expert] might disagree, there is now nearly universal scientific consensus that Bendectin has not been shown to be a teratogen, and, the issue being a scientific one, reasonable jurors could not reject that consensus without indulging in precisely the same speculation and conjecture which the multiple investigations undertook, but failed, to confirm.* That [the plaintiffs' expert] remains an unbeliever and was willing to testify to his disbelief "with reasonable medical certainty" does not mandate that this case be left as the jury decided it. *Without a genuine basis "in or out of the record," even his expert "theoretical speculations" are insufficient to sustain the plaintiffs' burden of proving, by a preponderance of the evidence, that Bendectin not only causes congenital defects generally, but that, in particular, it caused those limb reduction defects with which Carita Richardson was most unfortunately born.*

In *Lynch v. Merrell-National Laboratories*,[28] the most recent Bendectin decision, the court dealt masterfully with several key principles of teratology and epidemiology. The court first acknowledged the issue that only epidemiology could address in resolving an allegation of teratogenesis—the high "background incidence" of birth defects. It then noted that, as a result of the thalidomide catastrophe of the 1960s, extensive epidemiologic studies were undertaken of drugs used in pregnancy, including Bendectin, and that "no correlation, much less a causal connection, has been demonstrated between the use of Bendectin and limb reduction." In view of the epidemiologic data, the *Lynch* court held that causation could not be established.

How did the court deal with the testimony of the plaintiffs' experts to the contrary? The court first recognized its responsibility to carefully scrutinize the *substance* of their testimony:

> The ignorance that prevails as to the etiology of most birth defects does not mean causation in the given case could not be proven; it does mean that there is a large *terra incognita* where gossip and guesswork abound, and that *courts must carefully control the basis for testimony pointing to a particular cause.*

The court rejected the opinion of the plaintiffs' primary expert—which was predicated on his "reanalysis" of the data underlying previously published studies—because it had "never been refereed or published in any scientific journal or elsewhere."

The Antiintellectual Premises of the Ferebee Phenomenon

The argument that proof of causation in law differs from proof of causation in science starts with the erroneous premise that science demands certainty but the law needs only probability. The appellate court in *Wells*, for example, wrote that "a cause-effect relationship need not be *clearly* established by animal or epidemiological studies before a doctor can testify that, in his opinion, such a relationship exists," and that causation can be established in the courtroom even if "the medical community might require more research and evidence before *conclusively* resolving the question." These courts have reasoned that: "In a courtroom, the test for allowing a plaintiff to recover in a tort suit of this type is not scientific certainty but legal sufficiency."

Commentators have embraced this mythical distinction between "scientific certainty" and "legal sufficiency." Wagner espouses the use of "trans-science" to establish causation on the ground that justice should not wait for the "scientific certainty" that epidemiology offers:

> To determine whether exposure to a substance is a statistically significant factor in the cause of a disease, epidemiologists must compare a significant number of subjects exposed to the substance of unexposed populations. . . .
>
> Scientific quantification requires both that an epidemiological study be conducted, a highly expensive and time-consuming undertaking, and that the study be successful in distinguishing injuries caused by the product from those induced by the general environment. These scientific barriers not only insure that very few substances will be studied adequately to meet existing legal requirements, but

> also make it difficult, or even impossible, for a manufacturer to predict liability. . . . The standard of liability must be revised.[29]

Nesson likewise maintains that "requiring statistical proof substantially insulates companies from the consequences of negligently exposing persons to toxins. Making proof by statistical study a requisite for plaintiffs in toxic tort litigation hamstrings the ability of the judiciary to play a constructive role in future controversies."[30]

Based on this premise, Wagner and Nesson contend that epidemiologic evidence should never be required to prove causation in the courtroom, regardless of what science has to say. Instead, Wagner's proposal for trans-science—what others might call "semi-scientific evidence"—would permit a finding of causation based on "a qualitative showing of causation," one that entails "proof of substantial exposure to the substance and injury consistent with the substance."[31] She is at a loss to define "substantial exposure" or explain the meaning of "injury consistent with the substance." The fact is that "trans-science" needs science to address those questions.

Like Wagner, Nesson would permit a "medical diagnostician . . . to give his opinion that [a substance] caused a particular plaintiff's cancer, even though his opinion is based on a proposition to which scientists have not yet subscribed."[32] He would permit the courts to rely on a treating physician's clinical judgment because the clinician

> . . . assesses the significance of experiments and studies . . . in an intuitive way. He anticipates what the scientist would be able to prove if he would structure the perfect study, the perfect experiment. Lacking complete information, the diagnostician gives his best judgment. By its nature this judgment is not, of itself, scientific proof, but it may nonetheless constitute legal proof.

Despite his premise that clinical judgment suffices for legal proof, Nesson ultimately acknowledges that *scientific* judgment is an indispensable bulwark against irrational outcomes. He observes:

> There is, of course, a rational linkage between scientific and individual clinical diagnosis. How can a doctor know that given symptoms result from a particular cause in the absence of empirical data? Since causation cannot be directly observed in a case of cancer (contrast a statement that bleeding was caused by a cut at the location where the blood appeared), how can the doctor's clinical judgment, to the extent that it goes beyond what has been scientifically proven, be based on rational inference? At best, the doctor has observed or heard about an unscientific sample of patients, or is extrapolating from the data reported in scientific studies. One can easily imagine the sample the doctor has observed being so limited and disparate that a trial judge could consider the doctor's opinion speculative and hence inadmissible. . . . If many carefully controlled studies showed that eating carrots had no conceivable connection to cancer in humans or animals regardless of dose, a judge would certainly be justified in granting summary judgment or directing a verdict in favor of a defendant carrot

> company, notwithstanding a medical diagnostician's opinion that the cancer was caused by plaintiff's carrots.

Thus, the courts need *science* to decide whether "the doctor's opinion [is] speculative and hence inadmissible." What if no study has yet explored the issue? Can we equate the *absence* of reliable evidence of causation with *proof* of causation? Surely even Nesson would not permit a jury to condemn carrots as carcinogens without any scientific data apart from a physician's clinical judgment.

Gold's flexible approach[33] to the central problem of toxic tort causation gets to the heart of the matter. In order to "assure more compensation, more deterrence, and more opportunities to vindicate rights," he explicitly argues for a standard that

> contemplates a judgment which rests not solely on the factual existence of causation, but also on whether, given uncertainty about causation, imposing liability for certain conduct makes sense. Thus there is the possibility that *the culpability of defendant's conduct will actually become part of the fact finder's thinking on the causation issue.*

The notion that culpability (which already presupposes causation) should affect a determination of causation is contrary to a central premise of American law: "No policy can be strong enough to warrant the imposition of liability for loss to which the defendant's conduct has not *in fact* contributed."[34] Before proceeding to questions of culpability, therefore, we must first decide the question of causation in fact. Unless we first decide the question of causation, talk of "deterrence" and the "vindication of rights" makes no sense.

Like Gold's flexible approach, proposals for trans-science and the like are simply prescriptions for injecting prejudice into the determination of causation. Chemical and pharmaceutical companies would not stand a chance; a finding of causation would be a foregone conclusion in most toxic tort cases. To minimize the danger of prejudice, courts must strive to separate, not commingle, the factual and policy issues in toxic tort actions. As one court recently noted:

> Probably there are many Americans who find drug companies in general to be objects they love to hate. This being so, it is the special responsibility of courts to see to it that cases against them at least are fairly presented, and defense not unduly hobbled. At least we should not make matters worse than they already are. It was the same way with railroads a century ago, and no doubt there will be some now unforeseen scapegoat for public ire in A.D. 2084, at which time drug companies will be the objects of commiseration that railroads are today.[35]

The Coincidence of Scientific and Legal Reasoning

William James once observed that "we have to live today by what truth we can get today and be ready tomorrow to call it falsehood." Schlesselman, in his recent article entitled " 'Proof' of Cause and Effect in Epidemiologic Studies,"[36] notes:

> Scientific truth . . . is often thought of as the goal of a scientist's work, though "asymptote" would be the better word, for there can be no apodictic certainty in science, no finally conclusive certainty beyond the reach of criticism.

Thus, as one court aptly noted, "no scientific facts are ever 'final,' for they are forever subject to further discoveries."[37]

Many courts and legal scholars unfortunately remain infused with the "superstition about the infallibility of science; of almost mystical faith in its nonmystical methods." Thus, Wagner would not require epidemiologic evidence because it aims for "statistical certainty of causation"; Nesson because it pursues "absolute certainty." These propositions manifest a complete misunderstanding of what epidemiology and indeed science itself are all about.

It is useful to note that science and law share many common intellectual orientations:

> Science is like law in that it is a mode of seeking agreement among different individuals with respect to certain [factual] questions. . . . The common elements in both have been an effort to be wholly rational, to organize and institutionalize the search for truthful data, and, above all, to seek truthful data as the basis for judgments. Science can equally accept the basic principles of the legal system: to accept only rationally probative evidence and to examine all relevant evidence.[38]

In this regard, scientific reasoning does not differ from legal reasoning or any other form of reasoning. In discussing the nature and practice of scientific argument, Professor Ziman observed:

> The terms and concepts that are used may be extremely subtle and technical, but they are put together in quite simple logical forms, with expressed or implied relations as the machinery of deduction. . . . The reasoning used in scientific papers is not very different from what we should use in an everyday careful discussion of an everyday problem.[39]

Thus, courts need not stand in awe of scientific logic as some complex and refractory process with which they are incapable of dealing.

In seeking agreement on factual questions, science does not aspire to certainty any more than the law does. Both science and law seek to determine what *probably* occurred based on *all* of the relevant evidence. In other words, both seek to ascertain the facts to a *reasonable* degree of probability. When that degree of conviction has been reached, we are prepared to say that a hypothesis has been "proven." As a leading epidemiologic text notes:

> It is not possible to prove causal relationships beyond any doubt. It is only possible to increase one's conviction of a cause and effect relationship, by means of empirical evidence, to the point where, for all intents and purposes, cause is established.[40]

By recognizing this proposition, courts could also insure that parties not make a game of scientific issues. For example, a defendant confronted with overwhelming epidemiologic data in support of the plaintiff's causal hypothesis could seek to confuse the jury by parading a list of other "possible causes"—whether or not supported by evidence of actual exposure and the harmfulness of that exposure. In these instances, courts might be warranted in precluding the argument. As Jerome Cornfield observed in an analogous context:

> [The vaccinated group] may all have been vegetarians, or nonsmokers, or red-headed, and all or any of these things may render them less likely to contract cholera; but we do not see why objections which no sensible man would allow to influence him in the ordinary affairs of life should suddenly acquire scientific importance when the question is one of interpreting statistics.[41]

Consequently, the distinction between proof in science and other domains may "be neither good statistics, good science, nor good philosophy—though it may be good red herring."

Ferebee's distinction between "scientific certainty" and "legal sufficiency" appears to derive primarily from a misunderstanding of "statistical significance," and confuses the *type* of evidence that will be considered to support an argument (hypothesis) with the *level of comfort* (probability) required before it is accepted. Furthermore, the proponents of trans-science misconstrue the role of epidemiology as one merely designed to quantify otherwise known risks. In most instances, we *first learn* that a substance may be potentially hazardous through preliminary epidemiologic data and can often only substantiate that proposition through confirmatory epidemiologic data. Consequently, the argument for trans-science assumes the very conclusion it seeks to reach.

In the final analysis, trans-science would simply liberalize recovery at the expense of rationality. As Professor Allen cogently observed:

> The theory underlying these assertions seems to be that if a party can get someone with medical training to give an "opinion" no matter how unreasonable that opinion may appear to rational human beings attempting to determine what most likely happened in a case, then that opinion ought to be allowed to go to the jury. Thus, the issue no longer seems to be to structure mechanisms that will advance the difficult task of reconstructing reality. Rather, the task is to get to a jury no matter how unimpressive and unconvincing the evidentiary basis may be. This argument seems to rest on the principle that plaintiffs have a right to the "lottery" effect. Their case should be allowed to go to a jury to see what the jury wishes to do even if rational people could not find that the defendant violated the plaintiff's legal rights. On occasion one hears such theories explicitly espoused in

> remarks such as: "You want experts? I'll give you experts. How many do you want? I'll have them lined up on the courthouse steps tomorrow." This is the commodity theory of expertise. Expertise is not something to assist the jury. It is a commodity that is to be bought in order to generate the right to have the jury return an irrational verdict in one's favor.[42]

Thus, trans-science has no place in a court of law because an expert's opinion should be admitted only when it is likely to increase the rationality of the process.

A Proposed Reconciliation

In reaction to the *Ferebee* phenomenon, some commentators have argued that the law should *never* permit a toxic tort case to go to the jury "if positive [epidemiological] studies do not exist."[43] We disagree. We believe that it is not for the courts to state, as a matter of law, what scientific evidence may or may not be necessary for a scientific determination of causation. That question resides in the domain of science. *A court need only determine whether or not science, as opposed to the veneer of science, has been brought to bear.*

The correct approach was taken in *Marder v. G.D. Searle & Co.*[44] The court first dealt with the scientific constraints on a plaintiff's use of epidemiology. Noting that "proof of causation must be presented in scientific and medical terms," the court observed that "reliable evidence of a strong association between a product and an injury may lead a reasonable juror to conclude that a causal relationship is 'more probable than not.' " But the court rejected the premise that plaintiffs might rely on epidemiologic data that are not statistically significant to establish the existence of a causal relationship:

> The Court recognizes that evidence or absolute scientific "certainty" may be impossible for either plaintiffs or defendant to obtain in a products liability case of this nature, as it is difficult to isolate one of a variety of factors which may have caused an injury. [Citations omitted.] . . . Nevertheless, when presenting evidence of an association, just as with any other expert testimony, there must be some basis beyond mere theory and speculation for the opinion.

The *Marder* court then sensibly rejected the defendant's contention that, in toxic tort litigation, epidemiologic evidence is "required in order to state a case." As the court correctly observed:

> Rather than focusing on whether plaintiffs have provided a specific type of proof, the inquiry should be whether reliable scientific evidence, which is based upon sound methodology, has been presented, and whether through that evidence plaintiffs arguably have satisfied their burden of proof. The scientific evidence need not prove an absolute certainty of causation but must be sufficient to support a finding of a reasonable probability of causation.

If the scientific community requires epidemiologic data to evaluate a question scientifically, and there is simply no epidemiologic data available, there is nothing to litigate. If it does not, then a credible scientific case can be made for causation without it. In all events, however, courts should not go beyond the limits of our knowledge and render arbitrary decisions based on trans-science. At times courts must deny a recovery because "the state of the pertinent art or scientific knowledge does not permit a reasonable opinion to be asserted even by an expert."[45]

Thus it is for the scientific community to say, in light of the specific scientific question before the court, whether epidemiologic evidence is essential to establish causation; and if not, what other data the scientific community would use to reliably evaluate the question of causation.

THE FACT-FINDING PROCESS IN *WELLS*: AN INTELLECTUAL EMBARRASSMENT

With the exception of the plaintiffs' experts in *Wells*, the scientific community does not hold the opinion that spermicides cause birth defects. Prominent researchers associated with the National Institutes of Health (NIH), the Centers for Disease Control (CDC), and Harvard University, among others, found no credible scientific evidence of an association between spermicides and birth defects. Likewise, two advisory panels of leading scientists appointed by the Food and Drug Administration (FDA) reached the same conclusion and decided that a warning of such a risk was not warranted by the scientific evidence.

The plaintiffs' experts, based on their interpretations of 3 of the 23 scientific studies in evidence, concluded otherwise. Judge Shoob reviewed the scientific studies in evidence. He concluded that they only "indicated a *possible* link between spermicides and birth defects" and therefore "found the studies to be *inconclusive* on the ultimate issue of whether the product caused Katie Wells' birth defects."

Despite this key finding, Judge Shoob nonetheless concluded that the plaintiffs established causation to "a reasonable degree of medical certainty." In so finding, he dealt with the scientific literature as an entity separate and apart from the experts' oral testimony, even though the vast majority of that oral testimony concerned their interpretations of the scientific literature. Consequently, he "paid close attention to each expert's demeanor and tone. Perhaps most important, the Court did its best to ascertain the motives, biases, and interests that might have influenced each expert's opinion." Judge Shoob thus found that spermicides cause birth defects "primarily because [he] found plaintiffs' experts to be far more credible than defendant's."

The intellectual embarrassment of *Wells* is not so much Judge Shoob's finding of causation but the *methodology* applied. One would have thought that a federal judge would not decide a scientific question on the basis of someone's tone, demeanor, and possible biases. In the discussion that follows, we examine the steps of Judge Shoob's thinking that apparently led him to do so.

The Assumed Existence of a Scientific Controversy

Judge Shoob emphasized that his task

> was not to presume the expertise to resolve, once and for all, the dispute within the scientific community about the safety of spermicides. Rather, the Court's function was to render a legal decision, not a medical one. That is, the Court's duty was to weigh carefully the evidence that *these* parties presented to *this* Court in the trial of this case and to determine with reference to the facts of the case at hand whether plaintiffs had satisfied their burden of proving that they were entitled to the relief sought.

In general, a court's mission is to resolve a litigation based on the evidence before it—not "to resolve, once and for all, [any] dispute within the scientific community." However, Judge Shoob used this premise in *Wells* as a springboard for two leaps of logic.

First, Judge Shoob *assumed* the existence of a dispute within the scientific community about the safety of spermicides. In fact, by the time of the *Wells'* decision, the scientific community had fairly well concluded that spermicides do not cause malformations. Thus, Judge Shoob ignored the current state of scientific knowledge to judicially reopen a scientific controversy which was essentially settled within the scientific community.

Second, Judge Shoob assumed that the circumstances of this particular case had nothing to do with scientific studies showing whether or not there is a statistically significant association between spermicides and congenital malformations in a large population. Yet, logic instructs that we cannot disregard scientific studies showing whether a substance causes birth defects *at all* in determining whether it did so in *any* particular case.

The Oral Testimony Evaluated as a Separate and Distinct Entity from the Inconclusive Scientific Literature

Judge Shoob found that the plaintiffs presented "competent and credible medical and scientific evidence [that proved causation] to a reasonable degree of medical certainty" because they presented testimony by "physicians who were well qualified to address the issue of causation." Consequently, Judge Shoob felt that he "did *not* need to consider as substantive evidence the studies offered by plaintiff to suggest causation." It was enough that "well qualified" experts were willing to express opinions.

What of the scientific literature? Judge Shoob apparently considered it pertinent only to *negate* the hypothesis of causation, not establish it. He wrote that Ortho "attempted to rebut plaintiff's evidence of causation through various scientific studies and reports. . . ." He found, however, that these scientific studies and reports could not rebut the plaintiffs' oral evidence because they did not "rule out *all possibility* that spermicides can cause birth defects." Consequently, these studies were equated with those "offered by plaintiff[s] to suggest causation, and all were then disregarded as "inconclusive on the ultimate issue of whether [spermicides] caused Katie Wells' birth defects."

Judge Shoob's analysis of the scientific evidence is clearly flawed because epidemiologic studies cannot be considered in isolation; rather, as other courts have recognized, we must consider the significance of the literature in its entirety. In this instance, Judge Shoob balkanized the literature into two camps: the studies offered by the plaintiff "to suggest causation" and those offered by Ortho "to rebut the plaintiff's evidence of causation." He then considered the first group of studies alone and found that they did "suggest causation." That was enough to sustain the oral testimony which relied on epidemiologic data as a linchpin.

But what of the negative studies? Judge Shoob neutralized that literature by characterizing it as "inconclusive." Like any other type of evidence, however, scientific evidence is not irrelevant simply because it does not absolutely prove a hypothesis or rule out all possibility. Criminal defendants are sent to jail and fortunes change hands every day on the basis of such "inconclusive" (but nonetheless highly probative) evidence. Thus, courts are accustomed to decisionmaking in the absence of perfect information. This, of course, is what drives science as well. As Schlesselman has observed:

> All scientific work is incomplete—whether it is observational or experimental. All scientific work is liable to be upset or modified by advancing knowledge. That does not confer upon us a freedom to ignore the knowledge we already have.

Judge Shoob took that liberty with the scientific literature, which collectively represents all that was scientifically known about the teratogenicity of spermicides. Other courts have not disregarded scientific literature based on this "all or none" fallacy.

Finally, we believe Judge Shoob erred because he held the scientific literature to a higher threshold standard than the oral testimony. Of course, he did not find that the experts' oral testimony would be conclusive or even more probative than the inconclusive scientific literature. But he nonetheless based his decision on the oral testimony because the scientific literature was "inconclusive." This cynical, antiintellectual approach to the scientific literature is most apparent in this passage quoting one of the plaintiffs' experts with approval:

> You can bring in a stack of studies and stack them here that says this product causes no birth defects and is not absorbed. You can bring in another stack of studies and say just the opposite here. You can line people up all day long [with studies] going [in] both directions: one is a negative study, one a positive. It doesn't negate each other.

Thus the premise that one stack of scientific studies "doesn't negate" the other ultimately led Judge Shoob to ignore the accepted scientific methodology for resolving questions of causation.

Disregard for Accepted Methodology

There are several consensible criteria for evaluating cause and effect relationships with the use of epidemiologic data. While these criteria do not codify interpretation by rote application, they do play a critical role by providing a framework for debate. The experts on both sides in *Wells* acknowledged that replication is one of the key guides we have to weighing study evidence and reaching an informed opinion. Ultimately, this guide rests on an elementary principle of logic: if an apparent relationship is "real," it will happen again; if it is not real, it will not happen again, and we may conclude, as Oechsli observed, that our initial finding is a "statistical fluke . . . not to be taken at face value."[46]

Judge Shoob did not give credence to the scientific importance of replication. While noting the testimony concerning replication, he ultimately adopted a pharmacist's view that later studies which cannot replicate earlier ones should not affect his opinion because their existence "does not establish conclusively that [the earlier studies] have no significance." Consequently, Judge Shoob upended the replicability criterion in finding that:

> the [earlier] studies by Jick and others that indicated a possible link between spermicides and birth defects further undermine any suggestions that the [later] studies relied on by defendant conclusively show that its Product does not cause birth defects.

Certainly, the later studies do not "conclusively show" that spermicide does not cause birth defects because epidemiology cannot "rule out all possibility that [any substance] can cause birth defects." However, the later studies "conclusively show" that there is no credible scientific evidence of causation.

The "Most Plausible" of the Potential Mechanisms

Courts have recognized that it is meaningless to discuss potential mechanisms of causation before there is evidence that one or more of them may be in play—in other words, that a substance actually causes the injury in question. In *Marder v. G.D. Searle & Co.*,[47] the plaintiffs' experts "presented a series of alternative unsubstantiated theories" regarding the way in which an IUD might cause pelvic inflammatory disease (PID). They cited no data to show that, in fact, the IUD actually caused those injuries. The court wrote:

> Plaintiffs offered a wide variety of experts who presented explanations to the jury about the features of the Cu-7 IUD. In conjunction with these descriptions, the experts described how the Cu-7 can cause a variety of disorders and complications, including those allegedly experienced by plaintiffs. *A preliminary issue to the one which seemed to dominate plaintiffs' case about how injuries could be caused is the issue which the Court defined for [the] litigants at an earlier stage in the proceedings: can the Cu-7 cause plaintiffs' injuries? Plaintiffs failed to provide the Court with any sound data to support their experts' guarded statements on causation.*

By focusing on speculative potential mechanisms, Judge Shoob subtly shifted the burden of proof. He asked whether Ortho came forward with a potential mechanism more "plausible" than those suggested by the plaintiffs' experts and found that Ortho failed to do so. Even assuming Ortho failed to do so, however, that failure did not entitle him to find in the plaintiffs' favor, because the fact that one explanation for an event is more probable than another does not mean that it is true. At best, Judge Shoob found that of the hypothesized etiologies, the one that assumed a causal role for spermicides was the most plausible. But it is well settled that a finding of causation must be based on more than a theory or hypothesis.

The Weight of an Examination: Laying Hands on the Subject

In the absence of a known marker or syndrome, a physician cannot ascertain the etiology of a birth defect by examining a child.[48] In *Wells*, Judge Shoob found otherwise. He was impressed by the fact that:

> [the plaintiffs' primary expert] had examined Katie Wells in person, as opposed to merely viewing her medical records. . . . [He] explained his findings as he reenacted portions of the examination in court.

The examination was preposterous showmanship. This expert first examined Katie Wells *one hour* before he expressed his opinion, to a reasonable degree of medical certainty, that spermicide caused her birth defects. He had never before seen an arm deformity like Katie's, and had *never* before seen *any* birth defect which he attributed to spermicide. Yet, within an hour, he ruled out all other known genetic and environmental causes and came to the definite conclusion that the spermicide caused her birth defects.

Other courts have not fallen for the theatrics of a reenacted examination.[49] Judge Shoob's willingness to do so set the stage for *post hoc ergo propter hoc* logic—the most common fallacy in the analysis of toxic tort causation.

Post Hoc Ergo Propter Hoc Logic

The plaintiffs' primary expert eliminated "other causation" and implicated spermicide in the following manner. First, although he found that Katie Wells' cleft lip was most probably of genetic origin, he ruled out that etiology for her arm and hand defects because there is "nothing genetic in the family." Second, with respect to Katie Wells' defective hand, he first ruled out amniotic banding but later admitted that amniotic banding could not be ruled out. Ultimately, he concluded that Katie Wells' limb anomalies definitely were caused by the spermicide because "we have a case [in] which [the mother] used a spermicide."

Dr. Stolley described this methodology as follows:

> It's a very primitive form of reasoning. It is not scientific reasoning. It may be the first start toward developing a hypothesis, but it is not at all conclusive. Furthermore, there are many things to which people are exposed and they don't know it. Nitrosomines in hotdogs that are toxic, all sorts of things which, using that

> primitive form of reasoning, you probably logically ought to . . . include. So, it is simply inadequate and in no way scientifically reasonable to attribute malformations to exposures that occur in individuals unless there are all kinds of supportive data from other studies, which in this case . . . we have not seen.

The courts agree. In *In re "Agent Orange" Product Liability Litigation*,[50] the court addressed the legitimacy of similar "attempts to overcome the unavailability of any general evidence of causation. . . ." In that case, the plaintiff's expert noted "that the incidence rate for deaths from lymphosarcomatous leukemia in the population at large . . . is relatively rare," and that "certain [other] factors, including geographic location, familial history, exposure to radiation, and immunosuppression, increase the risk of developing lymphosarcoma." Based on his examination of the medical records, he ruled out those factors and concluded that Agent Orange must have caused the decedent's cancer. The court flatly rejected this methodology as unscientific and illogical, writing:

> The uncertainty surrounding the etiology of lymphosarcoma underscores the central problem with Dr. Carnow's testimony: he applies a causal hypothesis without any scientific support and excludes other potential causes without any factual basis for doing so . . . It is impossible to pinpoint which of the many personal, familial and environmental factors alone or in combination is responsible.

The court concluded: "The unfounded assumptions and speculation underlying Dr. Carnow's testimony reduce its probative force to a point approaching zero."

The same was true of the plaintiffs' primary expert in *Wells*. He too applied a causal hypothesis without any scientific support and excluded other potential causes without any actual basis for doing so. In choosing to credit that reasoning, Judge Shoob fell for "the post-hoc-ergo-propter-hoc fallacy, recognized thousands of years ago as a fraud."[51]

The Need for Careful and Reasoned Evaluation of Credibility

In confronting complexities beyond our immediate comprehension, we often fall back on the tried and true. That is what Judge Shoob chose to do in *Wells*. He reduced the case to a simple credibility contest. Once he found the scientific evidence inconclusive, however, at best suggestive of a possibility of causation, the case should have been over. A possibility of *general* causation cannot, through oral testimony, produce a probability of *specific* causation. Because oral testimony cannot rise above its inconclusive foundation, the question of causation should not have depended on the oral testimony of the expert witnesses.

Even conceding for the sake of argument the propriety of Judge Shoob's fact-finding methodology, he did not apply it in a careful and reasoned manner. Courts have long stressed the need for careful and reasoned credibility choices.[52] In other words, in assessing credibility, there may not be "a rule for Monday, another for Tuesday, a rule for general application, but denied outright in a specific case."[53] The record shows beyond question that Judge Shoob applied his credibility criteria in just that manner.

Background, Training, and Experience (Qualifications)

Courts have now recognized that the average physician is simply not qualified to express a reasoned scientific judgment concerning the etiology of most toxic torts. Since *Wells* involved the causation of birth defects, the body of scientific knowledge that covers this subject matter—teratology—had to be most important in terms of background, training, and experience. In that regard, knowledge of epidemiology was critical because that science is an integral part of teratology. Certainly, none of the plaintiffs' experts disputed these propositions; indeed, epidemiologic data were the linchpin of their opinions. Yet, without exception, none had any meaningful background, training, or experience in epidemiology.

Consider the plaintiffs' primary expert, who relied heavily on epidemiologic data. During the course of his testimony, he explained the extent of his background, training, and experience in epidemiology as follows:

> I'm not an epidemiologist. If you are asking me is that [data] statistically significant . . . I don't know. I don't understand confidence intervals. I never use them. I remember [the Mills (1982)] study now. Because the major thing that hit me was that he showed some limb defects, and he had a number of 1.07 relative risk.
> Q. Which is not statistically significant, is it, Doctor?
> A. No, but it's not zero or one.

Judge Shoob found that this expert was "the most credible of all the witnesses in this case. . . . This witness could hardly have been more credible."

Logic dictates that an expert cannot be "most credible" if he relies on scientific literature he does not understand. Indeed, most courts will not credit an expert's testimony if he relies on a type of data he is not accustomed to using. Since the plaintiffs' primary expert in *Wells* nonetheless relied on epidemiologic studies in formulating his opinion, he could not have been "the most credible of all the witnesses presented in this case."

Familiarity with the Circumstances (Data Base)

During the trial, Judge Shoob questioned the reliability of one of the plaintiffs' experts because "he did not, according to his testimony, review the defendant's studies when he gave an opinion." Judge Shoob apparently forgot about this criterion later. The witness he found most credible had not even read a majority of the scientific studies in evidence, including the two latest epidemiologic studies and the three FDA scientific reviews.

Courts have held that an expert's opinion is entitled to little or no weight if he has ignored data relied upon by experts in the field in reaching his conclusion. This is particularly true if one side's experts have selectively failed to consider scientific evidence inconsistent with their opinions. As one court explained:

> The conclusions Doctors Singer and Epstein reach are . . . insufficient as a basis for a finding of causality because *they fail to consider critical information, such as the most relevant epidemiologic studies and the other possible causes of disease*. . . . Neither doctor analyzes the epidemiological studies conducted on Vietnam Veterans. *The doctors' failure to consider and discuss the studies that address the actual population and amount of exposure involved in this lawsuit confirms the conclusion that their opinions are legally incompetent.*

Since the plaintiffs' experts in *Wells* also ignored data relied upon by experts in the field in reaching their conclusions, their opinions were necessarily inadequate for a finding of causality. Consequently, Judge Shoob erred in crediting their testimony and utilizing it in finding causation.

Tone, Demeanor, and Possible Biases (Gestalt)

Both the nature of the *Wells* opinion itself and other record evidence strongly suggest that Judge Shoob based his decision on subjective credibility criteria in order to render it unassailable on appeal. Yet his evaluation of those credibility criteria—each witness's "tone and demeanor" and "possible biases"—was remarkably inconsistent. Several examples suffice to make this point.

1. Judge Shoob discredited Ortho's experts for the "absolute terms," "exaggeration," and "terse manner" in which they expressed the view that the scientific data do not support the allegation that spermicides cause birth defects. The premise here is that an expert is not to be believed if he expresses his views too strongly or is unwilling to concede the possibility of an "honest difference of opinion."

   Did Judge Shoob then fairly examine the testimony of the plaintiffs' experts in light of this premise? Absolutely not. Instead, he found their testimony *more credible* because of the "emphatic tone" in which it was expressed. Indeed, he found no exaggeration in the view that spermicide "may be dangerous enough that it is a matter of national security." The expert who expressed that view was not "dogmatic"; rather, "his manner suggested objectivity and openness . . . and he showed no sign of bias or prejudice."

2. Judge Shoob discredited the testimony of Ortho's employees *because* they were Ortho's employees. He also discredited the scientific studies they had published in peer-reviewed journals on the same basis. What is ironic is that these men spent the better part of their working lives studying spermicides. Judge Shoob denigrated their experience with the simplistic premise that, by virtue of their employment with the company, their testimony and scientific studies could not be credible.

Did Judge Shoob then look for similar "potential biases" in the plaintiffs' case? Absolutely not. He found *no* reason to question the "potential biases" of the plaintiffs' primary expert, even though his compensation had not been set in advance of his testimony and he was the director of the rehabilitation clinic where Katie Wells would be treated—should she prevail—at a cost well in excess of $1 million.

3. Judge Shoob discredited Dr. Stolley's opinion because he disagreed with Oechsli's premise that his unpublished study raised "a *serious* suspicion" of teratogenicity. Dr. Stolley felt that Oechsli's study only raised "a *small* suspicion." The disagreement was one simply of degree, not direction. Yet, the credibility of this preeminent epidemiologist suffered because he had the temerity to "disagree" with the "express conclusion" of a relatively unknown investigator's unpublished study.

   The "disagreement" criterion got lost when it came to evaluating the plaintiffs' experts. In support of their theory of teratogenicity, for example, they relied on an animal toxicity study that found spermicide "embryolethal and fetocidal but *non-teratogenic* in the rat at a dose approximately ten times higher than recommended for controlling conception in women." Judge Shoob found that this study supported the teratogenicity theory "notwithstanding the author's stated conclusion." He discredited Ortho's experts for disagreeing with the plaintiffs' experts on the meaning of this study—even though their view was diametrically opposed to "the author's stated conclusion."

4. Based on Judge Shoob's view of possible biases, he disregarded the conclusions of the FDA's expert panels. On what basis did he do so? He simply accepted at face value the unsupported view of one of the plaintiffs' experts, a pharmacist, who opined that members of the FDA's panels "are readily swayed, I think, by other interests, including pharmaceutical manufacturers." Judge Shoob apparently concluded that paid partisans in a courtroom have fewer "potential biases" than preeminent scientists serving on FDA advisory panels.

These are but a handful of the many examples of arbitrariness available in the *Wells* record. They suffice to show that a scientific factual finding should not, under any circumstances, rest on an evaluation of tone, demeanor, and possible biases.

CONCLUSION AND RECOMMENDATIONS

Federal courts have observed that "there is not much difficulty in finding a medical expert to testify to virtually any theory of medical causation short of the fantastic."[54] Most recently, the United States Attorney General's Tort Policy Working Group[55] expressed its concern about the "increasingly serious problem" involving "reliance by judges and juries on noncredible scientific or medical testimony, studies or opinions." The Committee's Report noted:

> It has become all too common for "experts" or "studies" on the fringes of or even well beyond the outer parameters of mainstream scientific or medical views to be presented to juries as valid evidence from which conclusions can be drawn. The use of such invalid scientific evidence (commonly referred to as "junk science") has resulted in findings of causation which simply cannot be justified or understood from the standpoint of the current state of credible scientific and medical knowledge. Most importantly, this development has led to a deep and growing cynicism about the ability of tort law to deal with difficult scientific and medical concepts in a principled and rational way.

In a recent article addressed to the legal community, we noted the devastating social consequences that junk science portends:

> Quite clearly, product liability law carries the regulatory power to alter both the price and availability of most consumer products. [Citation omitted.] This power can serve society well when focused on defective products. Significantly, however, it can also deprive society of necessary products if product liability judgments are based on erroneous scientific or medical evidence. . . . For example, product liability judgments have had the effect of forcing the withdrawal of drug products from the market and inhibiting their introduction in the first instance.[56]

We therefore urged courts to take expert testimony in hand by carefully scrutinizing (1) the expert's qualifications, (2) the expert's data base, and (3) the expert's scientific methodology. While mistakes are as inevitable in law as in science, courts must sharpen the regulatory focus of tort law by screening out unsound expert testimony more effectively.

There is a role that the pharmacoepidemiologic community must play as well. Indeed, of all areas of science, epidemiology is perhaps the most integrally related to social regulation.[57] Unlike astrophysics, which may some day satisfy our cosmological curiosity about such profound questions as whether we live in an expanding or contracting universe, epidemiology could not be justified (and certainly would not be funded) unless we intended to *act* on the information it reveals.

We believe that epidemiologists can make three important contributions to combat junk science in the courtroom. First, the community of epidemiologists could establish standards that courts might use to determine whether someone is qualified as an expert in epidemiology. Second, the community of epidemiologists could subject expert testimony based on epidemiologic data to peer review. Third, the community of epidemiologists could bear in mind the regulatory consequences of their work and be responsible for them.

Standards for Qualification

Black and Lilienfeld noted four years ago that "no court has yet determined the qualifications necessary for a witness to offer expert testimony about epidemiology."[58] In *Wells*, Judge Shoob correctly noted that he could read and probably interpret epidemiologic literature as well as a general surgeon. Another court recently excluded the testimony of "a plastic surgeon with relatively little, if any, scientific knowledge regarding Bendectin, its components or its effects."[59] But the fact remains that no court has yet catalogued the signals of competence.

It is time for the epidemiologic community to help the courts do so. Courts have often looked to board certification as an indication of special competence.[60] The American College of Epidemiology (ACE) has published criteria to govern a membership process akin to board certification. The courts would be helped if that college, or those attending the next International Conference on Pharmacoepidemiology, either endorsed the ACE's criteria or set down others that courts could use to gauge claims of expertise.

Posttestimonial Peer Review

In the course of rejecting junk science, one court wrote that it was

> disappointed with the apparent fact that these so-called experts can take such license from the witness stand; these witnesses say and conclude things which, in the Court's view, they would not dare report in a peer-reviewed format. It has been as if no one else is listening.[61]

We believe that most experts would not dare espouse junk science in the courtroom if they *knew* that their peers were listening. Justice Brandeis once observed that "sunlight is . . . the best of disinfectants." Scientists, like other professionals, seek out and treasure the esteem of their peers. Few would not take care to avoid suffering within their professional circles an "intellectual embarrassment."

To enhance the quality of epidemiologic testimony in the courtroom, we propose a system of posttestimonial peer review.[62] Under this system, a professional society of epidemiologists would establish a standing committee of prominent members to review the nature and quality of expert testimony based on epidemiologic premises in significant toxic tort actions. A rigorous system of posttestimonial peer review may well be the most efficacious therapy yet devised for this "painful canker in the body of the law of evidence."[63]

Responsible Science

Alfred North Whitehead once said: "Duty arises from the power to alter the course of events." We have previously demonstrated the tremendous harm that junk science can do and believe that scientists have an obligation to take a stand against it. In this regard we suggest that epidemiologists might (1) exercise greater care in reporting the results of their studies, and (2) be more willing to participate as experts in the resolution of toxic tort suits.

Publication

Publication is the lifeblood of modern science. Through publication, private information is transmitted to the body of science and evaluated for its potential contribution to our consensible knowledge. But in the field of epidemiology, as perhaps no other, the publication of a study often has far broader social ramifications. Indeed, the *Wells* litigation itself was prompted by the publication of Jick (1981).[64]

Epidemiologists have recognized that, to insure the integrity and credibility of their science, greater care must be exercised in deciding *what* data to report and *how* to do so. In David Sackett's article "Bias in Analytical Research,"[65] for example, the author identifies several types of bias we regularly confront in toxic tort cases: "one-sided reference bias," in which authors "restrict their references to only those works that support their position"; "positive results bias," in which authors "are more likely to submit, and editors accept, positive than null results"; and "hot stuff bias," in which "neither investigators nor editors . . . resist the temptation to publish additional results, no matter how preliminary or shaky." These biases not only make for bad science, they can also result in ill-founded legal judgments with adverse regulatory consequences.

In response to a flurry of criticism following *Wells*, Lewis Holmes, one of Jick's co-authors, wrote that "our article should never have been published. It would have been much more appropriate for our findings to have gone through the more traditional process of being discussed among colleagues at scientific meetings."[66] Schlesselman also has asked:

> Could [the recent spermicide controversy which] now appears to be a false alarm have been prevented by use of the epidemiologic criteria for judgment?. . . Had Jick and colleagues reflected carefully on the [Surgeon General's five] epidemiologic criteria and their implications, they might have reconsidered their findings before publishing their report in a major medical journal. At the very minimum, the discrepancy between their results and those reported earlier . . . should have been addressed, the anomaly of reporting no increased rate of congenital malformations among women using spermicides in their study population compared with that among U.S. women in general should have been discussed, and a greater effort at assessing internal consistency and dose response should have been extended.[67]

Jick rejects this view. He feels that scientists should not "get involved in how our data are used. . . . What happens in the courts is the courts' business." We believe this view is untenable. As one clinician observed, Jick (1981) was "one of the most destructive things that has happened in the field of contraception within recent memory." We believe that both the credibility of epidemiology as a science, and the social ramifications of the science, demand that epidemiologists care about what happens in the courts and elsewhere as a result of their work.

Participation

We urge epidemiologists to participate as qualified, honest, objective experts in the resolution of toxic tort claims. Epidemiologists are actively engaged in the regulation of public health. While most think of the FDA when they think of regulation, scientists must recognize that a toxic tort action is designed to be, and is in fact, a powerful tool for regulating private conduct. Those who care to play a role in the regulation of public health must care about what happens in the courts.

Too often scientists tell us that they do not have the time or simply do not want to be bothered with testifying as an expert witness. This leaves the field open to those less qualified and less honest. Given the profound societal stakes involved in toxic tort litigations, those who would be responsible regulators of the public health must participate. As Ralph Nader once noted: "This is where the decisions are going to be made."

NOTES

1. 615 F. Supp. 262 (N.D. Ga. 1985), aff'd in part, rev'd in part, 788 F.2d 741 (11th Cir.), cert. denied, 107 S. Ct. 437 (1986). The authors of this chapter represented Ortho Pharmaceutical Corp. in the appeal process.
2. See, e.g., Neibyl, Jennifer R., "Drugs in Pregnancy and Lactation," in Obstetrics: Normal and Problem Pregnancies 249 (S. Gabbe ed. 1986):

   > Clearly, the consensus of the scientific community is that vaginal spermicides are not associated with increased malformations when women use them either just before or during pregnancy.

3. As a matter of policy, the FDA does not comment on the merits of pharmaceutical product liability actions. However, on June 24, 1986, the FDA issued a Talk Paper entitled "Spermicide Safety." The FDA noted that "[r]ecent lawsuits have attempted to show a link between spermicides and an increased risk of birth defects." The Talk Paper concludes by reaffirming the FDA's view that the available epidemiological data "did not support a link between vaginal spermicide exposure and an increased risk of birth defects" and, accordingly, "a warning was not warranted" with respect to that risk.
4. Mills, James L. and Alexander, Duane, "Teratogens and Litogens," 315 New England Journal of Medicine 1234, 1235 (Nov. 6, 1986).
5. Godfrey Oakley, quoted in Epidemiology Monitor (Jan. 1987), at 3.
6. See Authors Debate Validity of Work on Spermicides, Birth Defects, 8 Contraceptive Technology Update 57 (May 1987). The principal study relied on by the plaintiffs' experts was Jick, et al., Vaginal Spermicides and Congenital Disorders, Journal of the American Medical Association 1329 (April 3, 1981).
7. 52 Fordham L. Rev. 732 (1984).

8. The term "toxic tort" is commonly used to refer to cases in which the plaintiff's exposure to some chemical entity is suspected of causing a latent or chronic condition whose etiology is uncertain.
9. In re "Agent Orange" Product Liability Litigation, 611 F. Supp. 1223, 1239 (E.D.N.Y. 1985) ("epidemiologic studies on causation assume a role of critical importance").
10. Angel v. Rand Express Lines, Inc., 66 N.J. Super. 77, 85, 168 A.2d 423, 427 (App. Div. 1961).
11. An expert is qualified if he has sufficient "knowledge, skill, experience, training, or education" to "assist the trier of fact to understand the evidence or determine a fact in issue." Fed. R. Evid. 702.
12. For the determination of reliability, the court will focus on the expert's data base. Thus, Fed. R. Evid. 703 requires that an expert base his opinion on "facts or data perceived by him" or "of a type reasonably relied upon by experts in the particular field in forming opinions or inferences upon the subject."
13. An expert's conclusion is not admissible unless "the basic methodology employed to reach such a conclusion is sound." Ferebee v. Chevron Chemical Co., 736 F.2d 1529, 1535–36 (D.C. Cir.), cert. denied, 469 U.S. 1062 (1984).
14. United States v. Baller, 519 F.2d 463, 466 (4th Cir.), cert. denied, 423 U.S. 1019 (1975), citing United States v. Addison, 498 F.2d 741 (D.C. Cir. 1974).
15. New England Coalition on Nuclear Pollution v. United States Nuclear Regulatory Commission, 582 F.2d 87, 100 (1st Cir. 1978).
16. Miller v. FCC, 707 F.2d 1530, 1539 (D.C. Cir. 1983).
17. W. Gelhorn & C. Byse, Administrative Law 1056 (4th Ed. 1960).
18. See Prosser & Keeton, The Law of Torts 189 (1984) ("The standard of conduct becomes .... what is customary and usual in the profession.").
19. 724 F.2d 613 (8th Cir. 1983), aff'g, 580 F. Supp. 890 (D. Iowa 1982).
20. Id. at 619 (emphasis added).
21. 6 Wigmore, Evidence in Trials at Common Law § 1692, at 7 (Chadbourn rev. ed. 1976).
22. 649 F. Supp. 799 (D.D.C. 1986).
23. See, e.g., Nesson, Agent Orange Meets the Blue Bus: Factfinding at the Frontiers of Knowledge, 66 B.U.L. Rev. 521 (1986); Wagner, Trans-Science in Torts, 96 Yale L.J. 428 (1986); Gold, Causation in Toxic Torts: Burdens of Proof, Standards of Persuasion, and Statistical Evidence, 96 Yale L.J. 376 (1986).
24. 736 F.2d 1529 (D.C. Cir.), cert. denied, 469 U.S. 1062 (1984).
25. 506 A.2d 1100 (D.C. 1986).
26. In Ealy v. Merrell-Dow Pharmaceuticals, Inc., a jury found that Bendectin causes birth defects and awarded the plaintiffs $95 million. The trial judge eliminated the punitive damages award but sustained the compensatory damages award of $20 million. The decision, which has not yet generated a published decision, will almost certainly be appealed.
27. 649 F. Supp. 799 (D.D.C. 1986).
28. 830 F.2d 1190 (1st Cir. 1987).
29. Wagner, supra note 23, at 429–30.
30. Nesson, supra note 23, at 537.

31. Wagner, supra note 23, at 430.
32. Nesson, supra note 23, at 523.
33. See Gold, supra note 23, at 393.
34. J. Fleming, The Law of Torts 170 (6th ed. 1983) (emphasis added).
35. Deitchman v. E.R. Squibb & Sons, Inc., 740 F.2d 556, 565–66 (7th Cir. 1984).
36. 16 Preventive Medicine 195 (1987).
37. Ellis v. International Playtex, Inc., 745 F.2d 292, 302 (4th Cir. 1984).
38. Thomas, Scientists in the Legal System 22 (1974).
39. J. Ziman, Public Knowledge 8 (1968).
40. Fletcher, et al., Clinical Epidemiology: The Essentials 192 (1982).
41. Cornfield, Statistical Relationships and Proof in Medicine, 8 American Statistician 19, 20 n.2 (1954).
42. Allen, Rationality, Mythology, and the "Acceptability of Verdicts" Thesis, 66 B.U.L. Rev. 541, 558 n. 69 (1986).
43. McElveen, Reproductive Hazards in the Workplace, 20 The Forum 547, 578 (1985).
44. 630 F. Supp. 1087, 1092 (D. Md. 1986), aff'd sub nom. Wheelahan v. G.D. Searle & Co., 814 F.2d 655 (4th Cir. 1987) (per curiam).
45. Dyas v. United States, 376 A.2d 827, 832 (D.C. App.), cert. denied, 434 U.S. 973 (19077), quoting McCormick on Evidence §13, at 29–31 (2d ed. 1972).
46. Oechsli, Studies of the Consequences of Contraceptive Failure (unpublished paper 1976).
47. 630 F. Supp. 1087 (D. Md. 1986), aff'd sub nom. Wheelehan v. G.D. Searle & Co., 814 F.2d 655 (4th Cir. 1987) (per curiam).
48. See, e.g., Heyman v. United States, 506 F. Supp. 1135 (S.D. Fla. 1981) (Clinicians generally cannot determine "whether a relationship exists between an illness and a preceding event such as a vaccination [and] without at least some reference to epidemiological studies, plaintiff's position that her illness was caused by the swine flu shot amounts to nothing more than speculation.").
49. See, e.g., Carter v. United States, 593 F.Supp. 505, 508 (W.D. Mich. 1984) (an examination may be helpful in determining whether the plaintiff has a disease but not "in explaining to the Court the various processes involved in the origin of the diagnosed disease or diseases").
50. 611 F. Supp. 1267 (E.D.N.Y. 1985).
51. Royal, The Defense of Medical Causation, 23 Trial 40, 41 (Oct. 1987).
52. Corley v. Jackson Police Department, 566 F.2d 994, 1004 (5th Cir. 1978).
53. Mary Carter Paint Co. v. FTC, 333 F.2d 654, 660 (5th Cir. 1964) (Brown, J., concurring), rev'd on other grounds, 382 U.S. 46 (1965).
54. Stoleson v. United States, 708 F.2d 1217, 1222 (7th Cir. 1983).
55. See Report of the Tort Policy Working Group on the Causes, Extent and Policy Implications of the Current Crisis in Insurance Availability and Affordability (February 1986).
56. Epstein & Klein, The Use and Abuse of Expert Testimony in Product Liability Actions, 17 Seton Hall L. Rev. 601, 605 n.18 (1987) (citation omitted).
57. This is made plain by the stated goals of the Third International Conference on Pharmacoepidemiology:

> The goals of this conference are to provide a forum for the exchange of information between academic researchers, medical care practitioners, health care administrators, the pharmaceutical industry, and *regulatory agencies on pharmacoepidemiological approaches to studying the efficacy and safety of pharmaceuticals and the contributions of pharmacoepidemiology to developing public health policy.* [Emphasis added.]

58. Black & Lilienfeld, supra note 7, at 775.
59. Will v. Richardson-Merrell, Inc., 647 F. Supp. 544, 548 (S.D. Ga. 1986).
60. See, e.g., Buck v. St. Clair, 108 Idaho 743, 702 P.2d 781 (1985) (medical expert as to standard of care need not be from the specific locality if board-certified); Scheytt v. Industrial Comm'n of Arizona, 135 Ariz. 25, 653 P.2d 375 (1982) (same).
61. Johnston v. United States, 597 F.Supp. 374, 415 (D. Kansas 1984). Judge Higginbotham of the United States Court of Appeals also recently observed that:

    > [M]any experts are members of the academic community who supplement their teaching salaries with consulting work. We know from our judicial experience that many such able persons present studies and express opinions that they might not be willing to express in an article submitted to a refereed journal of their discipline or in other contexts subject to peer review.

    In re Air Crash Disaster at New Orleans, La. On July 9, 1981, 795 F.2d 1230, 1233–34 (5th Cir. 1986).
62. We wish we could claim to be the first to propose this idea or something like it. Regrettably, we cannot. Several years ago Dr. Robert Brent wrote:

    > Depositions and court testimony should be treated as scholarly endeavors. Academic medical scientists should be encouraged to report all medico-legal activities to the chairman of their department and review their expert opinion and analysis with their supervisors, colleagues, or peers. If employed in an industry, the expert should be encouraged to submit his testimony for review by his or her supervisor and peers. Practicing physicians should be encouraged to submit their case analysis to their colleagues for peer review. *I call this the 'light of day phenomenon' inasmuch as I believe that, if experts learn to consult with their peers, their testimony will become more accurate and scholarly.*

    Brent, The Irresponsible Expert Witness: A Failure of Biomedical Graduate Education and Professional Accountability, 70 Pediatrics 754, 761 (1982) (emphasis added).
63. Myers, "The Battle of the Experts": A New Approach to an Old Problem in Medical Testimony, 44 Neb. L. Rev. 539, 543 (1965).
64. Katie Wells' mother, Mary Maihafer, apparently learned through the media of Jick (1981). This study was "given wide coverage in the U.S. press" and "led to alarm among women who were pregnant or using spermicides at the time."
65. 32 J. Chron. Dis. 51 (1979).
66. Authors Debate Validity, supra note 6, at 59. He also wrote: "I had expected the vast amount of data contradicting our study would bury it. The court decision made it clear that our study had played a role in the thinking of the legal community and the public." Id.
67. Schlesselman, supra note 36, at 203.

SECTION THREE

Drug Surveillance

Introduction

Section Three contains a series of chapters which describe resources for observational data on drug safety.

One of the best known spontaneous reporting systems in the world is the "yellow card" system in the United Kingdom. Drs. Burton and Mann of the DHSS trace the history of the yellow card system since its inception in 1964. Included are discussions of current reporting requirements, an insight into data assessment, problems with the use and interpretation of spontaneous reports, and examples of major contributions of the system in documenting adverse drug reactions (ADRs).

Dr. Bruppacher et al. follow with a provocative discussion of the difficulties of quantitative analyses of spontaneous reports. They illustrate how European reporting rates are dependent on the life cycle effect (age of the product), secular trends, kind of adverse event, and route of administration for four Ciba-Geigy products.

The U.S. Food and Drug Administration funded a number of pilot projects through state health departments to address the problem of physician under-reporting of adverse drug reactions. Dr. Rogers et al. describe the first year's experience in Maryland to improve reporting by comparing modalities of physician education versus direct reporting (by telephone). Results of a pre- and post-intervention physician attitude survey are presented.

The Centers for Disease Control (CDC) has conducted surveillance for adverse effects of immunization since 1976 through its Monitoring System for Adverse Events Following Immunization (MSAEFI). Drs. Livengood and Mullen briefly describe MSAEFI and present information from the surveillance of DTP and measles vaccines. The article provides an insight into the strengths and limitations of the data and how the data has been used to establish policy.

Premarketing clinical trials provide initial profiles of adverse events associated with a drug and estimates (based on small numbers) of the relative frequency of individual events. Wallander et al. suggest that it is productive to continuously monitor adverse experiences differently than effect variables during clinical trials. ASTRA established an ADE group to continuously monitor adverse experiences using standardized coding procedures. Data is presented on the impact of this approach to identifying important information in the safety assessment of two new chemical entities.

In an effort to collect information within hospitals on the safety and effectiveness of drugs under actual clinical conditions, a nationwide drug surveillance program involving clinical pharmacists has been established. Dr. Grasela describes this network and reports on a pilot project conducted to obtain a cross-sectional view of antibiotic utilization vis-a-vis a nationwide prospective study.

Though the majority of U.S. hospitals now operate management information systems (MIS), few were designed to provide detailed data on in-hospital drug exposure and clinical outcome. Dr. Stryker describes progress in developing a record linkage system designed for use as a pharmacoepidemiology data base at the Brigham and Women's Hospital in Boston. Results from a study of theophylline use are presented.

Poison control centers in the United States have established a nationwide network to collect and report their experiences on the characteristics and outcomes of drug overdoses. Dr. McElwee et al. provide a description of this system and describe a pilot study of patients with accidental or intentional overdose of ibuprofen.

One of the best known resources for conducting population-based studies of drugs is the health care data from the Province of Saskatechewan. Large data bases permit linkage of prescriptions, hospital data, physician claims and cancer registry data. The Prescription Drug Plan has collected information on 90% of prescriptions in the Province since 1975. Ms. Downey describes how changes in coverage and data processing could limit the usefulness of this unique resource.

In the United States, the Computerized On-Line Medicaid Pharmaceutical Analysis and Surveillance System (COMPASS) provides access to Medicaid billing data on millions of beneficiaries. Dr. Carson provides a thoughtful review of the strengths and limitations of COMPASS or any Medicaid data base for performing epidemiologic studies, and a useful discussion of efforts to validate the data.

In Scotland, all prescriptions dispensed by community pharmacies are sent to the Prescription Pricing Division in Edinburgh for reimbursement. Mr. Beardon describes a record linkage study of NSAIDs conducted in Tayside, Scotland. Prescription data was linked to hospital discharge data, maternal discharge diagnoses, neonatal discharge diagnoses, psychiatric diagnoses, and mortality records.

6. *A Brief Review of the Yellow Card Adverse Reaction Reporting Scheme in the United Kingdom*

GRAHAM H. BURTON
RONALD D. MANN

INTRODUCTION

In June 1963, the Health Ministers of the United Kingdom established the Committee on Safety of Drugs and appointed Sir Derrick Dunlop as Chairman. The Committee's adverse reaction reporting system was instituted when the Chairman wrote to all doctors and dentists in May 1964, requesting reports of "any untoward condition in a patient which *might* be the result of drug treatment" and enclosing a small supply of yellow, reply-paid postcards for reporting these suspected reactions. A secretariat was established to run the scheme, and the reports received were recorded on a computerized register. A major piece of legislation, the Medicines Act of 1968, formalized the establishment of a Licensing Authority to control the marketing, manufacture, development, and importation of medicinal products intended for human use in the United Kingdom. A Medicines Commission was formed to advise on policy matters and to act as an appeals body. In 1971 under the auspices of the Medicines Commission, the Committee on the Safety of Drugs was subsumed into the Committee on Safety of Medicines (CSM). The CSM then took over the role of advisory body to the Licensing Authority on matters relating to the quality, safety, and efficacy of medicines intended for administration to man. From that time the Licensing Authority has administered the yellow card adverse reaction reporting system on behalf of the CSM. From the day the register of adverse reactions was set up, all reports and correspondence have remained confidential between the reporting doctor or dentist and the Committee and its secretariat. A copy of the current yellow card which is used in the United Kingdom is shown in Figure 1.

IN CONFIDENCE – REPORT ON SUSPECTED ADVERSE REACTIONS

1. Please report all suspected reactions to recently introduced drugs (identified by a black triangle in the British National Formulary), vaccines, dental or surgical materials, IUCD's, absorbable sutures, contact lenses and associated fluids, and serious or unusual reactions to all agents.
2. Record all other drugs etc, including self-medication, taken in the previous 3 months. With congenital abnormalities, record all drugs taken during pregnancy, and date of last menstrual period.
3. Do not be deterred from reporting because some details are not known.
4. Please report suspected drug interactions.

NAME OF PATIENT (To allow for linkage with other reports for same patient. Please give record number for hospital patients.)	Family name Forenames	SEX	AGE or DATE OF BIRTH	WEIGHT (Kg.)

DRUGS, VACCINES (Inc. Batch No.), DEVICES, MATERIALS etc. (Please give Brand Name if known)	ROUTE	DAILY DOSE	DATE STARTED	DATE ENDED	INDICATION
Suspected drug, etc.					
Other drugs, etc. (Please state if no other drug given.)					

SUSPECTED REACTIONS	STARTED	ENDED	OUTCOME (eg. fatal, recovered)

ADDITIONAL NOTES	REPORTING DOCTOR (Block letters please)
	Name:
	Address:
	Tel. No: Specialty:
	Signature: Date:

If you would like information about other reports associated with the suspected drug, please tick box – ☐

AR/20 250M/10/82 51-2836/PRINT PROCESSES LTD

Figure 1. The yellow card.

REPORTING REQUIREMENTS

The reporting requirements for doctors and dentists are similar: *all* suspected adverse reactions (ADR) to *new* drug products and serious reactions to established products should be reported. In this context, *serious* is defined as fatal, life-threatening, disabling or incapacitating, or resulting in hospitalization or prolongation of hospitalization. A new drug product can generally be identified in the United Kingdom by an inverted solid black triangle alongside its name in the product data sheet, product literature, and in other publications, including the *British National Formulary* and the industry's own *Data Sheet Compendium*. A *new drug* is generally a novel chemical entity or a major novel formulation of an existing drug. The adverse reaction reporting requirements for pharmaceutical companies are summarized in Table 1, which includes details for reporting ADRs to drugs undergoing clinical trials.

Table 1. Adverse Reaction Reporting by Industry

Reactions Occurring In the United Kingdom	All Serious Reactions* or Effects	Minor Reactions
Licensed products		
Spontaneous reports (new drugs)†	A	A
Spontaneous reports (other drugs)	A	N
Clinical studies after marketing (within terms of current data sheet or summary of product characteristics)	A	B
Products under trial		
Products under CTC or CTX or CTMP	A	B

Reactions Occurring Abroad (including those in clinical studies after marketing)	All Serious Reactions or Effects	Serious and Unpredictable‡ Reactions or Effects	Minor Reactions
Products licensed in the UK	n/a	A*	N
Products under CTC or CTX in the UK (i.e., usage not covered by a product license	A or A*	n/a	C

Source: From Medicines Act information Leaflet (MAIL 49) March 1987.

Note: A = report immediately on company yellow card form; A* = report immediately on CIOMS form; B = report in summary at conclusion of trial or study; C = report in summary at conclusion of the UK trials or at the time of a product license application; N = not required; n/a = not applicable.

**Serious reactions or effects* means all suspected adverse reactions which are fatal, life-threatening, disabling, incapacitating, or which result in hospitalization or prolong hospitalization.

†*New drug* means a medicinal product for which a black triangle V must be shown in the data sheet and promotional material.

‡*Unpredictable* means not previously referred to in the warnings, precautions or contraindications section of the data sheet; the summary of product characteristics or the product license.

MANAGEMENT OF THE YELLOW CARD SCHEME

All adverse reaction reports originating in the United Kingdom from doctors and dentists in clinical practice or from the pharmaceutical industry are given a unique registration number, acknowledged, and medically assessed. During this assessment, culpability is assigned to the suspect drug or product, and if more than one adverse reaction has been reported, the most important reaction (MIREA) is identified. The outcome of the reaction is ascertained, and where the outcome is death, the relation of the death to the adverse drug reaction is assessed on the available information.

The following information on the suspected adverse drug reaction is then added to the computer data base:

- report number
- age or date of birth
- sex
- reaction(s)
- suspect drug with start and stop dates, dose, and route of administration
- other drug(s) with start and stop dates, doses, and route of administration
- duration of drug administration
- drug-reaction interval
- outcome

In addition, the medical assessor may include further relevant information in a comments field (for instance, biochemical and hematological values).

DATA ASSESSMENT

The chief function of the yellow card spontaneous reporting scheme is to provide a means by which early warnings of adverse drug reactions are identified. During the routine daily assessments of the yellow cards, the medical assessors can be alerted by a report of any unusual, severe, or unpredictable adverse reaction. The assessor can then make enquiries of the adverse reactions data base to find out if there have been other similar reports. These enquiries can be directed specifically at alerts or queries regarding a particular drug or product, or they can arise directly from a routine *drug analysis print*.

Each such drug analysis print summarizes all of the data relevant to a drug or product. The standard print represents a summary of the most important reaction in each patient in which the drug concerned is the suspect cause in the opinion of the reporting doctor. Thus each yellow card counts once only, and the total shown for the drug equals the number of yellow cards received. These prints are available to the medical assessors for all licensed medicinal products.

A further way in which the data base is used to assess adverse reactions is by the means of the *F16 printout*, a computer printout produced every two weeks. It provides an update of reported reactions added to the register in the previous two weeks for all marketed and licensed drugs. This printout is carefully reviewed by the medical secretariat every two weeks. An example from this printout is shown in Figure 2. The F16 represents a prime alerting mechanism and is subject to special scrutiny for new or unexpected reactions.

As a new drug is released on the market, it is entered into a prospective monitoring scheme. A monthly summary of the adverse drug reactions reported on such drugs is reviewed by the medical secretariat in conjunction with a special Sub-Committee of the Committee on Safety of Medicines. The discussions of this Sub-Committee, the Adverse Reactions Group of SEAR (ARGOS), may then be reviewed by the main Safety, Efficacy and Adverse Reaction (SEAR) Sub-Committee of the CSM which, in turn, will report its finding to the main Committee. All Committees meet monthly and provide a forum for discussion on suspected adverse drug reactions.

If a drug is suspected of being associated with a serious adverse reaction, then the original yellow card reports and any overseas or additional reports can be reviewed by the medical assessor. At any stage in the assessment procedure the assessor can undertake further follow-up and validation of serious and rare reactions by telephone, letter, or, in certain circumstances, by using the Part-Time Medical Officer (PTMO) system. Part-Time Medical Officers (of which there are about 250) are registered medical practitioners scattered throughout England and Wales who will undertake *ad hoc* assignments to follow up and provide further details and assessments on any suspected adverse drug reaction report. The medical assessor has other sources of information available; these include the published literature, foreign reports of adverse reactions, data provided from other drug regulatory authorities, expert opinions, efficacy data, and data from the company (or companies) involved. The accumulated data can then be considered in conjunction with prescription data that are available on licensed medicinal products in the United Kingdom. These data provide an estimate based upon samples of prescriptions dispensed in retail pharmacies; they do not include hospital drug use.

Often the pharmaceutical company can provide prescription or sales data to assist the medical assessor. With this information, a risk-benefit assessment can be made in consultation with the advisory committees mentioned previously. The action then taken depends upon the nature and variety of the ADRs under discussion. The CSM can make available advice to the medical profession through its own *Current Problems* publication, through articles and letters to journals or, if necessary, by writing a letter to every doctor, dentist, and pharmacist in the United Kingdom. Negotiations, both formal and informal, can be undertaken with the relevant company to ensure the product literature and data sheets are in line with the conclusions reached. Extreme action (if necessary) can be undertaken to remove the product from the market. It must be said that the interaction with pharmaceutical companies in the United Kingdom is usually informal.

```
        Timeband - 26/09/87 TO 09/10/87 by MF-Date                                     Page no 21
Sus Const             MF-Date    AR Name
IBUPROFEN cont                                             CI Dth   Sex        Age       Age < 1 yr  Ex DI  Regno
SDcode 158120         Conscode   A0783
                      300987     OEDEMA PERIORBITAL

Total reports for above Product          -     16          B         M                                      188029
Total reports in 1986                    -     91
Total reports in 1987 to date            -    198
INDOMETHACIN
Sdcode 159110         Conscode   A0787

                      071087     RENAL FAILURE             B         F          84       - - - - - -  -  -    188087
                      071087     ASTHMA AGGRAVATED         B         F          54       - - - - - -  -  -    188096
                      300987     HEADACHE                  B         F          34       - - - - - -  -  -    173502
                      300987     INTESTINAL PERFORATION    A         M          63       - - - - - -  -  -    187859
                      300987     CONFUSION                 B         M          32       - - - - - -  -  -    188135
Total reports for above Product          -      5
Total reports in 1986                    -    168
Total reports in 1987 to date            -    104
KETOPROFEN
Sdcode 158030         Conscode   A3897

                      071087     DIARRHOEA                 A         F          40       - - - - - -  -  -    174303
                      071087     HAEMORRHAGE RECTAL                  M          16       - - - - - -  -  -    187408
                      071087     HAEMATURIA                A         M          16       - - - - - -  -  -    187408
                      071087     DRUG INTERACTION                    F          57                       *    187853
                      071087     DYSPNOEA                            F          57                       *    187853
                      071087     CHEST PAIN                          F          57                       *    187853
                      071087     FLUID RETENTION           A         F          57                   .   *    187853
                      071087     WEIGHT INCREASE                     F          57                       *    187853
                      071087     HAEMATEMESIS              A         F          88       - - - - - -  -  -    188207
                      300987     HYPERKINESIA              B         M                   - - - - - -  -  -    180930
                      300987     CONSTIPATION                        F          61       - - - - - -  -  -    187836
                      300987     VOMITING                            F          61       - - - - - -  -  -    187836
                      300987     DIZZINESS                 B         F          61       - - - - - -  -  -    187836
                      300987     DUODENAL ULCER PERFORATED B         M          15       - - - - - -  -  -    188189
Total reports for above Product          -     14
Total reports in 1986                    -    162
Total reports in 1987 to date            -    131
MEFENAMIC ACID                                             B         F          33       - - - - - -  -  -    188199
Sdcode 158210         Conscode   A0854                     B         F          83       - - - - - -  - .-    172963
                      071087     RASH                      A         F          49       - - - - - -  -  -    173524
                      300987     ERYTHEMA MULTIFORME       B         F          78       - - - - - -  -  -    187843
                      300987     DIARRHOEA
                      300987     NEPHRITIS INTERSTITIAL
```

Figure 2. Single page from the fortnightly printout of additions to the register (the F16 print). CI = culpability index: A = probable; B = possible; C = unlikely; D = not assessable. Dth = death: 01 (death due to ADR); 02 (death not due to ADR); 03 (death cause uncertain). Ex = suspected excipient reaction. DI = suspected drug interaction

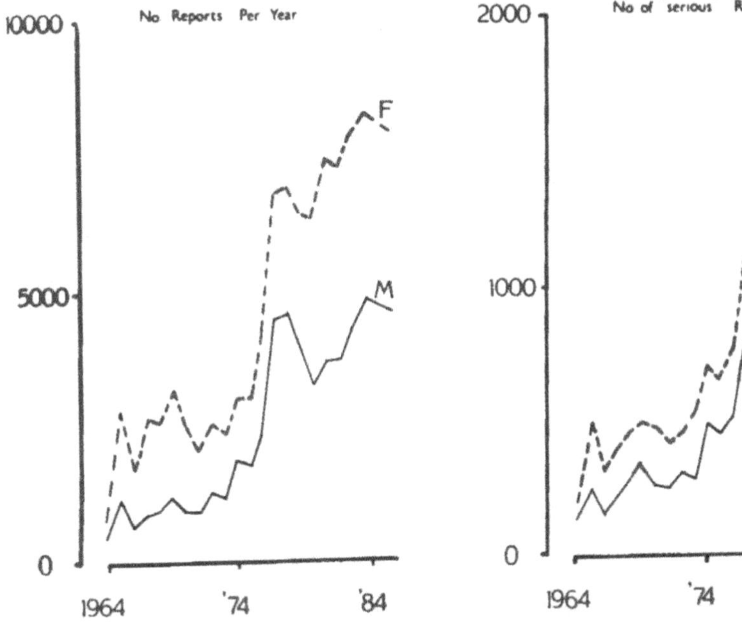

Figure 3. Total number of reports received per year for males and females. (A small number of reports do not identify the sex.) Males (M), solid line; females (F), interrupted line. (Adapted from Mann.[1])

Figure 4. Total number of serious reports received per year for males and females. Males (M), solid line; females (F), interrupted line. (Adapted from Mann.[1])

SOME DETAILS OF THE ADVERSE REACTIONS DATA BASE

An insight into some of the problems associated with the use of the spontaneous reporting scheme may be identified by examining the contents of the data base. Figure 3 shows the number of yellow cards received per year up to 1985. While the 1985 number was somewhat lower than 1984, reporting rates continue to rise.

Of these reports, approximately 30% are classified as serious, Figure 4 showing the increase in reporting rate for serious ADRs over the 21 years the system has been operating.

The figures show two main features of interest. Firstly, there was a steady increase in reporting rate early on in the scheme, and in 1977 there was a substantial increase, mainly as a result of the practolol incident and partly due to the wider availability of yellow slips in prescription pads. Secondly, there has been a consistently higher reporting rate for females than males, reflecting, among other factors, the increased use of drugs in women in the United Kingdom. More effort is presently being put into the development of ways and means to increase the reporting rate further, particularly in relation to serious

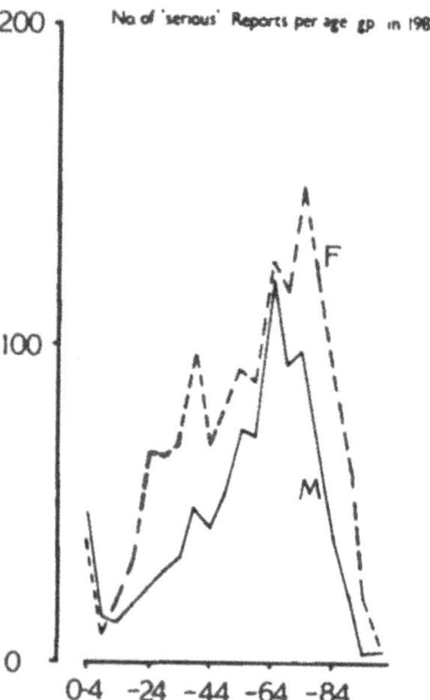

Figure 5. Number of serious reports received in 1985 according to age group. (A small number of reports do not identify age.) Males (M): solid line; females (F): interrupted line. (Adapted from Mann.[1])

ADRs. Such efforts include ensuring the yellow card is more widely available (in prescription pads and the *British National Formulary*) and by more frequent communication with the profession. Examples of such communications include the regular CSM "Update" series in the *British Medical Journal* and the *Current Problems* series issued by the Department of Health and Social Security.

Figure 5 shows the age breakdown of all serious reports received during 1985. There is a high number of reports in the age group 0–4 years, resulting from suspected adverse reactions following immunization. The figure also shows that a larger number of reports are received for females than for males throughout all age ranges and that a broad peak of maximum reporting for both sexes occurs in the 50–80-year-old groups. This peak may reflect prescription volumes and possible problems with the use of drugs in the elderly.

The number and nature of serious adverse reactions received in 1985 are shown in Table 2. In view of the nature and occurrence of gastrointestinal disease and the number and nature of the drugs most frequently used in the United Kingdom, it is perhaps not surprising that gastrointestinal reactions are

Table 2. Serious Adverse Reactions Reported in 1985

System and Type	Number of Reactions	
Gastrointestinal		470
ulceration, hemorrhage, perforation	417	
Blood		444
agranulocytosis and granulocytopenia	151	
thrombocytopenia	139	
aplastic anemia	69	
Central nervous system		331
convulsions	165	
Liver and biliary system		311
Skin		302
angioedema	134	
Anaphylactic reactions		189
Renal		150
Respiratory system		83
bronchospasm	52	
allergic or fibrosing alveolitis	30	
Cardiovascular		58
Other		77
TOTAL		2415

Source: Reproduced with permission from *Br Med J* 1986;293:688.

the most frequently reported. On the other hand, it is somewhat surprising that there are not more reports of suspected cardiovascular and respiratory adverse reactions, bearing in mind the incidence and nature of these diseases and the characteristics of the drugs used to treat them.

Table 3 lists the 10 drugs most frequently reported in association with serious reactions (during the period January to June 1986) and in which the medical assessor had considered the association to be probable or possible. While prescription numbers have not been taken into account, it is apparent that this table reflects the usage of the products throughout the United Kingdom.

Table 3. The 10 Drugs Most Frequently Reported as Suspected Causes of Serious Adverse Reactions

Suspected Drug Jan–June 1986	Number of Serious Reports
Piroxicam	100
Fenbufen	80
Enalapril maleate	78
Naproxen	77
Diclofenac sodium	59
Indomethacin	52
Co-Trimoxazole	44
Ibuprofen	41
Ketoprofen	41
Captopril	39

Source: From Mann.[1]

OTHER FEATURES OF THE ADVERSE REACTIONS DATA BASE

In 1984, the CSM secretariat published a survey of all the reports sent to the committee between 1972 and 1980.[2] The report showed that 19,749 doctors had sent in 53,685 reports, that about 45% of these doctors had sent in more than one report, and that general practitioners (being responsible for about 80% of prescriptions in the United Kingdom) sent in 80% of the reports. Thus only a small proportion of doctors in the United Kingdom sent in suspected ADR reports. In addition, the report documented several other features that had previously only been surmised:

1. Hospital-based doctors sent in more fatal or serious reports.
2. Serious adverse drug reactions comprised 10–20% of all reports (the definition of *serious* was later revised).
3. Fatal reports comprised 3% of all reports.
4. In only half the reports was only one drug mentioned; in slightly more than one-tenth of reports there were more than five drugs mentioned.

The findings did suggest that of all the doctors eligible to report throughout the period 1972–80 only 16% did so. The report was helpful as it indicated the directions in which future effort could be put to improve ADR reporting.

CONTRIBUTIONS OF THE YELLOW CARD SCHEME

Any spontaneous ADR reporting scheme has many limitations affecting the interpretation of data gathered. Nevertheless, the yellow card system has assisted in the documentation of adverse reactions. Recent examples where the scheme helped identify new drug hazards include zimeldine and the Guillain-Barré syndrome[3] and angioedema with angiotensin-converting enzyme inhibitors.[4] In terms of recognition of risk factors relevant in the development of ADRs, the yellow card system's most notable example is the recognition of the dose-dependency of thromboembolic disorders and the oral contraceptives.[5] The scheme has also identified age as being a risk factor in certain situations.

Examples include adolescents being at risk of developing acute dyskinesias with metoclopramide,[6] prochlorperazine, and haloperidol[7] and the elderly appearing to be more susceptible to blood dyscrasias with mianserin[8] and co-trimoxazole.[9] The third situation in which the yellow card scheme has helped has been in the provision of some estimate of the relative risk between drugs within the same therapeutic category. While interpretation of these kinds of data has to be very circumspect, such information concerning antidepressants helped identify the problem which led to the withdrawal of nomifensine.[10]

Comparisons between members of a therapeutic drug group have also provided a degree of reassurance about toxicity, especially when used with data from other sources. Such data helped establish the decision to permit the over-the-counter sale of loperamide and ibuprofen[11] in the United Kingdom. Finally the scheme may be used to help confirm suspicions that a product is associated with an adverse reaction by "prompting" reports from doctors and, while allowing for the bias introduced, observing the reporting rates following product changes. The publication by the Committee on Safety of Medicines of the suspicion that a bronchodilating nebulizer solution may have been associated with paradoxical bronchospasm[12] was followed not only by a large number of reports but also by controlled studies identifying the hypotonicity of the solution as being the main cause of the bronchospasm. The subsequent change in formulation led to a dramatic fall in the reports of paradoxical bronchospasm.

To conclude, the spontaneous "yellow card" adverse drug reaction reporting scheme has been the mainstay of adverse reaction surveillance since 1964 in the United Kingdom. The advantage of the CSM's yellow card scheme is that the data now cover the period 1964–1988, and this experience, now approaching a quarter of a century, has defined the uses and limitations of schemes concerned with spontaneous adverse reactions reporting.

It is clear that such schemes will be needed for the foreseeable future and that other methods of detecting, at reasonable cost, rare and important adverse drug effects are unlikely to become available.

REFERENCES

1. Mann RD: The yellow card data; the nature and scale of the adverse drug reactions problem, in Mann RD (ed): *Adverse Drug Reactions: the Scale and Nature of the Problem and the Way Forward.* United Kingdom, Parthenon Publishing, 1987.
2. Spiers CJ, Griffin JP, Weber JCP, et al. Demography of the UK adverse reactions register of spontaneous reports. *Health Trends* 1984;16:49–52.
3. Committee on Safety of Medicines: Zimeldine (Zelmid). *Current Problems* 1982; No. 11. HMSO.
4. Wood SM, Mann RD, Rawlins MD: Angioedema and urticaria associated with angiotensin converting enzyme inhibitors. *Br Med J* 1987;294:91–92.
5. Inman WHW, Vessey MP, Westerholm B, et al: Thromboembolic disease and the steroidal content of oral contraceptives. *Br Med J* 1970;2:203–206.
6. Bateman DN, Rawlins MD, Simpson JM: Extrapyramidal reactions with metoclopramide. *Br Med J* 1985;291:930–932.
7. Bateman DN, Rawlins MD, Simpson JM: Extrapyramidal reactions to prochlorperazine and haloperidol in the United Kingdom. *Quart J Med* 1986;59:549–556.
8. Committee on Safety of Medicines. Mianserin (Bolvidon, Norval). *Current Problems* 1981; No. 7. HMSO.
9. Committee on Safety of Medicines. Deaths associated with co-trimoxazole, ampicillin and trimethoprim. *Current Problems* 1985; No. 15. HMSO.

7. *Frequency Analysis of Spontaneous Reports from Different Countries: The Example of Continental Western Europe*

RUDOLF BRUPPACHER
RUDOLF BLATTNER
THOMAS FISCH
ROSEMARIE SIFT
GARY C. BERNEKER

QUANTITATIVE ANALYSIS: BASIC ELEMENT OF SCIENCE

Careful descriptions and definitions of events to be observed and related by hypothetic formulae and quantification of such relations are the basis of any scientific activity. There is a trivial but important statement we were taught as students: The first thing a scientist must learn to do is count. This is a long way from the sophisticated statistical analysis procedures we apply today in scientific work, procedures which have become so prevalent and so easy to do with our powerful computers that sometimes the basics of counting are forgotten.

The problems of counting and statistical analysis are exemplified in the topic of this chapter, frequency analysis of spontaneous reports of adverse drug reactions (ADRs).

In recent publications, Weber,[1] Speirs,[2] Sachs and Bortnichak,[3] and Rossi et al[4] have again demonstrated that comparisons of the frequencies of ADR reports must take into account many confounding factors and that great caution must be exercised in interpreting results.

These authors have confirmed and defined the concerns of many of us working with drug monitoring data in the pharmaceutical industry. They have focused on the nonsteroidal antiinflammatory drugs, and on the experience of two countries, the United States and the United Kingdom. Both have well-defined monitoring systems that are run by well-trained and experienced staff. They both apply quantitative methods to analyze the spontaneous ADR reports they receive. Although there are problems, this approach may be reasonable as long as it is confined to reports received under the fairly well known conditions of these countries. The problems, however, for pharmaceutical companies and pharmacoepidemiologists, have been accentuated by the formal requirement of U.S. authorities that frequency analysis of spontaneous reports be performed periodically on all reports of serious events by the holders of NDA (new drug application) licenses, not only on the national U.S. level but worldwide.

PHARMACOEPIDEMIOLOGY AT CIBA-GEIGY HEADQUARTERS

Ciba-Geigy, in its headquarters in Basel, Switzerland, has since the 1960s maintained a central drug monitoring department that supports and coordinates the efforts of its group companies all over the world.[5] In 1986 pharmacoepidemiologic activities were stepped up considerably, creating a separate section of pharmacoepidemiology that is relieved from the everyday efforts of case report analysis, documentation, and reporting to regulatory agencies. Its mission is to elaborate new concepts, develop and adapt methods, and support other functions of Ciba-Geigy so that the development and marketing of pharmaceutical products can better take into account the public health.

Currently our most important and very ambitious goal is to replace today's adverse reaction reports with public health balance sheets for pharmaceuticals. We call the action program to achieve that goal "CARE," which stands for comparative and alternative risk evaluation. *Alternative* in this context means "other therapeutic options."

It is obvious that to accomplish this goal we have to work with outside experts in this field. We need a pharmacoepidemiological relations network (PERN) including not only academic centers but also, as much as possible (and it is our conviction that quite a lot is possible and mutually useful), the analogous departments and colleagues of other research-based pharmaceutical companies and scientific experts in the regulatory agencies.

Efforts for both the CARE and the PERN programs have been considerably slowed down by the interference with work resulting from the above-stated requirement for periodic frequency analysis, a mandate which naturally has fallen onto the section of pharmacoepidemiology.

This mandate has led to a new project line: the program for quantitative analysis of spontaneous information (QUASI). The acronym reflects our ambivalent attitude to that type of activity. In the following we shall present some methodologic aspects of QUASI. With respect to the work already known, from the United States, the United Kingdom, and Sweden, we focus instead on continental western European countries (Germany, France, Italy, and Spain as well as Austria, Belgium, The Netherlands, and Switzerland). These countries together represent a pharmaceutical market of about the same size as the United States.

The situation will be illustrated using adverse drug reaction reports from the Ciba-Geigy ADR data base on four fairly widespread drugs used for different indications: carbamazepine, an antiepileptic marketed since 1963, diclofenac, a nonsteroidal antiinflammatory drug introduced in 1973, maprotiline, an antidepressant introduced in 1972, and metoprolol, a beta-blocking agent marketed since 1975. The period covered relates to the date of the occurrence of the ADR and goes from 1970 to 1985. Where small numbers are involved, we used a three-year running average to smooth the curves. The number of treatment days as the denominator for frequency calculation were derived from our own sales data and defined daily dosages based on our own experiences in different countries.

THE QUASI PROBLEM

The problem of quantitative analysis of spontaneous information is to estimate the "relative toxicity" of a drug. There are, however, many confounding factors. Most of them can be summarized by the formula

$$N = e \cdot i \cdot r$$

where N = number of ADR reports
e = exposure
i = incidence (definition) of ADRs
r = reporting rate

The drug's *exposure* can be estimated from sales, but it is also a function of drug utilization, meaning dosage and treatment duration, data that is only partially available through current marketing research. The *incidence of ADRs* is also dependent on the way a drug is administered, but we know from many examples that the vulnerability of a population, i.e., their susceptibility to certain diseases, may make a considerable difference. For the purpose of this chapter we assume that, of the factors described above, only sales have changed during the period covered.

According to our experience, the *reporting rate* differs from country to country mainly because of different medical care systems and physicians' attitudes, both of which also influence drug utilization. Different regulations and the local company's attitude to data collection are factors also. Another important element is the "climate of reporting," which is greatly influenced by public debate on drug policy or on specific drug problems and media coverage. Included in this "climate" is a secular trend toward generally increased reporting. Furthermore, experience shows that factors in the type of drug—not only its marketing age (life cycle effect) but also the route, the therapeutic class, and the reputation of the manufacturer—have a considerable effect on reporting rates. Finally, the type of event attributed to the drug and the characteristics of the victim make a difference. We must further acknowledge that all these influences do differ from one country to another and also may change over the years.

ILLUSTRATIONS OF FACTORS INFLUENCING ADR REPORTING FREQUENCIES

Life Cycle Effect

Starting with the better-known influences, Figure 1 shows the development over the years of ADR reporting rates for diclofenac tablets per million treatment days. It is obvious that these rates differ from country to country. However, they correspond to experiences in the United States and in the United Kingdom. Figure 2 presents the rates for the three-year periods of the

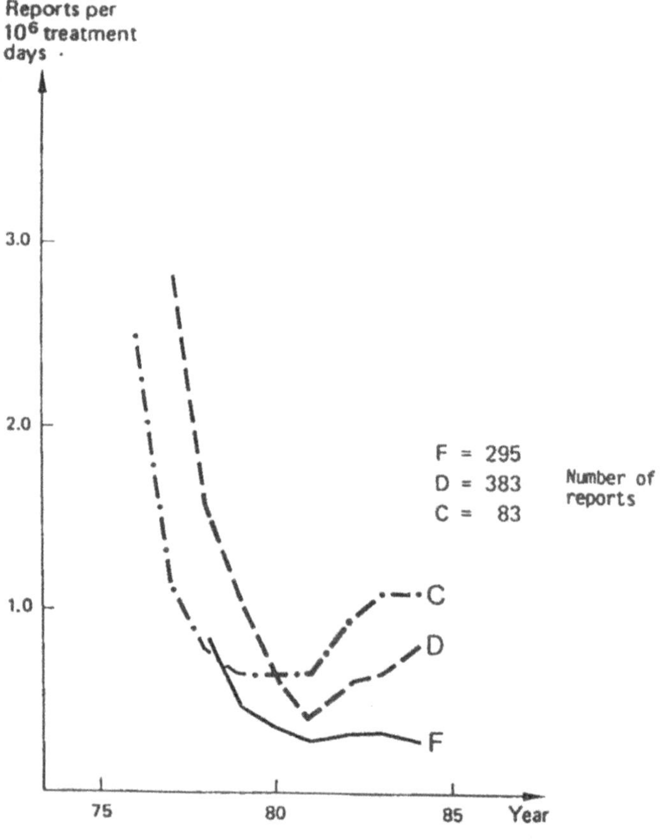

Figure 1. ADR reporting frequency for diclofenac tablets (France, Germany, Switzerland). *Legend*: C = Switzerland, D = Germany West, F = France.

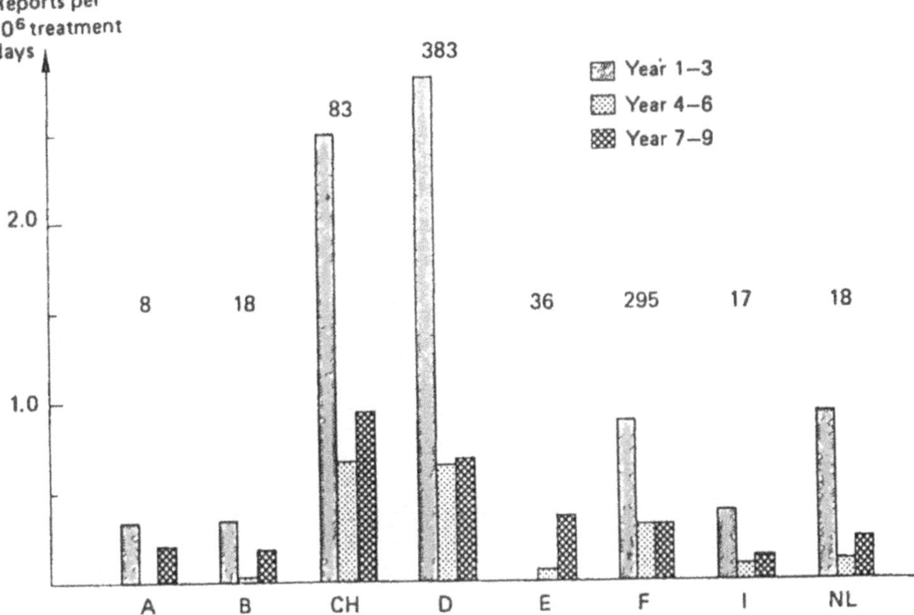

Figure 2. ADR reporting frequency for diclofenac tablets (three-year postmarketing periods in eight European countries). *Legend*: A = Austria, B = Belgium, CH = Switzerland, D = Germany West, E = Spain, F = France, I = Italy, NL - Netherlands. The figures over the bars represent the total number of reports from the respective country.

marketing of diclofenac in continental western Europe. Differences are apparent in the magnitude of the reporting rates as well as in development over time.

Comparing different drugs within a country also reveals considerable discrepancies. Figure 3 gives the example of diclofenac, maprotiline, and metoprolol in Germany. Surprising is the absence of a life cycle effect for the antidepressant maprotiline.

Secular Trend

Carbamazepine is a standard drug in western Europe for the treatment of epilepsy and neuralgias and provides a good basis for the analyses of the secular trend, since it was introduced long before the period covered by our analyses. Figure 4 demonstrates the development of ADR reporting rates in France, Germany, and Switzerland. Linear regressions for all the eight countries covered by our analysis suggest a grouping of countries with higher reporting rates (France, Germany, Switzerland) and lower reporting rates (Netherlands, Austria, Belgium, Italy, and Spain), and also a grouping of countries with more rapidly increasing reporting rates (France and The Netherlands) (Figure 5).

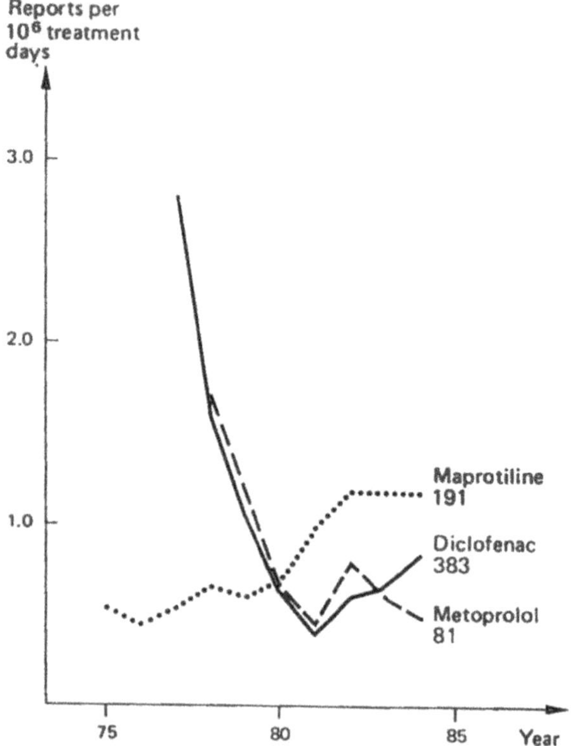

Figure 3. ADR reporting frequency for diclofenac, maprotiline, and metoprolol in Germany. *Legend*: The figures below the drug names represent numbers of reports.

Type of Adverse Event Reported

Reporting rates depend very much on the kind of adverse event attributed to the drug. Comparing recent intensive case surveillance studies by the International Agranulocytosis and Aplastic Anemia Study[6] and Schoepf (unpublished data, 1987) with our own files, we estimate that they are in the two-digit percent figures for severe cutaneous reactions and serious blood dyscrasias. They are probably lower than 1% for less severe events. Rates differ again for symptoms of other organ system reactions and develop in dissimilar ways in different countries. Proportional reporting rate analyses can be used to demonstrate this, for example, the astonishingly different pattern of the proportion of gastrointestinal adverse reaction reports to diclofenac (Figure 6).

Some of these differences result from the development of diagnostic procedures. One example is the proportional increase of reported ADRs to diclofenac identified by laboratory methods, mainly hepatic and hematologic (Table 1) with a corresponding decrease of ADRs identified by physical examination, observation, or history.

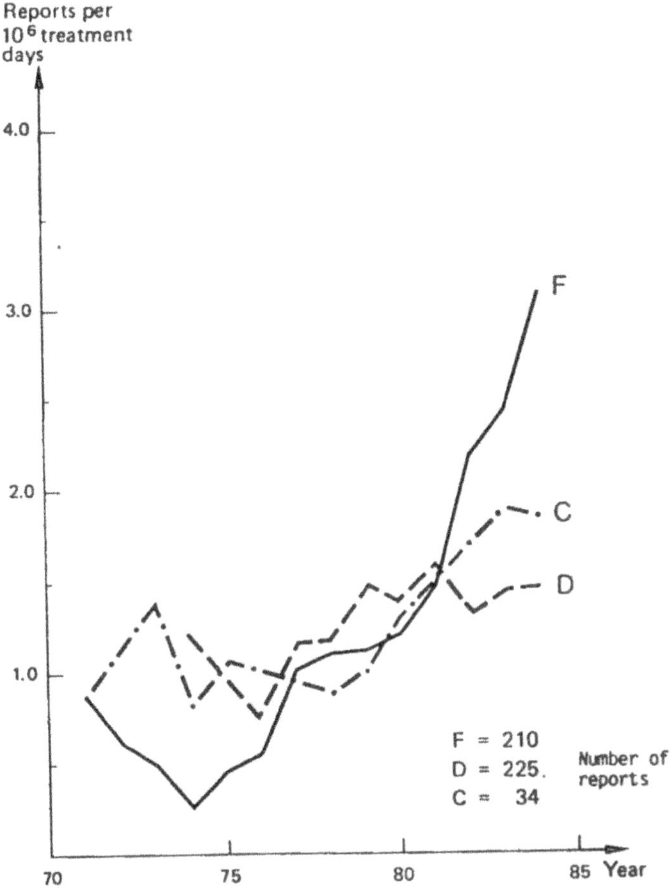

Figure 4. ADR reporting frequency for carbamazepine in France, Germany, and Switzerland. *Legend:* C = Switzerland, D = Germany, F = France.

Route of Administration

Parenteral administration produces more untoward reactions than oral administration. This has obvious pharmacokinetic causes. For most drugs, injection site reactions, as well as allergic or pseudoallergic reactions, account for a large proportion of the reports. These factors may not, however, explain the five- to tenfold higher reporting rate for most drugs (exemplified by Figure 7 for diclofenac in Germany). Confounders such as severity of the disease treated or obviousness of temporal relationship certainly play an important role.

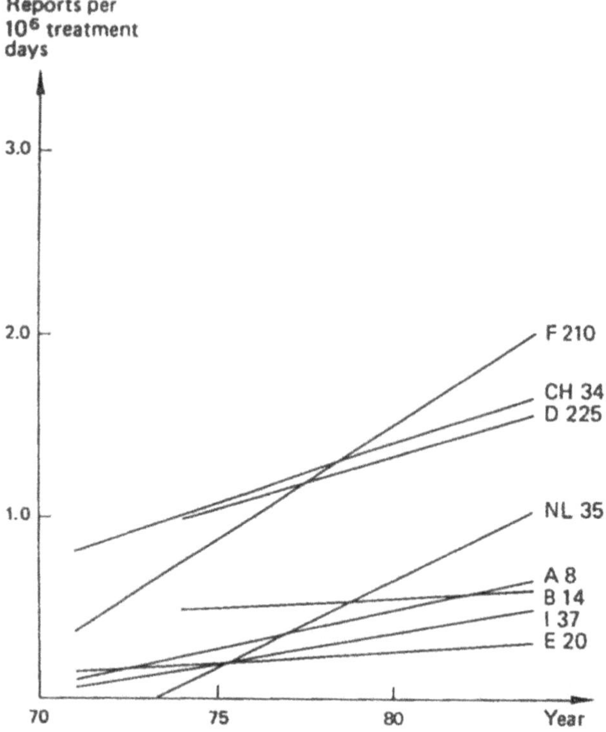

Figure 5. Linear regressions of reporting frequency for carbamazepine in eight Western European countries. *Legend:* A = Austria, B = Belgium, CH = Switzerland, D = Germany West E = Spain, F = France, I = Italy, NL = Netherlands. The figures behind these abbreviations represent the number of reports from the respective countries.

INTERPRETATION OF REPORTING RATES FROM DIFFERENT COUNTRIES

The example used here refers to a group of countries that are all considered "developed" and, as seen from the transatlantic distance, a rather homogeneous array of populations. We did not include South American, African, or Asian countries, but even so, the range of differences apparent in ADR reporting varies in a complex and practically unpredictable manner. Considering the factors at work, we should not be surprised. Quantitative analyses of spontaneous information remains a quasi-statistical enterprise, regardless of more sophisticated methods, because the foundation for probability statistics cannot exist for this sort of spontaneously offered information. On the other hand, the obligation to compile worldwide denominator figures and to relate them to the number of reports in an intelligent way has put a considerable

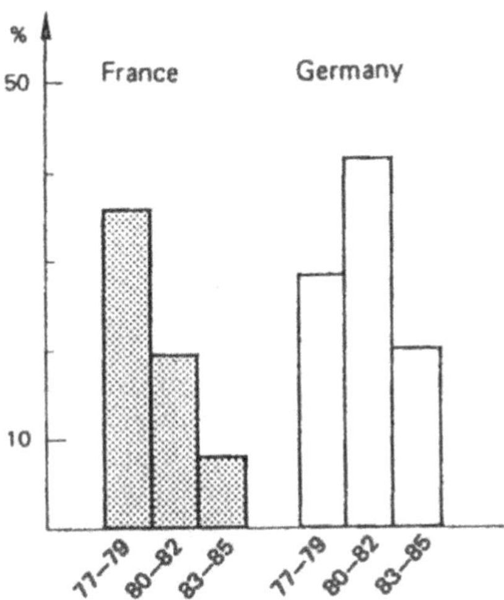

Figure 6. Patterns of ADR reports for diclofenac tablets; proportion ADRs on GI tract.

extra workload on groups that could be employed much more fruitfully. We understand the need for international reporting of serious adverse reactions and sincerely support these efforts. We also are very much in favor of up-to-date epidemiologic and statistical quantitative approaches to evaluate comparative and alternative risks of drug therapy. We have indeed been fascinated by the attempts to handle spontaneous reports in a quantitative way. However, we think the limitations and the comparative benefit of such an approach should be considered, for quantity and quality, as well as the merits of better founded epidemiologic activities such as record linkage studies or classic epidemiologic studies.

SUMMARY

Quantitative analysis of spontaneous reports by physicians to authorities or drug companies has been the basis of many regulatory decisions and requirements. It has considerably diverted the efforts of drug monitoring groups from

Table 1. Proportion of Adverse Reaction Reports to Diclofenac Tablets Based on Laboratory Diagnosis

	France		Germany	
Period	N (total)	% (lab.)	N (total)	% (lab.)
1977–1979	95	21.1	136	20.6
1980–1982	77	39.0	53	17.0
1983–1985	101	48.5	101	33.7

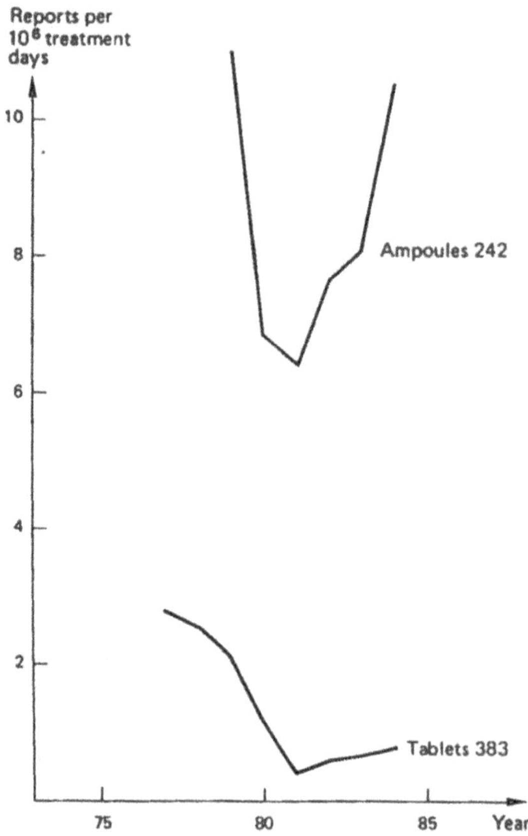

Figure 7. ADR reporting frequency for diclofenac tablets and ampoules in Germany.

other pharmacoepidemiologic activities in the research-based pharmaceutical companies, including Ciba-Geigy. The frequency of spontaneous reports is, however, not only dependent on the incidence of adverse reactions and on drug exposure, which are both quite difficult to measure, but also on the likelihood that an event is recognized as a suspected adverse reaction and is actually reported. This can be illustrated by the development of the number of reports, adjusted by drug sales, for four Ciba-Geigy products. The age of the product, the secular trend, the influence of type of event, and route of administration can produce wide differences in the reporting rate even between continental western European countries, which may be considered relatively homogeneous on a worldwide scale. Considering the work capacity bound by these QUASI efforts (quantitative analysis of spontaneous information) and the subsequent opportunities missed in record linkage projects and epidemiologic studies, the relative benefit of these analyses should be carefully considered.

REFERENCES

1. Weber JPC: Epidemiology of adverse reactions to non-steroidal anti-inflammatory drugs. In Rainsford KD, Velo GP (eds): *Advances in Inflammation Research*. New York, Raven Press, 1984, vol 6.
2. Speirs CJ: Prescription related adverse reaction profiles and their use in risk benefit analysis. In D'Arcy and Griffin (eds): *Iatrogenic Diseases*, ed 3. Oxford University Press, 1986.
3. Sachs RM, Bortnichak EA: An evaluation of spontaneous adverse reaction reporting systems. *Am J Med* 1986;81(Suppl 5B):49–55.
4. Rossi AC, Hsu JP, Faich GA: Ulcerogenicity of piroxicam: An analysis of spontaneously reported data. *Brit Med J* 1987;294:147–150.
5. Borda IT, Berneker GC: The pharmaceutical industry: Drug monitoring by Ciba-Geigy. In Inman WHW (ed): *Monitoring for Drug Safety*. Lancaster, MTP Press Ltd, 1986.
6. The International Agranulocytosis and Aplastic Anemia Study: Risk of agranulocytosis and aplastic anemia. *JAMA* 1986;256:1749–1757.

8. *Evaluation of First Year Experience of a State Pilot Project to Promote Physician Reporting of Adverse Drug Events to the Food and Drug Administration*

AUDREY SMITH ROGERS
EBENEZER ISRAEL
GERALD FAICH
CRAIG R. SMITH

INTRODUCTION

The U.S. Food and Drug Administration (FDA) has maintained a spontaneous, voluntary system for the reporting of adverse drug events for over three decades. Based on the experience of the American Medical Association registry for drug-related aplastic anemia, the current FDA spontaneous reporting system (FDA-SRS) was initiated following the public reaction to thalidomide-induced phocomelia.[1]

Viewed initially and naively as a method to guarantee drug safety for the public, the inability of the SRS to perform as such soon became apparent. In time, however, the public health utility of the SRS was recognized when it began to be viewed as an early warning system to monitor possible drug risk. In fact, recent critical evaluations of the SRS have concluded that it may be the most efficient and the only affordable method of detecting serious clinical events which occur less frequently than once per 10,000 drug exposures.[2-4]

The chief criticism of the SRS has been in the unrepresentativeness of its data: the SRS is voluntary, and reporting rates vary among physician groups, among drug classes, and according to the age of the drug. Furthermore, the reports are events out of context; there is no information on the population of equally exposed individuals from whom the adverse events emerged.

Since the SRS is entirely voluntary, its most serious problem is underreporting. The rate of adverse drug reaction reporting per 1000 physicians in the United States in 1982 was 57.6; this was one-third to one-half the rate in Denmark, Sweden, the United Kingdom, or Canada.[5] This low rate of reporting, while improving,[6] remains a problem.

Many hypotheses have been generated to explain physician underreporting, including mistaken belief in drug safety, fear of litigation, guilt due to patient harm, ambition to publish, ignorance of reporting system, diffidence about reporting mere suspicions, and lethargy.[7] While all these factors intuitively have merit, the degree to which any may actually contribute to underreporting is not known. Conversely, factors which may induce reporting have been proposed and include the severity of the reaction, the certainty of attribution of the reaction to the drug, the mechanism of the reaction (idiosyncratic or allergic events seem to be more likely to be reported than pharmacologic ones),[8] and previous publicity about the reaction.[9] Milstien et al[10] confirmed that the severity of the reaction is indeed an important factor when they surveyed physician reporters to the FDA to determine which factors induced reporting. However, their study provides no information on the factors involved in the failure of community physicians to report.

In order to improve the function of the SRS, the FDA contracted for a series of pilot projects conducted through state health departments to promote physician reporting of adverse drug events. The objectives of the project in Maryland were the assessment of community physician knowledge, attitudes, and reporting behavior relating to the FDA-SRS and the implementation of methods to improve each of these. This chapter presents an evaluation of the first year experience.

METHODS

The study area comprised the greater Baltimore region, in which 5139 physicians received licensure in 1986. Two control groups were chosen from Prince Georges and Montgomery counties, where 3104 physicians were licensed. These counties were selected as controls because they approximated the Baltimore area in physician and population density. To increase the likelihood of surveying community physicians, the areas of Rockville and Bethesda, where large government research facilities are located, were excluded. There were 1500 randomly selected physicians in Baltimore who received a baseline questionnaire in February 1986, the area intervention, and a termination questionnaire after nine months. The first control group consisted of 1500 randomly selected physicians who received both questionnaires but no intervention. The second control group comprised 500 randomly chosen physicians who received the termination questionnaire only (Table 1). The representativeness of the responders was assessed by comparing available demographic characteristics from the Maryland State Health Department statistics for physicians in the respective areas. These data are generated in the biennial licensing process and

Table 1. Design of Maryland Pilot Project to Assess Physician Knowledge, Attitudes, and Behavior About Adverse Drug Event Reporting and Intervention to Encourage Adverse Drug Event Reporting

	Baltimore City and Baltimore County (n = 5171)	Prince Georges County and Montgomery County (n = 3104)*	
	Study Group (n = 1500)	Control Group One (n = 1500)	Control Group Two (n = 500)
Baseline questionnaire (February 1986)	X	X	
Intervention	X		
Termination questionnaire (November 1986)	X	X	X

*Excluding Bethesda and Rockville.

represent all physicians in 1981–82 and a nonscientific half-sample in 1985. Comparison factors are limited to sex, medical specialty, and age (1985 only).

Undeliverable questionnaires or those returned from self-declared ineligible physicians (due to retirement or no direct patient care) were replaced by other randomly selected physicians from the same area. Physicians were guaranteed confidentiality. All forms were coded to facilitate second mailings. No follow-up beyond a second mailing was attempted for either questionnaire.

Questionnaires sought information in four areas: (1) demographic information about physician responders; (2) knowledge about the FDA-SRS; (3) attitudes toward the FDA-SRS and adverse drug event reporting, and (4) behavior related to its use during the previous calendar year.

The intervention targeted the study group area only and consisted of an educational component (direct mailings, medical staff and society presentations, grand rounds on ADE identification and surveillance) and a direct reporting component (local telephone number for reporting and communication with local hospital pharmacy and therapeutics committees to capture all events). In April 1986, a telephone line was initiated for direct physician reporting of adverse events; this was announced by mail to all study area physicians. From May to October, the reporting program was presented at medical staff meetings at eight community hospitals and to committees at two others. Brochures with updates about the program were mailed to 5200 community physicians every three months. An information booth was manned at the Maryland State Medical Chiurgical Society Meeting, and announcements appeared in the *Maryland Medical Journal*.

The analysis of the questionnaire results consisted of a before/after group comparison between the study group and the first control group. The second control group was included to assess the effect of the baseline questionnaire on subsequent knowledge, attitudinal, and reporting changes. Change in reporting behavior was examined by comparing reporting rates for Maryland physicians in 1985 (the year prior to the inception of the project) and 1986 rates.

Table 2. Response to Questionnaires, by Groups Returning Baseline Questionnaire Only; the Termination Questionnaire Only; and Both Baseline and Termination Questionnaires

	Baseline Questionnaire Only		Baseline and Termination		Termination Questionnaire Only
Study Group	246 (16%)	606 (40%)	360 (24%)	539 (36%)	179 (12%)
Control Group One	207 (14%)	516 (34%)	309 (21%)	493 (33%)	184 (12%)
Control Group Two	—		—		188 (38%)
TOTAL	N = 453 (15%)	1122 (37%)	N = 669 (22%)	1220 (35%)	N = 551 (16%)

McNemar and chi-square tests of association and tests for independent proportions[11] were employed.

RESULTS

The study and first control group were surveyed at two points in time. The numbers of responders to baseline-only, baseline and termination questionnaires, and termination-only are presented in Table 2. The numbers responding at each time are not different in study or control group categories (chi-square = 2.46, p = 0.29). These responder groups were examined for differences in relation to any outcome variable in either the baseline or termination questionnaire. Physicians who responded to both questionnaires had a statistically significantly higher level of knowledge about the SRS than those physicians who either responded at baseline alone or termination alone (Table 3). For those who answered both questionnaires, the study group demonstrated a statistically significant increase in knowledge about the SRS, while the first control group did not. There appeared to be little effect on knowledge level attributable to the receipt of the questionnaire alone.

The study and control groups differed substantially on a number of demographic characteristics as reported elsewhere.[12] Neither group demonstrated a difference in age or sex when compared to state statistics for physicians from the corresponding areas. While the groups were clinically and demographically different, there was no difference between physician groups on any outcome measure at baseline: no difference in knowledge, attitudes, or behavior related to the FDA-SRS.

Table 3. Percent of Physician Knowledge About the Spontaneous Reporting System, by Study Group and Respondent Status in the Questionnaires at Baseline and at Termination

	Baltimore City Baltimore County			Prince Georges County and Montgomery County			
	Study Group (n = 1500)			Control Group One (n = 1500)			Control Group Two (n = 500)
	BL Only	Both	TM Only	BL Only	Both	TM Only	TM Only
(Number)	(246)	(360)	(179)	(207)	(309)	(184)	(188)
Baseline	48%	* 64%		49%	* 61%		
Intervention		xxx *			*		
Termination		86%	* 66%		65%	* 44%	54%

*p< 0.001

Fifty-seven percent of the responders knew about the SRS. The attitudes of these Maryland physicians reflected beliefs that a single case can be important, serious drug reactions are well documented at the time of marketing, financial reimbursement for reporting should not occur, and that reporting will not much increase liability. They believed reporting to be a professional obligation and expressed little concern about governmental interference, time consumption, or the need for an easier method.

Thirty-seven percent of these physicians had detected a moderate to severe adverse drug reaction during the previous year in their practices and 18% had reported the event in some fashion. One of every five of these reports was directly to the FDA.

After the interventions had been conducted for nine months in the study area, the termination questionnaire was distributed to assess change. Both intragroup and intergroup change in knowledge of the SRS over time was examined (Table 4). There was a statistically significant increase in knowledge about the SRS in the study group in both comparisons. The level of knowledge in the second control group was not different from that in the first control group at study termination (54% vs. 57%), again suggesting the reception of the baseline questionnaire had little influence on subsequent knowledge of the SRS.

Attitudinal change is more difficult to induce and, as expected, few statistically significant differences from baseline were demonstrated. However, two distinct patterns were consistently observed: study group physicians developed more favorable attitudes while control groups remained unchanged, or study group physicians maintained baseline values while control group attitudes

Table 4. Proportion of Physicians Who Knew About the Food and Drug Administration Spontaneous Reporting System, by Group

Group	Baseline Questionnaire	Termination Questionnaire	χ^2 p value (intragroup)
Study Group	0.58	0.80	$p < 0.0001$
Control Group 1	0.56	0.57	$p = 0.80$
Control Group 2	—	0.54	—
χ^2 p value (intergroup)	$p = 0.63$	$p < 0.0001$	

became less positive. More favorable attitudes were demonstrated in study group physicians who felt that really serious adverse drug events are not necessarily well documented at the time of marketing, that reporting does not increase liability, and that reporting is a professional obligation. Two more favorable differences were statistically significant: reporting does not require financial reimbursement ($p = 0.05$) and reporting will not result in endless forms ($p = 0.006$). The other trend had the study group maintaining baseline values while those of the control group worsened. The control group felt more strongly at termination that the attribution of the adverse event to the drug was not possible, that single cases were unimportant, and that reporting was time-consuming.

The level of detection of adverse drug events in practice decreased at termination in all groups of participating physicians (Table 5). This decrease was statistically significant in the study group; however, the decrease in the study group was not different from that in the first control group. Both were comparable to the level of detection in the second control group, suggesting a general phenomenon independent of the intervention.

When the reporting rates were examined in the questionnaire responders, no statistically significant changes were demonstrated (Table 6), although trends in reporting supported an intervention effect. However, respondents from the sample of physicians surveyed represented only 10% of all physicians in the

Table 5. Proportion of Physicians Who Detected a Serious or Moderate Adverse Drug Event in Their Practices During the Previous Year, by Group

Group	Baseline Questionnaire	Termination Questionnaire	χ^2 p value (intragroup)
Study Group	0.37	0.28	$p = 0.0007$
Control Group 1	0.37	0.32	$p = 0.06$
Control Group 2	—	0.29	—
χ^2 p value (intergroup)	$p = 0.99$	$p = 0.37$	

Table 6. Proportion of Physicians Who Reported a Serious or Moderate Adverse Drug Event in Their Practices During the Previous Year, by Group

Group	Baseline Questionnaire	Termination Questionnaire	χ^2 p value (intragroup)
Study Group	0.15	0.18	p = 0.45
Control Group 1	0.16	0.11	p = 0.19
Control Group 2	—	0.11	—
χ^2 p value (intergroup)	p = 0.78	p = 0.15	

intervention area. When the 1986 reporting rate of the full area was evaluated (Figure 1), there were 135 reports, 90 of these through the project reporting line and 45 directly to the FDA. There were 26 reports from other areas of the state. This represented an increase 3.8 times over the rate in 1985, when direct reports from all Maryland physicians numbered 42.

Because factors influencing reporting are poorly understood and rates fluctuate, 1985 and 1986 rates observed in Maryland were compared to corresponding rates from contiguous states (Table 7). In 1985, the reporting rate for Pennsylvania physicians was 42 per 10,000, in Virginia 35, and in Maryland 35. There was no significant difference among these rates. In 1986, statistically significant differences were observed among the rates. In examining the changes within states, the decrease in the Pennsylvania rate probably indicated normal fluctuation. There was a 50% increase in the Virginia rate, which was statistically significant (p = 0.03). The change in Maryland rates represented almost a fourfold increase and was clearly the strongest factor in the difference among states' rates in 1986.

Table 7. Comparison of Numbers of Adverse Drug Event Reports and Reporting Rates Among Physicians in Pennsylvania, Virginia, and Maryland During the Calendar Years 1985 and 1986

	Pennsylvania Physicians (n = 25,000)	Virginia Physicians (n = 11,000)	Maryland Physicians (n = 12,000)
1985			
Number of ADE reports	106	39	42
Reporting rate	0.0042	0.0035	0.0035
1986			
Number of ADE reports	97	57	161
Reporting rate*	0.0039	0.0052	0.0134
Ratio $\frac{1986}{1985}$	0.93	1.49	3.83

*Differences among rates statistically significant: χ^2 = 120.8; p < 0.0001.

DISCUSSION

The SRS is essentially a method for safeguarding the public health. To perform as such, it is critical to have the participation of physicians in reporting serious adverse drug events in the patients they treat. Scattered, delayed, and biased reporting undercuts the capacity of the system to monitor and signal potential problems, timely definition of which benefits not only the public for whom the SRS was designed but all involved in drug development.

We planned an educational and promotional intervention to encourage physician reporting with a before/after assessment of randomly chosen physicians to evaluate the effect of the intervention. In addition to the study group of physicians, we chose two control groups, one receiving both assessments but no intervention and the other the termination assessment only. In this way, we believe we controlled for temporal trends and the effect of the questionnaire itself and thus were in a position to attribute observed differences to the effect of the intervention.

The response rate to both sets of questionnaires averaged 36% which, while it prevents broad generalizations to the entire physician community, is attenuated by the favorable comparison of physician respondents to available state statistics on a limited number of demographic variables.

We tailored an intervention based on two hypotheses: (1) that physicians do not have an adequately high level of suspicion about adverse effects of drug therapy when faced with untoward experiences in the patients they treat, and (2) when they may suspect an adverse drug event, the inconvenience of the reporting system discourages their best intentions to report. We have attempted to promote reporting by increasing knowledge about the SRS, providing a convenient and quick method of reporting, and changing physician attitudes about the SRS through educational offerings.

We examined change in knowledge, adverse drug event detection, and reporting in the randomly chosen physicians who were surveyed. While knowledge had increased significantly in the study group, detection had decreased in both groups, and reporting did not increase. Remarkably, 20% of the study group physicians, who had four mailings about the project, did not know about the SRS at termination.

In addition, we were able to determine which 1986 ADE reports from Maryland originated in our study area, permitting us to properly attribute source. Finally, we were able to compare the composite Maryland rate (since study area reports comprised 84% of all reports) to those from contiguous states to assess random variation or trends. We are confident the intervention increased physician knowledge and believe we produced a modest increase in reporting behavior.

While the physicians we surveyed support reporting in general as a professional obligation and expressed little concern over the time or perceived risk involved, their actual behavior resulted in only 1 in 20 cases (defined by them as moderate to severe clinical events) being reported to the FDA. We believe the discrepancy can be derived from the nature of clinical training which, because it focuses on the experience of one patient at a time, lacks a public health orientation. Few medical school curricula address issues involved in drug development, and few attending physicians model ADE reporting for students and residents. Thus, while physicians may intellectually acknowledge their role in promoting drug safety, reporting is not demonstrated in their education as an activity that a physician does.

Increased knowledge is an attainable short-term goal, but inducing behavioral change, particularly in a situation as complex as the medicolegal and clinical one, will require sustained and long-term efforts.

CONCLUSIONS

1. The pilot project has resulted in a statistically significant increase in the study group physicians' knowledge about the FDA-SRS.
2. The attitude of physicians in the study area concerning interacting with a governmental agency has improved and is statistically better than the attitude of physicians in the control areas.
3. Rejection of financial reimbursement and support for the professional obligation of reporting have increased among study physicians while decreasing among control physicians. These differences achieved only borderline statistical significance.
4. The level of concern about increased liability resulting from reporting was maintained in the study physicians, but increased in the control physicians. The differences were only of borderline statistical significance.
5. Direct physician reports to the FDA increased from 42 during the year prior to the project to 71 in the project year; an additional 90 reports were contributed through the project telephone reporting line. This represents nearly a fourfold increase in the number of statewide reports.

ACKNOWLEDGMENT

Research upon which this publication is based was performed pursuant to Contract Number 223-85-4267 from the Food and Drug Administration, Department of Health and Human Services. The authors thank John P. Juergens, Ph.D. for his invaluable assistance in this project.

REFERENCES

1. Faich GA: Adverse drug reaction monitoring. *N Engl J Med* 1986;314:1589–1592.
2. Rossi AC, Knapp DE, Anello C, O'Neill RT, et al: Discovery of adverse drug reactions. *JAMA* 1983;249:2226–2228.

3. Rossi AC, Knapp DE: Discovery of new adverse drug reactions. *JAMA* 1984;252:1030–1033.
4. Lasagna L: Discovering adverse drug reactions, editorial. *JAMA* 1983;249:2224–2225.
5. Griffin JP, Weber JCP: Voluntary systems of adverse reaction reporting. Part II. *Adv Drug React Ac Pois Rev* 1986;1: 23–55.
6. Faich GA, Knapp D, Dreis M, et al: National adverse drug reaction surveillance: 1985. *JAMA* 1987;257:2068–2070.
7. Inman WHW: The United Kingdom. In Inman WHW (ed): *Monitoring for Drug Safety*. Lancaster, MTP Press, 1980.
8. Koch-Weser J, Sidel VW, Sweet RH, et al: Factors determining physician reporting of adverse drug reactions. *N Engl J Med* 1969;280:20–26.
9. Wardell WM, Tsianco MC, Anavekar SN, et al: Postmarketing surveillance of new drugs. I. Review of objectives and methodology. *J Clin Pharmacol* 1979;Feb-Mar:85–94.
10. Milstien JB, Faich GA, Hsu JP, et al: Factors affecting physician reporting of adverse drug reactions. *Drug Inf J* 1986;20:157–164.
11. Fleiss JL: In: *Statistical Methods for Rates and Proportions,* ed 2. New York, John Wiley and Sons, 1981.
12. Rogers AS, Israel E, Smith CR, et al: Physician knowledge, attitudes, and behaviour related to reporting adverse drug events. *Arch Int Med* 1988;148:1596–1600.

9. *Monitoring System for Adverse Events Following Immunization: Risk Factors for Convulsions After Vaccination*

JOHN R. LIVENGOOD
JOHN R. MULLEN

Surveillance for adverse effects of immunization began at the Centers for Disease Control (CDC) in 1976–1977 with the A/New Jersey, Swine Flu Vaccination campaign. This surveillance effort successfully detected an increased incidence of Guillain-Barré syndrome (GBS), subsequently estimated at slightly less than one excess case of GBS attributable to the influenza vaccine for every 100,000 vaccinees, and stimulated the development of an ongoing system to collect reports of illness following immunization.[1,2] The basics of this system, the Monitoring System for Adverse Events Following Immunization (MSAEFI), have been previously described.[3] Briefly, MSAEFI is a stimulated passive postmarketing surveillance system for adverse events severe enough to require a visit to a health care provider which occur within 28 days of vaccination with public sector vaccine. Public sector vaccines, that is, vaccines purchased with federal, state, or local government funds, account for approximately half of all childhood immunizations in the United States. This proportion varies widely from state to state. Thus, MSAEFI complements the Spontaneous Reporting System of the Food and Drug Administration (FDA) in the surveillance of vaccine safety.

MSAEFI has three main purposes: first, to develop indices of rates of adverse events following immunization in order to provide information on the risks of present vaccines and assist in the ongoing evaluation of new vaccines as they are licensed by the FDA. Second, MSAEFI collects lot-specific information to monitor the safety of individual vaccine lots. And third, MSAEFI can be used to identify factors that increase the risk of adverse events following immunization, and thus may play an important role in modifying national immunization recommendations. In this chapter, we present data from

MSAEFI on the personal and family history of convulsions and the risk of neurologic events after vaccination with diphtheria/tetanus toxoids/pertussis vaccine (DTP) or measles-containing vaccines.

The Immunization Practices Advisory Committee (ACIP) and the Committee on Infectious Diseases of the American Academy of Pediatrics (AAP), commonly called the Red Book Committee, are the two main bodies which currently provide policy guidance on immunization recommendations for the United States. Vaccine manufacturers provide additional information on recommendations and contraindications in their product labels.

The ACIP is an advisory committee of the U.S. Public Health Service composed of nationally recognized experts in infectious diseases, immunology, virology, epidemiology, and public health from academic institutions and state and local health departments. In addition, liaison members from the American Academy of Pediatrics, the American Academy of Family Practitioners, the National Institute of Allergy and Infectious Diseases, the Food and Drug Administration, and the Canadian National Advisory Committee on Immunization participate in committee deliberations. Recommendations of the ACIP are published periodically in the *Morbidity and Mortality Weekly Report* (MMWR) and provide the main policy guidance in the public sector. The AAP Committee on Infectious Diseases is composed of prominent experts in pediatrics and pediatric infectious diseases who serve a similar advisory function for private sector pediatricians.

The ACIP recommended in 1985 that children with a prior personal history of convulsions have their DTP immunization deferred until a complete evaluation has been performed to determine that an evolving neurologic disorder is not present.[4,5] Children with controlled seizure disorders, however, should be vaccinated. Using these criteria, it was estimated that less than one-half of 1% of children would not complete their three-dose series of DTP because of a personal history of seizures.[6] This is similar to what was recommended by the AAP, but differs from the manufacturers' package inserts.[7] No specific recommendations were made for measles-containing vaccines.

For the ACIP and the AAP, this recommendation was based at least in part on data from MSAEFI which compared the personal and family history of convulsions of persons reporting neurologic adverse events following DTP immunization to those reporting nonneurologic events.[6] These data covered the first four years of operation of MSAEFI (1979–1982). In this analysis, persons reporting neurologic events after DTP were 7.2 times more likely to also report a personal history of convulsions than were those reporting nonneurologic events.[6]

Recently, the ACIP reviewed additional MSAEFI data comparing the history of convulsions in children reporting neurologic adverse events following DTP and measles-containing vaccines. The committee subsequently issued a supplemental statement on DTP immunization of children with family histories of seizures, and information on measles immunization of children with either a personal or family history of seizures was included in the recent revision of the ACIP measles vaccine statement.[8,9]

For these analyses, the group of persons reporting neurologic adverse events after immunization was compared to the group of persons reporting nonneurologic events in response to questions concerning a personal or a family history of convulsions. The resulting ratio (the odds ratio) approximates the increased risk of convulsions after immunization among persons with histories of seizures compared to the general population.

Neurologic events were defined as convulsions, encephalopathy, Guillain-Barré syndrome, Reye's syndrome, and other neurologic symptoms (symptoms or diagnoses neurologic in character not elsewhere classified, such as paresthesias, neuritis, or paralysis). Nonneurologic adverse events included all other reports. Neurologic events reported to MSAEFI are predominantly seizures, and nonneurologic events are mostly local reactions and fever.[10] In addition, we defined febrile convulsions as a report of a convulsion with a concurrent MSAEFI report of fever, either subjective (felt hot) or a measured temperature ≥ 100°F. Nonfebrile convulsions were all other reports of seizures. Therefore, certain of these convulsions may be misclassified. For example, convulsions without fever as reported to MSAEFI may have actually been febrile convulsions. This distinction is potentially of great importance in that febrile seizures are, in general, almost always benign.[11] We used MSAEFI data for the years 1979 through 1986 for personal history of convulsions and 1985 and 1986 for family history of convulsions. The data from 1986 are still provisional.

For DTP, we restricted the analysis to those events occurring within three days of DTP vaccination, given either alone or with trivalent oral poliovirus vaccine. For 1979–1986 there were a total of 1068 neurologic events and 4909 nonneurologic events following DTP which met these criteria; 800 (75%) of neurologic events were convulsions, and 661 (62%) were convulsions with fever (Table 1). Nine hundred thirty-eight (88%) of those reporting neurologic adverse events responded to the question on personal history of convulsions compared to 3971 (81%) of those with nonneurologic events. This difference in response rate, although small, is statistically significant ($p < 0.001$) and

Table 1. Personal History of Convulsions, by Adverse Event Type: DTP, 1979–1986

	Total Reports	Total Responders	Percent Responders	Percent Positive Response
Neurologic adverse events	1068	938	88	11
Febrile seizures	661	579	88	14
Nonfebrile seizures	139	118	85	14
Nonneurologic events	4909	3971	81	2

Note: Odds ratio (95% confidence interval): neurologic/nonneurologic, 6.6 (5.0–8.7); febrile seizures/nonneurologic, 8.9 (6.7–11.9); nonfebrile seizures/nonneurologic, 8.6 (5.2–14.2).

may indicate reporting bias. Percentages of persons with febrile and nonfebrile convulsions who responded to the personal history question were similar.

A personal history of convulsions was reported in 11% of persons with neurologic events following DTP compared to 2% of those with nonneurologic events, for an odds ratio of 6.6, or a 6.6-fold increased risk. For both persons with febrile and those with nonfebrile convulsions, 14% of responders reported a prior history of convulsions. When compared to responders with nonneurologic events, these persons had an increased risk (or odds ratio) of 8.9- and 8.6-fold, respectively. There were insufficient data to make any assessment of the risk of more severe neurologic events, such as encephalitis or encephalopathy. These data confirm results of the earlier analyses showing an increased risk of neurologic adverse events, primarily convulsions, following DTP for children with a prior personal history of seizures.[6]

Due to changes in the MSAEFI form, data on history of seizures in first-degree family relatives (i.e., siblings or parents) are only available for 1985 and 1986. Prior to 1985, the degree of relation of family members was not specified. For these two years the percentage of persons responding to the family history question did not differ between the neurologic and nonneurologic event groups (Table 2). However, 13% of responders with a neurologic event reported a history of convulsions in a first-degree family member compared to 6% of the comparison group (odds ratio = 2.4). Considering only those persons reporting seizures, persons with febrile seizures were 2.9 times more likely to report a family history of seizures than those with nonneurologic events, and those with nonfebrile seizures were 3.5 times more likely. Analysis by age at immunization or controlling for a personal history of seizures does not change these associations.

In summary, these data indicate an increased risk of neurologic adverse events after DTP for children with a history of convulsions in first-degree relatives, but the association is not as strong as that for personal history of convulsions. In addition, over 80% of seizures after DTP reported to MSAEFI are febrile seizures, a condition only rarely associated with subsequent epilepsy or impaired intellectual development.[11] Finally, exempting the 5–7% of all children with family histories of seizures would diminish overall DTP vaccination coverage, which might substantially increase the risk of acquiring pertus-

Table 2. Family History of Convulsions, by Adverse Event Type: DTP, 1985–1986

	Total Reports	Total Responders	Percent Responders	Percent Positive Response
Neurologic adverse events	556	448	81	13
Febrile seizures	308	260	84	15
Nonfebrile seizures	45	34	76	18
Nonneurologic events	1930	1577	82	5

Note: Odds ratio (95% confidence interval): neurologic/nonneurologic, 2.4 (1.7–3.4); febrile seizures/nonneurologic, 2.9 (2.0–4.3); nonfebrile seizures/nonneurologic, 3.5 (1.3–9.4).

sis in the general population.[12] Therefore, the ACIP did not recommend a change in the immunization policy for children with family histories of convulsions.[8]

There are several methodologic problems with these MSAEFI data.[10,13] First, a child with a personal history of seizures is more likely to have a seizure after any event than someone without a similar history (i.e., by temporal association alone). Therefore, causation cannot be inferred from this analysis. A second concern is recall bias. Although use of persons who report nonneurologic adverse events as a comparison group tends to decrease recall bias, a parent of a child who had a seizure following immunization may be more likely to remember or report a seizure disorder in other family members. Potentially a more severe problem is selection bias. MSAEFI receives reports on only a nonrandom sample of all adverse events, which may not represent the entire population. Finally, no attempts are made to verify the seizure histories with health care providers.

A similar analysis was performed for persons reporting neurologic adverse events and convulsions after receipt of measles vaccines. Only those persons who reported events after immunization with a measles-containing vaccine alone (MMR, MR, or single-antigen measles) were included. All persons who received multiple vaccines or reported onset of the adverse event before day 5 after immunization were excluded.

Over the eight-year period from 1979 to 1986, 222 neurologic events and 766 nonneurologic events were reported to MSAEFI following immunization with a measles-containing vaccine (Table 3). Over 85% of these neurologic events were febrile convulsions. The difference in response rates to the personal history of convulsions question between persons with and without neurologic adverse events, although not significant, was of the same order of magnitude as with DTP. Persons reporting a neurologic adverse event following a measles-containing vaccine were 5.2 times more likely to have a personal history of convulsions than those with a nonneurologic event. Persons reporting febrile convulsions were 5.6 times as likely to have a prior history of convulsions. There were insufficient data reported to make any assessment of risk of nonfebrile convulsions or more severe neurologic events.

In 1985–86, 34% of responders reporting neurologic events and 37% of

Table 3. Personal History of Convulsions, by Adverse Event Type: Measles-Containing Vaccine, 1979–1986

	Total Reports	Total Responders	Percent Responders	Percent Positive Response
Neurologic adverse events	222	186	84	13
Febrile seizures	192	167	87	14
Nonneurologic events	766	616	80	3

Note: Odds ratio (95% confidence interval): neurologic/nonneurologic, 5.2 (2.8–9.4); febrile seizures/nonneurologic, 5.6 (3.1–10.1).

persons with febrile convulsions had a history of convulsions in first-degree relatives (Table 4). Only 3% of responders with nonneurologic events had such a history, compared to an expected proportion of 5–7%.[12] While the risk of seizures is apparently greater in persons with a family history of seizures than those without this history, more data are needed to document the degree of risk in these persons.

In evaluating these data, the ACIP considered the risk of acquisition of natural measles among nonvaccinated persons, the generally benign outcome of febrile seizures (essentially all of the seizures after measles vaccine) and the effect on measles vaccine coverage of not immunizing persons with a personal or family history of convulsions. The committee concluded that the benefits of measles vaccination in these persons outweigh the increased risk of convulsions.[9] These persons should continue to be immunized with measles vaccine in a manner similar to children without such histories.

In summary, the ACIP continues to recommend that DTP be deferred at least temporarily in infants with a personal history of seizures and that a family history of convulsions not contraindicate DTP vaccination. For measles vaccine, the ACIP believes that neither a personal nor a family history of seizures is a contraindication to measles immunization.

Monitoring of adverse events following immunization is central to the ongoing assessment of the costs and benefits of vaccination.[3,10] Analysis of the data collected by MSAEFI can provide valuable information for those involved in establishing vaccination recommendations, such as the ACIP and the American Academy of Pediatrics, but limitations of these data and their applicability to public policy must be recognized. In the future, we will continue to utilize MSAEFI data and to examine alternate data sources to provide accurate and timely analyses of the risk and occurrence of adverse events following immunization for use in determining immunization recommendations for the United States.

Table 4. Family History of Convulsions, by Adverse Event Type: Measles-Containing Vaccine, 1985–1986

	Total Reports	Total Responders	Percent Responders	Percent Positive Response
Neurologic adverse events	85	71	84	34
Febrile seizures	71	62	87	37
Nonneurologic events	287	175	85	3

Note: Odds ratio (95% confidence interval): neurologic/nonneurologic, 14.4 (6.3–32.6); febrile seizures/nonneurologic, 16.6 (7.3–37.7).

REFERENCES

1. Schonberger LB, Bregman DJ, Sullivan-Bolyai JZ, et al: Guillain-Barré syndrome following vaccination in the national influenza immunization program, United States, 1976–1977. *Am J Epidemiol* 1979;110:105–123.
2. *Adverse Events Following Immunization,* surveillance report no. 1, 1979–1982. Atlanta, Centers for Disease Control, August 1984.
3. Stetler HC, Mullen JR, Brennan JP, et al: Monitoring system for adverse events following immunization. *Vaccine* 1987;5:169–174.
4. Immunization Practices Advisory Committee: Supplementary statement on contraindications to receipt of pertussis vaccine. *MMWR* 1984;33:169–171.
5. Immunization Practices Advisory Committee: Diphtheria, tetanus and pertussis: Guidelines for vaccine prophylaxis and other preventive measures. *MMWR* 1985;34:405–414,419–426.
6. Stetler HC, Orenstein WA, Bart KJ, et al: History of convulsions and use of pertussis vaccine. *J Pediatr* 1985;107:175–179.
7. Committee on Infectious Diseases of the American Academy of Pediatrics: *Report of the Committee on Infectious Diseases,* ed 20. Elk Grove Village, Illinois, American Academy of Pediatrics, 1986.
8. Immunization Practices Advisory Committee: Pertussis immunization: Family history of convulsions and use of antipyretics—supplementary ACIP statement. *MMWR* 1987;36:281–282.
9. Immunization Practices Advisory Committee: Measles prevention. *MMWR* 1987;36:409–418,423–425.
10. *Adverse Events Following Immunization,* surveillance report no. 2, 1982–1984. Atlanta, Centers for Disease Control, December 1986.
11. Nelson KB, Ellenberg JH: Prognosis in children with febrile seizures. *Pediatrics* 1978;61:720–727.
12. van den Berg BJ, Yerushalmy J: Studies on convulsive disorders in young children. *Pediatr Res* 1969;3:298–304.
13. Prensky AL: History of convulsions and use of pertussis vaccine. *J Pediatr* 1985:107:244–245.

10. *Application of a New Method for Adverse Experience Monitoring to Premarketing Studies on Two New Drugs: Some Experiences*

MARI-ANN WALLANDER
PER LUNDBORG

INTRODUCTION

Over the past 15 years the patient books—known as case record forms (CRFs)—used in clinical trials have become increasingly standardized to facilitate comparisons of results from different trials and to allow for computerized data handling. The CRFs register patient history, physical examination data, medications taken, effect variables, laboratory values, and adverse experiences at each or every second visit to the doctor.

When analyzing data from a clinical trial, the conventional method has been to treat effect variables and adverse experiences in a similar way. Thus, the total number of adverse experiences noted in the adverse experience (AE) form at each visit has been calculated and compared to corresponding figures for the reference drug(s) or placebo. In our view, this course of action does not give a true picture of the adverse experience profile of a drug.

Depending on many factors (e.g., the design of the CRF, the instructions to the investigator, and the underlying disease of the patient), an extensive amount of information on adverse experiences is noted not on the AE form but elsewhere in the CRF. By restricting analysis to the AE forms, as is the conventional method, valuable information is not taken into consideration when assessing the safety of a drug. Furthermore, although adverse experiences are measured at predetermined visits either by active questioning using a checklist or by spontaneous reporting, it should be noted that, regardless of method used, the recorded adverse experience is not directly related to a particular visit as is the value of an effect variable.

For instance, nausea is reported by patient NN at visits three and four during a clinical trial. This does not necessarily mean that patient NN was affected by nausea when he saw his doctor at visits three and four, respectively, but could just as well mean he had suffered from nausea for a very long period or that he had had a few attacks of nausea which passed very quickly. It is obvious that to get a clear picture of the patient's adverse experience, we have to look at it in relation to the total study period. Thus, the final adverse experience stored for this patient must be a judged summary of information noted at one or several visits. In most registers for clinical trial data, the nausea reported by patient NN would have been stored twice, once for visit three and once for visit four. We believe that this reaction should only be stored once, together with the necessary information on duration, outcome, and so on.

Differences Between Effect Variables and Adverse Experiences

A prerequisite for an effect variable is the existence of a measurable condition, e.g., blood pressure, heart rate, or ulcer size, in *all* patients taking part in the clinical trial. In general, such variables are measured either on predetermined occasions or continuously, as with angina attacks, during a given period of time by means of diary cards.

In adverse experience monitoring, we are interested not only in adverse experiences that are foreseeable and thereby measurable in a way similar to the effects of a drug, but also in those that are unknown to us. If it were possible to define as variables all symptoms/conditions that may occur, and if those were sure to be measurable at the time of the visit to the doctor, we would not need any specific technique to monitor adverse reactions to a drug.

However, we will never have a complete knowledge of what we seek, and therefore we must handle adverse experience monitoring differently from effect monitoring. When analyzing results from clinical trials, adverse experiences and effect variables should be treated differently due to the fact that the number of patients included in each separate trial is sufficient to calculate the effect of a drug, while a much greater number of patients is needed to evaluate the adverse effect profile of a drug.

Effect variables are visit-related, whereas adverse experiences are not. Thus, effect variables and adverse experiences demand different storing structures, i.e., different registers. Another reason for this is that the need for pooling adverse experiences from different trials is greater than the need for pooling effect variables.

It is also important to be able to assess adverse experiences continuously while a study is ongoing without destroying the blindness of it for the physician or the monitor. Thus, all data on adverse experiences should, in our belief, be handled by a staff separate from the monitoring of the trial.

The philosophy of computing at Hässle has previously been described[1] as well as the structure of our previous storing system for adverse experiences.[2] Five years ago, when we were just about to start the clinical program for some new chemical entities in our company, we were fully aware of the fact that careful documentation of drug safety is as important as the documentation of drug efficacy.

To overcome some of the difficulties above, our organization took the following steps:

1. formation of an adverse drug event (ADE) group with full responsibility for the handling of adverse experiences
2. standardization of data handling and reporting
3. standardization of terminologies used in adverse experience monitoring during clinical trials

Formation of an ADE Group with Full Responsibility for the Handling of Adverse Experiences and Standardization of Data Handling and Reporting

Within the clinical plan for a new drug project, studies are performed in a number of different countries. In order to enable an analysis of adverse experiences by the standards we have set, it is essential that all CRFs from these studies are reviewed by the ADE group in the parent company. This group is independent from the medical department and reports directly to the research director of our company.

Specially trained personnel, who deal with one single product at a time, scrutinize the complete CRFs for adverse experiences or symptoms that have occurred during the clinical trial. This means that not only the adverse experiences mentioned in the AE form are included in the analyses but also symptoms or signs noted elsewhere in the CRFs, e.g., in the forms for patient history, concurrent medication, and so on. This procedure requires an act of judgment and necessitates a highly specialized staff. Needless to say, the study code for the individual patient is not broken until the symptom is entered into the data base after classification and coding. Because completed CRFs are continuously sent to the parent company, one need not await completion of the study before entering data into the adverse experience data base. This enables interim analyses of the safety of the trial program.

To ensure the blindness of the studies, data on adverse experiences are stored in a data base separate from the clinical data base in the company. The accessibility and the structure of this adverse experience data base is different from the clinical data base. Only those few people working with a specific product in the ADE group can access and analyze the AE data on that product. The ADE group is responsible for the production of reports, tables, summaries, and analyses needed for the development and safety assessment of the drug. The data base is structured to allow analyses of single studies as well as various analyses of pooled data.

Standardization of Terminologies

Standardization of drug and adverse experience terminologies has been developed in collaboration with the other two product companies within the Astra group in Sweden. Standardized terminologies were previously used only for adverse experiences reported to marketed drugs, but today they are used also for clinical trial data. To ensure a high degree of consistency, all coding of adverse experiences is performed by the ADE group.

RESULTS

To serve as examples of this alternative handling of adverse experiences, we will report some results from phase II/phase III clinical programs with two new chemical entities, omeprazol and felodipine. They are briefly described below.

Omeprazol is a substituted benzimidiazole that suppresses gastric acid secretion by inhibiting the proton pump (H^+, K^+ -ATPase) located in the secretory membrane of the parietal cell. In the phase I program, the drug was found to cause a dose-dependent, long-lasting inhibition of gastric secretion, and later the drug was found to be more effective than H_2 blockers in, for example, the rate of healing of duodenal ulcers.

At the start of the clinical program, no pharmacodynamic properties of omeprazol other than effect on gastric secretion had been seen in either animal or human pharmacologic studies. Thus, no adverse symptoms could be predicted. The initial clinical program consists mainly of short-term studies in duodenal ulcer patients and esophageal refluxes. These patient categories have, in general, a variety of different symptoms that can be attributed to their disease, and rapid relief of symptoms generally occurs at this institution of active treatment. Presence or absence of ulcer symptoms are generally used as effect variables in ulcer trials and do not appear on the AE form in the CRF. It is possible that this could prevent the detection of drug-induced symptoms of similar character. Thus, the occurrence of new "ulcer symptoms" or aggravation of previously existing symptoms are stored as adverse experiences in our system.

Felodipine is a calcium antagonist with high selectivity for resistance vessels. Animal studies as well as human pharmacologic studies have shown that the drug is a potent vasodilator. Thus, various symptoms could be predicted at the start of the clinical program, e.g., headache, flushing, tachycardia, and ankle edema attributed to vasodilation.

Although the efficacy of felodipine is often assessed in short-term studies, long-term follow-up studies are common. The drug is mainly used in treating hypertension, in combination with other drugs, beta-blockers and/or diuretics, or as monotherapy. Many of the patients in the trial program have other diseases, and their hypertension has been poorly controlled while on other

Table 1. Totals of Adverse Experience Reports

	Felodipine	Omeprazol
No. of patients	1200	2685
No. of AEs	2041	972
Patients		
AEs	669 (56%)	650 (24%)
serious AEs	44 (3.7%)	39 (<2%)

drugs. Disease-related symptoms are not as frequent in hypertension as in, for example, duodenal ulcer.

The differences between the two drugs in pharmacodynamic properties, indications for treatment, length of treatment/number of visits, as well as dissimilarities in decisions taken by the two project groups, led to some differences in the handling of adverse experiences. Thus, in the omeprazol program only spontaneous reporting of adverse experiences has been used, whereas in the felodipine program both active questioning and spontaneous reporting have occurred. Information on adverse experience reporting is summarized in Tables 1 and 2.

Of 1200 hypertensive patients treated with felodipine, 669 (56%) reported 2041 adverse experiences. Noted on the AE form were 82%, while 18% were noted elsewhere in the CRFs.

Serious adverse experiences (as defined by the FDA) were reported by 44 patients. Only 34% of these were found on the AE form; 66% were in other places on the CRFs. Of 2685 patients treated with omeprazol, 650 patients (24%) reported 972 adverse experiences, of which 73% were noted on the AE form. Serious adverse experiences were reported by <2% of the patients, i.e., 39 patients reported 54 serious adverse experiences. Only 60% of these were on the AE form. Thus, a substantial number of adverse experiences were noted not in the AE forms but elsewhere in the CRFs.

A preliminary analysis indicates that the profile of adverse experiences not noted on AE forms is essentially the same as for the total material. For felodipine, the predicted adverse experiences dominate, namely, symptoms related to its vasodilating properties like headache, flushing, tachycardia, and ankle edema.

For omeprazol, the gastrointestinal drug, most of the spontaneously reported symptoms adhere to the gastrointestinal tract, such as obstipation,

Table 2. Distribution of Adverse Experiences in the Case Record Forms

	No. of AEs	On AE Form (%)	Elsewhere in CRF (%)
Felodipine			
all AEs	2041	82	18
serious AEs	56	34	66
Omeprazol			
all AEs	972	73	27
serious AEs	54	60	40

diarrhea, and flatulence. Most noteworthy is the considerable number of serious events that were not noted on the AE forms, in spite of the fact that the investigators were informed about the procedures required. The most common explanation given by the investigators, when they were contacted for further information, is that they did not consider the event to be related to the drug treatment.

COMMENTS

In our opinion, there are several separate aims that are satisfied with a careful handling of adverse experience information during clinical trials.

1. **A continuous safety assessment during the course of the clinical program.** This aim is achieved through the continuous flow of CRFs to the ADE group at the product company. Interim analyses can be performed at regular intervals, and changes in the adverse experience profiles detected at an early stage. Serious adverse experiences not previously reported by the investigator are identified rapidly and, if necessary, further information requested without delay.
2. **Identification of unusual or unexpected symptoms with possible implications for drug safety.** To detect such symptoms, it is important to have a standardized terminology and a centralized coding of the adverse experiences.
3. **Presentation of relevant adverse experience profiles and subanalyses.** The easiest way to achieve this aim is to use a data base designed to allow calculation of incidence and subanalyses of data with regard to age, sex, concurrent diseases, simultaneous medication, length of treatment, and so on.

Our results indicate that using conventional methods for adverse experience monitoring will omit important information in the safety assessment of a new drug. The steps taken in our organization, which have been discussed above, have led to a considerable improvement in this respect. However, we have also identified some important issues which should be further considered.

1. **Study design**—Studies should be designed not only for the registration of effect variables, but also for an optimal documentation of safety and tolerability.
2. **Case record forms**—The ADE group should be involved in the construction of case record forms.
3. **Clinical monitors**—All clinical monitors should be carefully informed about the aim of adverse experience monitoring.
4. **Investigators**—The investigator and his/her staff should also be thoroughly informed about the aim of adverse experience monitoring. This information must always include definition and handling of serious events.

It is our belief, then, that the knowledge and experience which emanate from daily work on problems in adverse experience assessment should be taken into account when addressing the above issues.

REFERENCES

1. Wallander M-A, Palmer LS: A monitoring system for adverse drug experiences in a pharmaceutical company: The integration of pre- and post-marketing data. *Drug Information J* 1986;20:225–235.
2. Palmer LS: Computing in a pharmaceutical company: Hässle's unconventional approach. *Drug Information J* 1986;20:43–50.

11. *A Nationwide Drug Surveillance Network*

THADDEUS H. GRASELA, JR.

INTRODUCTION

In the early 1960s, widespread use of thalidomide by pregnant women resulted in an epidemic of phocomelia, a previously rare birth defect. Although this problem was mainly centered in Europe, the response to this tragedy was worldwide. In the United States regulatory action was taken in the form of the 1962 Harris-Kefauver amendment to the Federal Pure Food and Drug Act.[1] The amendment established the investigational new drug application (IND) and the three extensive phases of clinical testing designed to provide sufficient evidence of drug safety and efficacy to warrant FDA approval and subsequent release of the drug to the marketplace.

In order to satisfy these regulations and demonstrate drug safety and efficacy, pharmaceutical companies have come to largely rely on randomized clinical trials. Although this methodology has proven to be very effective in demonstrating drug efficacy, the high cost of clinical trials imposes limitations on the scope of these trials, rendering such studies less effective in determining the safety of a new medication.[2]

The consequences of the limitations of the new drug approval process have surfaced in a number of unfortunate and highly publicized cases. Ticrynafen, benoxaprofen, zomepirac, suprofen, and nomifensine successfully completed the new drug approval process, but were subsequently found to produce adverse reactions serious enough to warrant removal from the marketplace. These experiences have fueled initiatives to monitor the clinical experience with a drug in the postmarketing period in an attempt to detect previously unsuspected adverse drug reactions.

The Food and Drug Administration Spontaneous Reporting System,[3] the Boston Collaborative Drug Surveillance Program,[4] and computerized data bases[5,6] are examples of systems that have been developed to address the issue of drug safety and efficacy in patient populations. Although each of these has substantial strengths, there are also significant limitations, and an important need exists for an alternative system capable of performing prospective and targeted surveillance in a variety of clinical settings. This chapter describes the goals, methodology, advantages, and limitations of the Drug Surveillance Network that has been organized to meet this need by The Pharmacoepidemiology Research Center at The State University of New York at Buffalo. In addition, the results of a pilot project performed to assess the feasibility of this approach is provided as an example of the data-generating capabilities of this network.

THE DRUG SURVEILLANCE NETWORK

The limitations inherent in previously attempted approaches to postmarketing surveillance of drugs suggest the need for alternative, innovative approaches to this problem. Ideally, this approach would use trained observers to evaluate patient outcome in a carefully structured manner to facilitate pooling of data. The program would permit rapid response to the identification of a potential problem and support studies of multiple drugs and/or disease states within specific patient populations of interest.

Recognizing the need for such a system and the increasing role of the clinical pharmacist in the Joint Commission for the Accreditation of Hospitals mandated quality assurance program for drug therapy, the Pharmacoepidemiology Research Center has organized a nationwide network of clinical pharmacists to perform postmarketing surveillance of drugs. These pharmacists are actively involved in patient monitoring activities and are able to obtain clinically relevant information regarding patient demographics, drug therapy, and outcome, both beneficial and adverse, for a variety of drugs and/or disease states. The number of individuals involved in the network permits the rapid collection of desired information from large patient populations specifically targeted for surveillance.

Goals and Objectives

The overall goal of this program is to study the acute effects of drugs, both beneficial and adverse, in targeted patient populations by utilizing the drug therapy monitoring activities of clinical pharmacists actively involved in inpatient quality assurance programs.[7] The specific objectives of this program are: (1) to assess the relation between drug exposures and specific clinical and laboratory outcomes, and (2) to investigate and quantitate the risk of previously known or suspected drug-associated events in targeted populations.

Methodology

The approach to postmarketing surveillance to be used by this network is schematically represented in Figure 1. The signal to initiate a surveillance project can arise from the Food and Drug Administration Spontaneous Reporting System, published case reports of adverse drug reactions, preliminary findings from preapproval clinical trials, or from hypotheses generated from the known pharmacologic effects of drugs, such as the precipitation of congestive heart failure from beta-blockers.

The identification of a potential problem prompts the notification of partic-

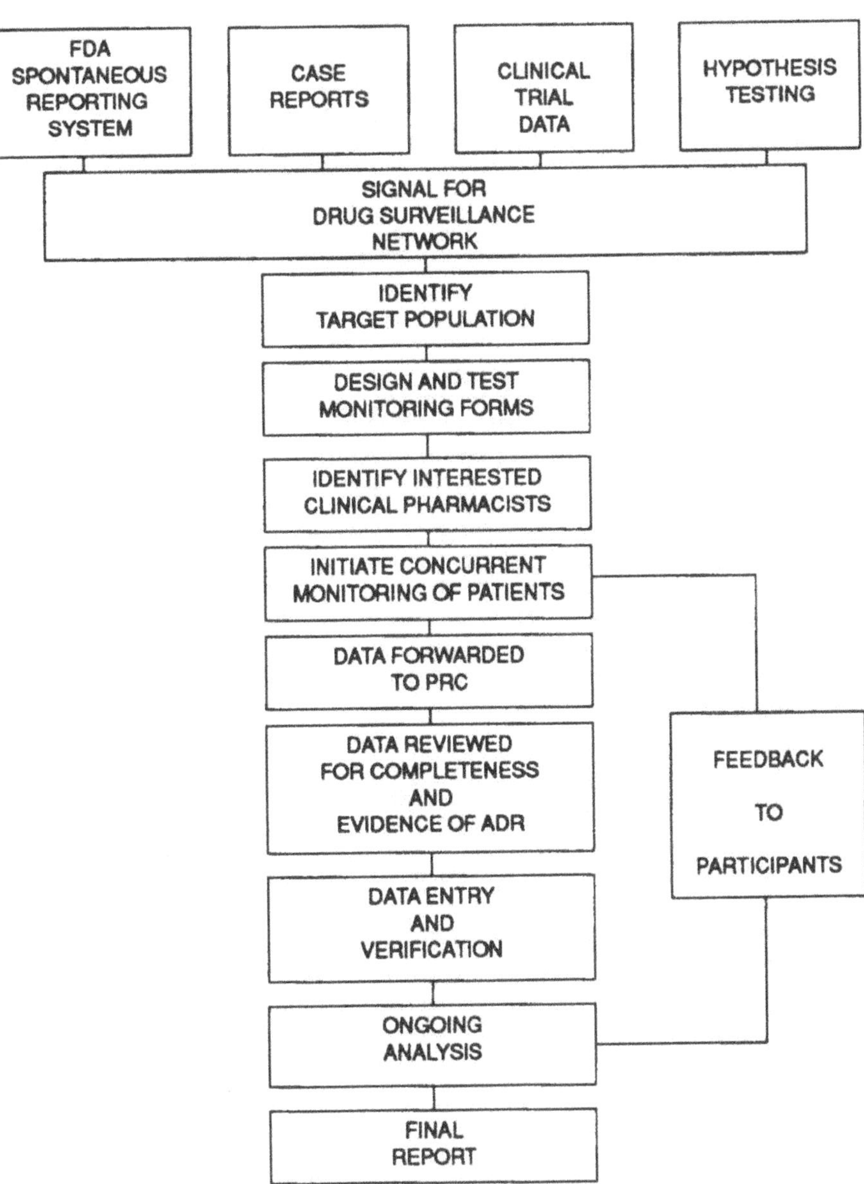

Figure 1. Schematic representation of Drug Surveillance Network operation. Identification of a problem initiates a targeted surveillance program using clinical pharmacists to concurrently evaluate patient outcome. From Grasela TH, Schentag JJ.[7] Reprinted with permission of Harvey Whitney Books.

ipating clinical pharmacists, thus increasing the index of suspicion. Case report forms specifically constructed to query outcomes of interest are developed and tested to ensure validity. The use of these case report forms is a valuable component of this program, since it can be structured to capture the presence or absence of significant positive or negative findings. For example, it is important to determine the frequency of failure to follow serum creatinine concentrations in patients receiving aminoglycosides, since the intensity of testing will affect the incidence of reported nephrotoxicity.

Clinical pharmacists on the Drug Surveillance Network mailing list are sent notification of initiation of a project and invited to participate. Participation in a given project is voluntary and generally based on an individual's interest in the project and ready access to the targeted patient population.

The case report forms are then distributed and used to record observations made as the clinical pharmacist concurrently follows the course of drug therapy in the targeted patients. Completed forms are forwarded to the Pharmacoepidemiology Research Center, where they are immediately reviewed for completeness and evidence of adverse drug reactions. This permits immediate follow-up with the clinical pharmacist who completed the form in order to obtain additional information if necessary. The data are then entered into a data base using a customized dbase III Plus program (Culver City, CA, Ashton-Tate, Inc., 1986), and the accuracy of the entered information is verified. Ongoing analysis of the data base permits early trend analysis with subsequent feedback to participants.

Network Demographics

A recruitment program to enroll clinical pharmacists in the network was initiated in September 1986. Interested individuals were asked to complete a brief questionnaire requesting descriptive information regarding the clinical responsibilities of the practitioner, the clinical practice site, and available resources, e.g., availability of computers and extent of clinical pharmacy services.

As of January 1, 1988, a total of 429 clinical pharmacists from 306 acute care hospitals have enrolled in this program. The participants are distributed across the United States and practice in a variety of clinical settings. Figure 2 is a map of the United States indicating the number of participants in each state. At the present time there is at least one participant in each of the 50 states and several in Canada.

The hospitals involved range in size from 38 beds to more than 1000 beds. Fifty-eight of the 306 hospitals are nonfederal government; 176 are nongovernment, nonprofit; 13 are for profit, 23 are federal government, and 36 are unspecified. The majority of hospitals involved provide general medical and surgical services. Figure 3 is a histogram showing the distribution of hospital bed size in institutions represented on the network as compared to the distribution of all acute care hospitals in the United States.

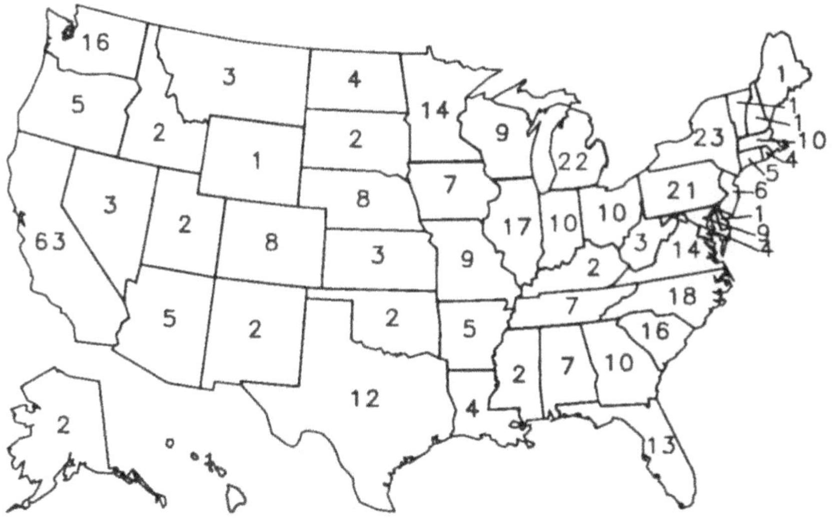

Figure 2. Map of the United States indicating the number of participants in each state. From Grasela TH, Schentag JJ.[7] Reprinted with permission of Harvey Whitney Books.

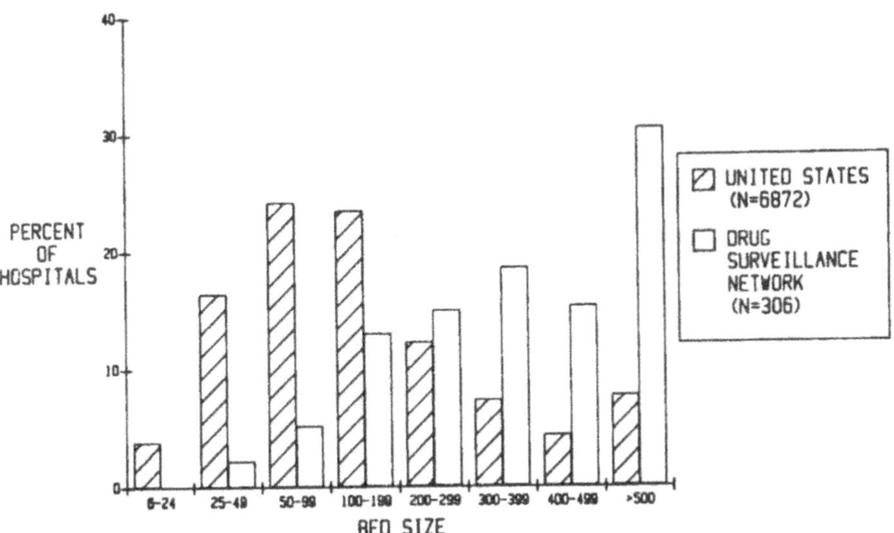

Figure 3. Distribution of hospitals by bed size in 306 institutions represented on the network.

Results of the Pilot Project—A Nationwide Survey of Antibiotic Utilization in Bacterial Infection

To assess the feasibility of this innovative approach to drug surveillance, a pilot project was initiated in February 1987. The two goals of this project were to (1) obtain a cross-sectional view of antibiotic utilization in bacterial infection from a variety of patient care settings, and (2) identify the potential problems inherent to expansion of this network. The results of this study have been recently published, and the following is a summary of the methodology and findings of this project.[8]

Methods

As a broad-based test of the network, participants were requested to concurrently monitor 20 consecutive patients receiving antibiotic therapy for the treatment of a bacterial infection. If possible, the pharmacist was requested to use the entire hospital population as a basis for the survey. Patients receiving antibiotics for antimicrobial prophylaxis prior to surgery were excluded from the survey. No other exclusion criteria were established. Participants entered all data on preprinted forms for subsequent analysis upon completion of the study. For each patient surveyed, information regarding patient demographics, infectious diagnosis, antibiotic therapy, microbiologic response, and clinical outcomes was collected. In addition, the following information was recorded: (1) the date of admission; (2) location of treatment (outpatient versus inpatient); (3) site of infection or reason for initiating antibiotic therapy; (4) source of infection (community acquired, nosocomial, postoperative); and (5) identity of the suspected pathogen if an organism was isolated.

Information extracted for each antibiotic in the treatment regimen included the antibiotic name, dose, dosing interval and total number of doses given, date started, and date stopped for each antibiotic. At the end of antibiotic therapy or 14 days of treatment, whichever came first, the microbiologic and clinical outcomes of therapy were recorded. Each patient was also evaluated for the presence of an adverse drug reaction that was possibly or probably related to the antibiotic regimen. In an attempt to standardize the adverse drug reaction data collected, definitions obtained from *Drug Evaluations* were used regarding the relation to the agent (i.e., possibly or probably related) and reaction severity.[9] Adverse events to any concomitant medication the patient was receiving that was not attributable to the antibiotic regimen were not included. The information collected for patients with an adverse event included a description of the event, the date of onset, severity, action taken to deal with the event, and the resolution, if any.

The completed forms were returned to the Pharmacoepidemiology Research Center, and the data were entered into a data base using a specially developed dBase III Plus program (Culver City, CA, Ashton-Tate, Inc., 1986). Summary and analysis of the data were performed using SPSS (*SPSSX User's Guide*, ed 2. Chicago, SPSS Inc., 1986.)

Results

Network Demographics. One hundred nine clinical pharmacists from 35 states and two from Canada participated in the survey. Information was collected from 100 acute care hospitals and 11 ambulatory care or long-term care facilities. Data were collected from 20 consecutive patients by 91 of the pharmacists and intermittently, as time permitted, by the remaining 20. In the 100 acute care hospitals, the entire hospital was used as a basis for the survey by 71 pharmacists, while 29 pharmacists collected data from selected patient care areas. The hospitals ranged in size from 38 beds to greater than 1000 beds, with the majority of hospitals having between 200 and 500 beds.

Data on the course of therapy of 2310 patients with bacterial infections were collected over approximately a three-month period (February–April 1987). Since the majority of data collected for this survey originated from an inpatient setting, this report will focus on this population. Outpatient data are excluded. Also excluded from this analysis are all antimicrobial courses administered by other than IV, IM, or oral routes of administration.

Patient Demographics. In the population of 2038 patients treated on an inpatient basis and surveyed by the network, 47.9% of the patients were female and 52.1% were male. Seventy-eight percent of the patients were white, 13.6% black, 4.8% Hispanic, 2.5% unknown, and 1.1% Asian. Most patients, 1335 (65.5%), acquired the infection in the community. Nosocomial infections were reported for 703 patients (34.5%). Two-hundred-sixty-four patients (12.9%) developed infections following a surgical procedure. The mean (SD) age for patients with a nosocomial infection was 60.9 (24.4) years, while the mean age for patients with a community-acquired infection was 51.3 (26.9) years. The age ranged from premature infants to approximately 100 years of age for both groups.

Specific sites of infection or reasons for treatment were classified into 11 general categories, including the following types (sites) of infection: pulmonary; genitourinary; skin and soft tissue; abdominal; blood; eyes, ears, nose, and throat; cardiovascular; immunocompromised patients; bone and joint; central nervous system; and miscellaneous. The most common types of infections—pulmonary, genitourinary, skin and soft tissue, and abdominal infection—accounted for 77.2% of the nosocomial infections and 76.2% of the community-acquired infections. Table 1 lists the frequency of sites of infection for patients with nosocomial and community-acquired infections surveyed by this program.

Table 1. Frequency of General Sites of Infection for Nosocomial and Community-Acquired Infections

Site of Infection	Nosocomial Infection Number of Pts (%)	Community-Acquired Infection Number of Pts (%)
Lung	217 (30.9)	469 (35.1)
Genitourinary	192 (27.3)	241 (18.1)
Skin and soft tissue	88 (12.5)	184 (13.8)
Abdomen	46 (6.5)	123 (9.2)
Blood	52 (7.4)	79 (5.9)
Eyes, ears, nose, throat	23 (3.3)	63 (4.7)
Cardiovascular	10 (1.4)	14 (1.1)
Immunocompromised patients	10 (1.4)	27 (2.0)
Bone and joint	7 (1.0)	27 (2.0)
Central nervous system	0 (—)	13 (1.0)
Other	58 (8.3)	95 (7.1)
Total	703 (100)	1335 (100)

Source: Grasela TH, Edwards B, Raebel M, et al.[8] Reprinted with permission of Harvey Whitney Books.

Antibiotic Utilization

The 2038 hospitalized patients surveyed by this project received a total of 58 different antibiotics encompassing almost all of the currently available antibiotics. The antibiotics were classified into 19 general drug categories using the American Hospital Formulary Service Pharmacologic-Therapeutic Classification Scheme.[10] Table 2 lists the frequency of antibiotic use according to general drug category and Table 3 shows the use of specific antibiotics in four selected general drug categories. Single-agent therapy was used to treat 1207 (59.2%) patients, 570 (28.0%) were treated with two antibiotics, and the remaining 261 (12.8%) were treated with a combination of three or more antibiotics.

Duration of Antimicrobial Therapy. The mean (SD) duration of therapy for all nosocomial and community-acquired infections was 7.8 (4.8) and 6.9 (5.0) days, respectively. Table 4 shows the mean (SD) duration of therapy in days for nosocomial and community-acquired infections classified by general site of infection.

Microbiologic Response. The microbiologic response to drug therapy was based on review of cultures as reported in the patient's medical records. An assessment was made as to whether the organism was eradicated or persisted, or a new organism was isolated during treatment. Lack of follow-up was also recorded.

The infecting organism was identified in 914 (44.3%) patients. Three-hundred-eighty-two of these patients had a nosocomial infection and 532 had community-acquired infection. Of the 382 nosocomial infections, the organism was eradicated in 120 patients, it persisted in 55 patients, a new organism was isolated during treatment in 31 patients, and follow-up cultures were not obtained in 164 patients. In the 532 community-acquired infections, the orga-

Table 2. Usage of Antibiotics in Hospitalized Patients, by General Drug Category

Antibiotic Category	Number of Drug Exposures*	Percent	Cumulative Percent
aminoglycosides	610	19.3	19.3
1st-generation cephalosporins	490	15.5	34.8
aminopenicillins	401	12.7	47.5
2nd-generation cephalosporins	323	10.2	57.7
3rd-generation cephalosporins	295	9.4	67.1
antianaerobic antibiotics	170	5.4	72.5
sulfamethoxazole/trimethoprim	165	5.2	77.7
erythromycin	133	4.2	81.9
extended-spectrum penicillins	125	4.0	85.9
vancomycin	108	3.4	89.3
penicillinase-resistant penicillins	104	3.3	92.6
natural penicillins	96	3.1	95.6
tetracyclines	74	2.3	98.0
other	64	2.0	100.0
Total	3158	100.0	100.0

Source: Grasela TH, Edwards B, Raebel M, et al.[8] Reprinted with permission of Harvey Whitney Books.

*More than one antibiotic was given, yielding a column total greater than the number of patients enrolled.

nism was eradicated in 165 patients, it persisted in 57 patients, a new organism was isolated during treatment in 27 patients, and follow-up cultures were not obtained in 265 patients. Most of the patients without follow-up cultures had a satisfactory clinical response, suggesting a good microbiologic response.

Clinical Response. The clinical reactions of the patients, as defined by the outcome of drug therapy, were divided into these nine categories: satisfactory, unsatisfactory, switched to an oral drug and discharged, deceased, greater than two weeks' duration of therapy, discharged on original regimen, regimen adjusted based on bacteriology results, satisfactory response with recurrence, and unspecified.

Overall, a satisfactory response was noted for 61.4% of patients, and 12.6% were switched to an oral drug and discharged from the hospital. If these two groups are combined, an overall satisfactory response was observed in 74% of the patients. An unsatisfactory response requiring a change in drug therapy regimen was reported in 8.5% of patients, and 4.8% expired. Drug therapy was adjusted based on bacteriology results in 1.7% of patients, 1.5% had an initial satisfactory response with subsequent recurrence of the infection, 2.3% of patients were discharged on the original regimen, 4.3% were treated for greater than two weeks, and outcome was indeterminate in 3.0% of patients. Table 5 summarizes the clinical responses noted for nosocomial and community-acquired infections.

Table 3. Frequency of Use of Specific Antibiotics in Hospitalized Patients

General Drug Category	Specific Agent	Frequency	Percent
aminoglycosides	gentamicin	422	69.2
	tobramycin	139	22.8
	amikacin	42	6.9
	netilmicin	5	.8
	other	2	.3
	Total	610	100.0
2nd generation	cefoxitin	129	39.9
	cefuroxime	113	35.0
	cefotetan	34	10.5
	cefaclor	29	9.0
	cefamandole	10	3.1
	cefonicid	8	2.5
	Total	323	100.0
3rd generation	ceftazidime	105	35.6
	cefotaxime	68	23.1
	cefoperazone	52	17.6
	ceftriaxone	50	16.9
	ceftizoxime	20	6.8
	Total	295	100.0
extended-spectrum penicillins	piperacillin	47	37.6
	mezlocillin	41	32.8
	ticarcillin	19	15.2
	Timentin	14	11.2
	carbenicillin	3	2.4
	azlocillin	1	.8
	Total	125	100.0

Source: Grasela TH, Edwards B, Raebel M, et al.[8] Reprinted with permission of Harvey Whitney Books.

Table 4. Comparison of Mean (SD) Duration of Therapy, in Days, for Nosocomial and Community-Acquired General Sites of Infection

General Site	Nosocomial Mean (SD)	Community-Acquired Mean (SD)
Lung	8.1 (4.4)	6.8 (4.4)
Genitourinary	6.9 (3.9)	6.8 (4.3)
Skin and soft tissue	9.5 (7.7)	7.7 (6.8)
Abdomen	8.2 (4.2)	5.7 (3.6)
Blood	6.6 (4.4)	7.6 (4.8)
Eyes, ears, nose, throat	8.8 (3.3)	6.1 (4.4)
Cardiovascular	6.4 (3.4)	13.0 (12.4)
Immunocompromised patients	8.9 (4.7)	6.1 (4.2)
Bone and joint	12.0 (4.4)	7.8 (5.8)
Central nervous system	0 (—)	8.6 (5.3)
Other	6.9 (4.1)	6.6 (5.1)
Overall	7.8 (4.8)	6.9 (5.0)

Source: Grasela TH, Edwards B, Raebel M, et al.[8] Reprinted with permission of Harvey Whitney Books.

Table 5. Clinical Responses for Nosocomial and Community-Acquired Infections

Clinical Outcome	Nosocomial Infection n (%)	Community-Acquired Infection n (%)
Satisfactory	435 (61.9)	748 (56.0)
Unsatisfactory	70 (9.9)	106 (7.9)
Switched to oral drug and discharged	58 (8.2)	279 (20.9)
Deceased	45 (6.4)	64 (4.8)
>14 days of therapy	31 (4.4)	50 (3.7)
Regimen adjusted based on bacteriology results	14 (2.1)	21 (1.6)
Satisfactory response with recurrence	16 (2.3)	13 (1.0)
Other	34 (4.8)	54 (4.1)
Total	703 (100%)	1335 (100%)

Source: Grasela TH, Edwards B, Raebel M, et al.[8] Reprinted with permission of Harvey Whitney Books.

Adverse Drug Reactions. A total of 161 adverse events, possibly or probably related to antimicrobial therapy, were reported in 153 patients for an overall incidence of 7.5%. The majority of these adverse events were minor and consisted of 58 reports of gastrointestinal complaints, (nausea, vomiting, diarrhea), 39 reports of allergic reactions, primarily rashes, and 10 reports of phlebitis, or irritation of the vein at the site of infusion.

Other, more serious, reports of adverse events included 18 cases of increased serum creatinine, primarily in patients receiving aminoglycosides; 12 reports of hematologic toxicity, including eosinophilia, neutropenia, and megaloblastic anemia; 12 cases of superinfection with *Candida* sp.; 5 reports of elevated liver function tests and 3 cases of pseudomembranous colitis documented with isolation of *Clostridium difficile* toxin.

Discussion

The results of this pilot project demonstrate the data collection capabilities of a nationwide network of clinical pharmacists and suggest this network to be a potentially valuable source of clinically relevant drug experience data. Although this was not a true probability sampling of all U.S. hospitals, the variety of hospitals included and the distribution across the country provided a representative sample. It is important to note, however, that the hospitals included in this drug surveillance network have, by definition, an active clinical pharmacy program. The impact of this requirement is the overrepresentation of larger hospitals, which are most likely to support clinical pharmacy services, as seen in Figure 3. Moreover, extensive involvement of the clinical pharmacist can have a marked effect on drug utilization. Thus the results may not be reflective of drug utilization in smaller institutions without clinical pharmacists. Nevertheless, the unrestricted sampling used for this survey allowed the accumulation of data on a wide variety of patients with a broad range of infectious diagnoses and provides an overview of current antibiotic prescribing patterns in typical patients treated under actual clinical conditions.

The major sites of infection for both nosocomial and community-acquired infections involved the lungs, genitourinary tract, skin and soft tissue, and the abdomen. These infections account for over 75% of the infections surveyed by the network and conform to a similar profile demonstrated by previous surveys.[11,12]

The drug utilization data obtained by this survey reveal some important patterns regarding drug therapy selection. As seen in Table 2, the aminoglycosides, first-generation cephalosporins, and the aminopenicillins are the most commonly used antibiotics encountered and represent approximately 50% of antimicrobials used in the surveyed population. The aminoglycosides are frequent choices for treating both nosocomial and community-acquired infections. These drugs are maintaining their usage patterns in 1987, in spite of intensive marketing pressures from competing products. Interestingly, gentamicin continues to be used to a much greater extent than tobramycin, 69.2% versus 22.8%, respectively (see Table 2), in spite of the widely published information suggesting tobramycin is less nephrotoxic than gentamicin.[13] The high cost of tobramycin may be one reason for the disparity of use. Many hospitals have established guidelines for restricting tobramycin usage in patients at high risk for aminoglycoside nephrotoxicity, e.g., elderly patients. We found no difference, however, in the mean (SD) age of patients receiving gentamicin, 54.1 (26.3) years of age, as compared with the mean age of those receiving tobramycin, 52.7 (28.1) years of age.

The combined usage of the second- and third-generation cephalosporins do not equal the usage of first-generation cephalosporins and the aminoglycosides. This perhaps indicates the adherence of many hospitals to use of combination therapy, older antibiotics, or both. Use of imipenem and aztreonam was not encountered in the survey. This is somewhat surprising in view of their broad spectrum of activity. This perhaps suggests a conservative view toward new antibiotics, with continued reliance on the aminoglycosides alone and in combination.

An important trend detected in this survey is a potential decline in the duration of therapy for common infections and an increasingly popular practice of switching a patient to oral therapy and discharging the patient from the hospital. In this survey the average duration of therapy was approximately seven to eight days, regardless of infection site. This is much shorter than the often quoted recommendations to treat infections for 10–14 days.[14] Further, 12.6% of patients were switched to oral therapy and discharged from the hospital. These data must be interpreted carefully, however, since they include both culture-positive and culture-negative patients. Fully 38.4% of culture-positive patients were treated for more than eight days, compared with 21.8% of culture-negative patients (excluding bone/joint infections).

These are important trends that can be expected to continue and perhaps accelerate once the quinolones are introduced into the marketplace. The impact of decreasing length of stay and early discharge on quality of care has been discussed, but the issue remains to be decided. As currently structured, this survey did not involve postdischarge follow-up of patients to determine the eventual outcome. This will be an important factor to measure in future studies.

The major problem encountered in the pilot study concerns the identification of patients and the validity of pooling data collected under various clinical conditions. For 29 of the 100 participating pharmacists who practice in an acute care institution, using the entire hospital as a patient population proved to be difficult. This difficulty was primarily encountered by pharmacists practicing in large (more than 400 beds) hospitals that were not computerized to allow easy identification of patients. This can also be a problem for hospitals with pharmacy computer systems because the system may not provide the necessary information, i.e., a listing of all patients with a specific diagnosis receiving a specific drug or drugs. In these cases, the pharmacist used his/her specific site of practice, frequently primary patient care areas served by a satellite pharmacy, as the basis for the sampling. This remains an important issue to be resolved, since the ability to perform a complete population survey is an important prerequisite for studies aimed at determining the incidence of adverse drug reactions.

The ability to perform population surveys is expected to improve as hospitals continue to computerize all aspects of patient care information management facilitating the identification of patients. In addition, future studies will target a specific disease state or drug for study, and this should simplify identification and recruitment of patients.

Primary consideration in the interpretation of these results is the well-recognized problem of pooling data from patients with a wide range in severity of illness. The surveyed population represents both ambulatory patients with community-acquired infections and severely ill, mechanically ventilated patients with polymicrobial infections. Classifying patients according to severity of illness has been identified as a major problem with the prospective payment system, and a number of rating scales have been prepared to address this issue.[15,16] None of these has achieved widespread acceptance, however, and implementation of a scaling system across the network would be difficult under present conditions. Classification of patients according to severity of illness should become possible as this area of research evolves and hospitals begin widespread implementation of a widely accepted rating scale.

Advantages of the Drug Surveillance Network

The approach to postmarketing surveillance taken by this network is an attempt to develop a system with the strengths of the approaches used previously while avoiding the weaknesses. The use of trained clinical pharmacists to concurrently monitor patient drug therapy, similar to the approach used by the Boston Collaborative Drug Surveillance Program, allows for clarification of the significance of patient signs and symptoms in terms of outcome, and subsequent investigation, when necessary, into the reasons for treatment and patient outcome. Moreover, the observation of patients by someone other than the physician allows for potentially more objective and unbiased assessments.

The number and distribution of clinical pharmacists participating in the network permits the rapid collection of data from a large number of patients all over the United States. The amount of patient data that can be quickly accrued by this network is dependent upon the number of patients with a particular disease or receiving a specific medication(s) of interest and the number of clinical pharmacists interested in participating in a given project. As the number of participants increases, the network will develop the ability to quickly capture information from progressively greater numbers of patients in diverse clinical settings.

The ability to target a specific patient population is an important advantage of the network. By focusing on specific patient populations at risk for an adverse drug reaction, the (presumed) higher incidence of the adverse drug reaction will improve chances for detection. The clinical experience with cimetidine is an excellent example of the advantage of targeted surveillance. During the preapproval clinical trials and the Phase IV surveillance study conducted by Smith Kline and French Laboratories, the incidence of mental confusion was very small.[17] A subsequent case report in *Lancet*[18] prompted Cerra et al and others to investigate this problem further in critically ill patients.[19] The results of these targeted surveillance studies have demonstrated that mild degrees of cimetidine-associated mental confusion occur in 30–60% of patients in the intensive care unit. Clearly the relatively frequent occurrence of confusion in critically ill patients was being diluted by the overwhelming nontoxic experiences with cimetidine in relatively healthy patients.

The studies performed by the Drug Surveillance Network are prospective cohort studies that can potentially be population-based and thus allow the calculation of incidence rates for adverse drug reactions. Moreover, if an appropriate control group is added, this design allows one to calculate the relative risk of developing an adverse event. Prospective cohort studies also permit the comparison of outcomes from different drug treatments for the same disease process. While not as statistically powerful as a randomized clinical trial, a prospective cohort study has a number of important ethical and logistical advantages when one desires to study patients in the clinical setting.

The Role of the Clinical Pharmacist in the Drug Surveillance Network

Over the last decade, the role of the pharmacist has evolved from traditional dispensing functions to a greater emphasis in patient monitoring activities. One clear barometer of the extensive involvement in adverse drug reaction surveillance is the increasing number of adverse drug reactions submitted by pharmacists to the FDA Spontaneous Reporting System. Sills et al recently found that one-third of adverse drug reactions reported directly to the FDA by health care providers were submitted by pharmacists.[3]

Hospital accreditation standards established by the Joint Commission for the Accreditation of Hospitals (JCAH) have been an important influence on the practice of hospital pharmacy. In recent years these standards have expanded and progressed from a drug delivery focus to include more comprehensive requirements regarding the evaluation of quality of care and patient outcome. JCAH has recently adopted regulations that require both the medical staff and the pharmaceutical department to implement a "planned and systematic process for the monitoring and evaluation of the quality and appropriateness of patient care services and for resolving identified problems."[20] These JCAH-required activities, in fact, represent the foundation upon which the Drug Surveillance Network is established.

The incorporation of network projects into the quality assurance programs has a number of important benefits for all parties involved. The development of a well-designed case report form will assist the Department of Pharmacy in satisfying the institution's requirements for quality assurance data. Moreover, by harnessing the drug therapy monitoring activities of clinical pharmacists, data collection for specific projects becomes an extension of daily routine and thus reduces the cost of data collection. In addition, the subsequent use of collected data for internal purposes provides more incentive to ensure data accuracy and reliability.

Obstacles

As with any new and innovative approach to a problem, various obstacles and challenges must be satisfactorily addressed in order to achieve widespread acceptance and implementation. The obstacles facing the drug surveillance network include the following.

Funding

The long-term success of this program requires funding from various sources to support the efforts of the participants and to maintain interest in the network. Funding can come from three major sources – the federal government, the pharmaceutical industry, and philanthropic organizations.

The Food and Drug Administration is acutely aware of the existing limitations on premarketing clinical trials, particularly in regard to drug safety. The FDA continues to seek sources which provide rapidly accessible information regarding the safety of marketed medications. A request for applications recently published in the *Federal Register* details the interest of the FDA in postmarketing surveillance. The Drug Surveillance Network described herein provides many of the characteristics desired by the FDA for a postmarketing surveillance system.[21]

Pharmaceutical manufacturers have an interest in evaluating the comparative performance of a newly marketed medication in terms of both efficacy and safety. This information allows the company to identify a specific clinical situation(s) in which the drug has definite therapeutic advantages. This is a benefit not only to the company but also to the physician and ultimately the patient, since selection and utilization of optimal therapy is a common goal. Moreover, there is a tremendous cost to the pharmaceutical manufacturer, in terms of both dollars and reputation, when a drug must be withdrawn from the market for previously unrecognized adverse drug reactions. An aggressive postmarketing surveillance system that can rapidly identify a problem and the associated risk factors may allow labeling changes that can circumvent the problem, i.e., cautionary statements or recommendations for dosage adjustments in specific patient populations.

Finally, there are a number of national philanthropic organizations that have made a serious long-term commitment to health care information technology, particularly as this affects on national cost-containment and quality of care to special, at-risk patient populations.

Maintaining the Interest and Support of Clinical Pharmacists

The clinical pharmacist involved in patient care is the central figure in this network. In order to sustain the level of interest and enthusiasm demonstrated to date, the projects conducted by the network must be clinically relevant and within the scope of activities performed by the majority of participating pharmacists. Funding must be available to justify the time and effort required, and there must be sufficient recognition for the individuals involved. Procedures have been established to provide public recognition of participation and, when warranted, coauthorship on publications. All individuals who contribute data to a project are acknowledged in the publication. Finally, all participants in the network are encouraged to suggest potential projects for study by the network. Individuals who develop a protocol and case report form for a study that is completed using the network have the option of becoming a primary author on the publication.

Institution Approval

An essential element of this program is institutional approval of network participation by the clinical pharmacists. This includes both administrative approval and Institutional Review Board (IRB) approval when appropriate. Administrative approval is essential since endorsement minimizes intramural political resistance to participation. In addition, the formal request for approval enhances the visibility of the pharmacy department within the institution and allows for recognition of participation in the network.

It is also essential that all participants in a drug surveillance project adhere to federal and local institutional regulations governing the activities of the Drug Surveillance Network. The exclusive focus of this network is the observation and recording of patient outcomes from marketed medications being used for therapeutic purposes. Within this framework two general types of studies may be conducted. In the most commonly performed studies, participation will be limited to abstracting patient medical records, monitoring for drug effects, and recording observations on a monitoring form. These studies are completely naturalistic. Only data generated as part of the routine clinical care of patients are collected, and no attempt is made to alter patient care for the purposes of the Drug Surveillance Project. All decisions regarding drug therapy selection and patient monitoring procedures are made on the basis of the usual medical practice at an institution. In this situation the only risk to the patient is a breach of confidentiality (see section below). Such studies are eligible for expedited review by the IRB and, depending on the institution, may not require signed informed consent. A second, more active, approach to drug surveillance involves the procurement of clinical data, laboratory studies, in particular, which are performed for the purposes of the drug surveillance project and which would not be obtained as part of routine clinical care. In all such cases IRB approval is mandatory, and informed consent must be obtained.

Patient Confidentiality

The maintenance of patient confidentiality is an important consideration whenever data are collected and forwarded to a central processing site. The Pharmacoepidemiology Research Center is aware of its responsibility in this area and has established a mechanism for protecting the privacy of patients enrolled in drug surveillance studies. All studies employ a coding system to mask the identity of the patient and the institution. Each patient is assigned a sequence number upon enrollment into a study, and this number, along with the patient's initials, if permitted, is recorded on the monitoring form. In no case does the patient's name appear on the form. Thus it is not possible for personnel at the Pharmacoepidemiology Research Center to associate a particular case report form with a specific patient at any institution.

Challenges for the Network— A Nationwide Quality Assurance Program

The results of the pilot study performed by 113 members of the Drug Surveillance Network suggest that most, if not all, of the above obstacles can be satisfactorily addressed. The major challenge to the network at this point is to continually improve and document the quality of the information collected. A critical factor in maintaining the scientific integrity of the Drug Surveillance Network is the gradual implementation of a rigorous quality assurance program developed with sensitivity to the voluntary nature of participation. This process will be accomplished, in part, by developing educational programs focused on specific projects, which will provide network participants with insight into the rationale for requesting specific data items. The instructional material can be distributed prior to the initiation of a specific study and allow for participant feedback regarding the nature and significance of a project.

Several additional steps have been taken to improve the quality of the data collected by the network, including (1) careful design of the case report forms, to minimize errors and speed data collection; (2) identification of regional coordinators responsible for assisting in review of case report forms and quality control; (3) development of specific instructions for completion of case report forms and definitions to be used in completing the case report form; and (4) establishment of a toll-free number (1-800-248-4244, 9 A.M.-5 P.M. EST) to facilitate communications with network participants. As the network matures and sophistication of projects increases, a system for performing random comparisons of case report forms and patient charts could be implemented.

SUMMARY

The availability of reliable postmarketing drug utilization information is a high priority of the Food and Drug Administration, pharmaceutical manufacturers, and individual hospitals. Such information is essential for developing guidelines for drug therapy selection, establishing criteria for appropriate use, designing educational programs and marketing strategies, and health care planning purposes. The nationwide Drug Surveillance Network organized by the Pharmacoepidemiology Research Center seeks to provide these data by utilizing the drug monitoring skills of clinical pharmacists to concurrently monitor patients and collect information regarding drug therapy outcome, both beneficial and adverse, in patients receiving a drug under actual clinical conditions.

REFERENCES

1. Ziporyn T: The Food and Drug Administration: How "those regulations" came to be. *JAMA* 1985;254:2037–2046.

2. Temple RJ, Jones JK, Crout JR: Adverse effects of newly marketed drugs. *N Engl J Med* 1979;300:1046–1047.
3. Sills JM, Tanner LA, Milstien JB: Food and Drug Administration monitoring of adverse drug reactions. *Am J Hosp Pharm* 1986;43:2764–2770.
4. Slone D, Jick H, Borda I, et al: Drug surveillance utilizing nurse monitors. *Lancet*. 1966;2:901–903.
5. Jick H, Madsen S, Nudelman PM, et al: Postmarketing follow-up at Group Health Cooperative of Puget Sound. *Pharmacotherapy* 1984;4:99–100.
6. Strom BL, Carsen JL, Morse ML, et al: The computerized on-line medicaid pharmaceutical analysis and surveillance system: A new resource for postmarketing drug surveillance. *Clin Pharmacol Ther* 1985;38: 359–364.
7. Grasela TH, Schentag JJ: A clinical pharmacy oriented drug surveillance network. I. Program description. *Drug Intelligence and Clinical Pharmacy* 1987;21:902–908.
8. Grasela TH, Edwards, B, Raebel M, et al: A clinical pharmacy oriented drug surveillance network. II. Results of a pilot project. *Drug Intelligence and Clinical Pharmacy* 1987;21:909–914.
9. *Drug Evaluations*, ed 6. Chicago, American Medical Association, 1986, pp 31–40.
10. *AHFS Drug Information '87*. American Hospital Formulary Service, American Society of Hospital Pharmacists, Inc., 1987, pp xiv-xvi.
11. Shapiro M, Townsend TR, Rosner B, et al: Use of antimicrobial drugs in general hospitals. II. Analysis of patterns of use. *J Infect Dis* 1979;139: 698–706.
12. Horan TC, White, JW, Jarvis WR, et al: Nosocomial infection surveillance. MMWR 35:1755–2955,1984.
13. Schentag JJ, Plant ME, Cerra FB: Comparative nephrotoxicity of gentamicin and tobramycin: Pharmacokinetics and clinical studies in 201 patients. *Antimicrob Agents Chemother* 1981;19:859–866.
14. Mandell GL, Douglas RG, Bennett JE (eds): *Principles and Practice of Infectious Diseases*, ed 2. New York, John Wiley and Sons, Inc., 1985.
15. Horn SD: Measuring severity of illness: Comparisons across institutions. *Am J Public Health* 1983;73:25–31.
16. Garg, ML, Lorris DZ, Gliebe WA, et al: Evaluating inpatient costs: The staging mechanism. *Med Care* 1978;16:191–201.
17. Gifford LM, Aerigle ME, Myerson RM, et al: Cimetidine Postmarket Outpatient Surveillance Program: Interim Report on Phase 1. *JAMA* 1980;243:1532–1535.
18. Grimson TA: Reactions to cimetidine, letter. *Lancet* 1977;1:858.
19. Cerra FB, Schentag JJ, McMillen M, et al: Mental status, the intensive care unit and cimetidine. *Ann Surg* 1982;196:565–570.
20. *Accreditation Manual for Hospitals*, 1987 ed. Chicago, Joint Commission for the Accreditation of Hospitals, 1987, pp 175–187.
21. Studies of reported adverse effects of marketed drugs. *Federal Register* 1987;52:26086–87.

12. *The Pharmacoepidemiology Data Base of the Brigham and Women's Hospital*

SCOTT STRYKER

The Harvard Medical School Brigham and Women's Pharmacoepidemiology Program has been a collaborative effort to develop a linkage system specifically for use as a pharmacoepidemiology data base. As a hospital-based system it has been designed to incorporate all the data available within the hospital files. The philosophy has been to stress flexibility of data base searches and analyses. Patients can be selected by any set of characteristics, such as a particular combination of diagnoses, drug exposures and lab test results. The data base is designed to make searches and analyses fast. This requires intensive work initially in organization of the different types of data records. The issue of data quality was expected to be a straightforward one, such as recognizing and matching drug names and numeric codes; however, we went through a period of discovery finding out how recorded data could deviate from reality.

This chapter will provide an overview of the information in the data base followed by details of the sources of the data, paying particular attention to the elements of drug exposure, some flaws in the system, and then an example of use of the data base to explore some potential drug interactions.

The greatest effort has been directed toward the development and use of the computerized pharmacy. Primary goals have been to develop an archive that captures the prescription as written by the physician and the details of drug exposure. Drug exposure information currently is based on what is dispensed from the pharmacy. All drug items in the data base are classified by chemical name as well as brand name. They are also coded according to both the National Drug Code (NDC), which identifies a particular product of a manufacturer, and the American Hospital Formulary Service (AHFS), which classifies drugs into therapeutic groups. Drug exposure of patients is retrievable by any of these classifications.

A data base on drug exposure requires detailed information about the individuals in order to be useful in epidemiologic research, especially so, considering the selected nature of drug prescribing. The computerized information on Brigham and Women's patients is extensive. Complete demographic information is captured as the details of hospitalization such as admitting service, payor, and DRG classification. For infants, it includes birth weight, gestational age, and Apgar scores. The results of all laboratory tests also are available. In practice the data base can be searched by any of the patient characteristics. However, not all information has been recorded in detail since 1982. Detailed information on drug exposure such as dates and drug amounts has been available since April 1987. The detailed results of laboratory tests have been recorded since mid-1986.

The kinds of patients and drug exposures in the data base are dependent on the hospital that is the source for patients. The Brigham and Women's Hospital is a 720-bed teaching hospital affiliated with Harvard Medical School. During the past five years, with computerized information, there have been approximately 187,000 admissions. The total population recorded 1.5 million drug exposures, or eight different drugs per person, on average. This figure includes any exposure to a drug during the hospitalization, counting oral and injectable exposures separately. The range in mean number of drug exposures extends from 0.5 for newborns to 16 for patients over 65 years of age.

There are also separate specialized automated data bases maintained within the hospital, including files from surgical and autopsy pathology, microbiology, and obstetrics that can be merged with ours for specific purposes. In addition to the automated data base, complete medical records are available for review.

For some 25% of the Brigham and Women's patients, it is possible to link the inpatient data set to outpatient events and drug prescriptions that precede or follow the hospitalization. The Brigham and Women's Hospital is the principal inpatient facility for the Harvard Community Health Plan, a 250,000-member health maintenance organization that maintains a computerized medical record system. This linkage is a very attractive one for epidemiologic research. It combines the plan's advantage of extended follow-up over time of a large population with the very detailed information such as laboratory results and diagnostic observations that are present in the hospital system. To facilitate such linkages, the data base is designed to allow rapid merging of these data with other pharmacoepidemiology data sets and to allow export of records for populations of interest to other investigators.

The basic information is derived from the on-line data of the hospital's computerized information system, which includes an automated pharmacy and an automated laboratory. Prescriptions are filled daily by pharmacists who use a computer record of the prescription to dispense inventory items of the pharmacy formulary. In most cases, the laboratory devices download the results directly to the computer. Results of laboratory tests performed during an individual's hospitalization are grouped together and archived on computer tape at monthly intervals based on the patient's discharge date. Each laboratory test is captured as a separate record that contains the test name (such as hemoglobin concentration), the test results and comments, the total number of tests, the sequence number (e.g., the fourth hemoglobin), the date, and an indicator if the test result is abnormal or a large change from the previous measured value. The other information on patients is entered directly into the computer records created by the admitting office to which are added discharge, diagnostic, and procedure information by the medical records department. The drug exposure data in complete detail is cumbersome and not directly useful for determining exposure to drugs on a generic basis. Three types of records based on the on-line pharmacy are written to tape each month: a copy of the pharmacy formulary itself, the daily dispensing activity at the formulary item level, and a summary of the patient prescriptions. An additional type of record called the admission drug summary is maintained on the computers on-line.

The admission drug summary is a compilation of drug exposure by chemical name and the basic route of administration during the patient's hospitalization. The chemical or generic name is the drug name that the pharmacoepidemiology unit maintains. The pharmacists preferred different sets of names, such as generic fiorinal or triple sulfa, to assist them in dispensing. Similarly, the "rollup route" was created to classify drugs as oral, injectable, topical, etc., as the pharmacy had an extraordinary range of routes of administration.

Each prescription is summarized as a single record. This includes information taken directly from the physician's orders and additional information taken from the on-line formulary based on the formulary inventory item used to fill the prescription. We record what the physician orders. These orders can be highly complex, such as a sliding scale for insulin given subcutaneously.

The rest of the prescription is derived from the dispensing data of the automated pharmacy. This includes the chemical name, rollup route, and other items, as described for the admission drug summary. If only a fraction of the formulary package item was used to make up the prescription, the total amount of drug from the formulary package item is multiplied by that fraction so that the total amount reflects what the patient was intended to receive. For completeness, daily dispensing records are maintained for each formulary item. Even at this level of automation, data integrity is still at risk. There is one known highly automated pharmacy system where pharmacists, instead of making a new prescription on the computer, simply edited old prescriptions. By updating the patients' prescriptions in this manner they wiped out the history of the previous prescriptions.

All the drug exposure data is ultimately derived from the pharmacy formulary—a dictionary of drug items with associated details and classifications. As mentioned, the chemical names and rollup routes are maintained separately to ensure data quality. The formulary dictionary is also copied to tape each month along with the prescription records created from it. This maintains an audit trail and avoids some of the problems resulting from using records created mostly by pharmacists accustomed to systems designed for billing. Pharmacists and accounting personnel take actions to simplify their work. Records of drug charges were found that looked clean but were not consistent over time. In one instance, three different barbiturates were alternated over time for the same use and recorded identically for billing purposes. In another, elderly men, to the best we could discern, were getting charged for contraceptive diaphragms. Apparently the coding scheme for charging the anti-Parkinson drug Sinemet had duplicated the one for a diaphragm. It has taken investigation to discover these lapses in data quality. It has taken persuasion and software modification to try to prevent them.

A few problems with the data on drug exposure are noted here. The automated pharmacy computer system currently serves all patient care areas of the hospital except the operating rooms, the labor and delivery suites, and the department of radiology. The operating rooms will join the computerized pharmacy on October 1, 1987. The timing of drug exposure is dependent on drug dispensing and thus may be one day off for some prescriptions. Currently, a simple search by a chemical name does not find the combination drugs. There are a few other areas where the structure of the data was awkward, but we have been able to work around these.

The imperfections of the patient information are largely a result of the limited time patients are hospitalized. This is potentially remedied for patients belonging to the Harvard Community Health Plan.

The organization of the data has been most difficult. However, the compensation for the overhead in maintenance is the ease and speed of analysis. In short order, the patients can be selected by any number of criteria, and records exported to statistical software.

An example illustrating use of the data base is a preliminary study of the theophylline levels. For inpatients and outpatients, theophylline is commonly prescribed with other agents. Theophylline has a relatively narrow therapeutic range and toxicity is a potentially dangerous event. If physicians are unaware of the potential for interactions with specific agents, they may coadminister drugs without dosage adjustment, leading to theophylline toxicity. This has public health implications, particularly since on an outpatient basis physicians may add a drug to a patient's maintenance theophylline therapy without measuring levels. In the hospital, levels are usually measured. Because levels are directly related to toxicity, a study of theophylline levels has direct clinical usefulness.

Prescription information for theophylline products lists a number of drug interactions leading to increased levels. Specific drugs mentioned include cimetidine but none of the calcium channel blockers. In light of cimetidine's effect on serum concentration of theophylline there has been debate about whether ranitidine causes an increase. Several case reports suggest an increase in theophylline levels after nifedipine exposure. One report associated verapamil, another calcium blocker, with increased serum theophylline concentrations. There have been no reports about diltiazem, yet another calcium channel blocker.

Goals of the theophylline study are as follows: (1) to evaluate drugs for interactions with theophylline, (2) to determine frequency of toxic levels, (3) to estimate differences in levels that may be due to drug interactions, and (4) to estimate the increased risk of toxic levels from drug exposure.

Between May 1986 and June 1987, we identified 1347 patients who were prescribed theophylline. Of these, 724 were prescribed injectable medications. Patients under the age of 18 years were excluded, leaving 547 adults who received intravenous aminophylline. Eighty-three percent had measured plasma theophylline levels. These 454 patients are the basis of the following analyses. Nineteen patients received cimetidine; 136, ranitidine; 43, diltiazem; 64, nifedipine; and 28, verapamil. Median ages were similar for persons exposed to the five different drugs.

The preliminary analysis of theophylline levels was performed using the highest level or peak level measured over each patient's admission. The median number of theophylline concentrations was 6 for cimetidine, diltiazem, and nifedipine, 5 for rantidine, and 9.5 for verapamil. We defined theophylline toxicity as a peak level greater than 20 mcg/mL. The percentage of each group that had a toxic level was 36% for verapamil and 15-21% for the others.

Because we wished to control for potential confounding by age and gender, we used multivariate models in the rest of our analyses. We estimated the relation between peak theophylline level and exposure to one or more of the histamine antagonists or calcium blockers by linear regression modeling. We used the peak theophylline level for each patient as the dependent variable. Independent predictor variables were indicator variables representing exposure to each of the five drugs under study and gender. Age was included as a continuous variable. We had separately determined that diagnosis (represented by 27 DRG strata) was not associated with the occurrence of toxic theophylline levels and so did not include this variable.

This model indicated the average peak theophylline level for verapamil recipients was 2.5 mcg/mL higher than average ($p = 0.03$). Differences for the other four drugs were less than 0.8 mcg/mL and were not significant.

A second analysis was performed using logistic regression to estimate the risk of having a toxic drug level. The odds ratio for verapamil was 2.2 (95% CI = 0.9, 5.2). The odds ratio for nifedipine was 1.2; for diltiazem, 0.6; for cimetidine, 1.1; and for ranitidine, 1.0 (each with wide confidence intervals).

These analyses have some limitations. The timing of administration and the dosage of drugs were not considered because this information has been recorded only since April. At the time of analysis this complete information was available on 121 persons and, when included, did not materially change results.

In this preliminary analysis, the theophylline levels in the toxic range were frequent. The data suggest potentially important increased theophylline levels occur among verapamil recipients. We did not observe increased levels with nifedipine as had been reported, nor was there any support in these data for risk of increased levels with cimetidine or ranitidine. Further analyses will consider the timing of administration and dosing to evaluate possible dose-response relationships. In particular, we will focus on the dosing of theophylline and the calcium channel blockers up to the time that the toxic levels are measured.

The usefulness of this data base is supported by the ease and speed of this demonstration, bringing forth evidence that it is worth looking closer at theophylline levels and calcium channel blockers. The great body of work has been to harness a computerized system and its main users and coax them into recording information in a way useful for quick studies and general epidemiologic research. Since this has largely been accomplished, the data base can be explored for other potential adverse reactions and doing more refined analyses.

13. *Overcoming Limitations of Routine Surveillance of Drug Overdose*

NEWELL E. MCELWEE
JOSEPH C. VELTRI
MARY CATHERINE SCHUMACHER

INTRODUCTION

Drug overdose, either accidental or intentional, is inevitable in today's society and represents a serious public health problem. Yet the problem of drug overdose is studied much less rigorously than drug toxicity at therapeutic dosage levels. For newly marketed drugs, the overdose knowledge base often consists of at most a few isolated case reports and extrapolations from animal studies, usually done with rodents. Clinicians who treat cases of drug overdose may lack information characterizing toxicity at high dosage levels which, at best, results in unnecessary admissions to health care facilities for observation. Conversely, some cases may be discharged too early and later suffer a serious or fatal consequence. Our goal has been to develop a system capable of prospectively monitoring overdoses of specific drugs that will allow us to provide detailed descriptions of the observed effects.

There are several potential sources of data for detailed descriptive studies of drug overdose. Because the effects are usually acute and dose-related and must be described in detail, clinical trials would probably afford the most ideal study design for evaluating the effects of drug overdose. Obvious ethical considerations preclude administering massive doses to human volunteers. Although there may be isolated cases of overdose during clinical trials, human experience with drug overdose must generally come after the drug has been marketed. Postmarketing surveillance techniques tend to focus on events resulting from chronic use at therapeutic dosage levels.[1,2] The information available on drug overdose has come from three primary sources: poison control centers, retrospective reviews of hospital and death certificate records, and isolated case reports. Although each source provides necessary and useful information, they all have limitations.

Poison control centers (PCCs) in the United States have established a

Table 1. Data Routinely Collected by the National Data Collection System

General data	Date and time of call Reason for exposure (accident, intentional, etc.)
Caller characteristics	City and state of caller Site of caller (residence, workplace, etc.)
Patient characteristics	Age and sex Initial symptom assessment Pregnancy status
Exposure characteristics	Substance (up to 2, by product-specific code) Route of exposure Site of exposure (residence, workplace, etc.)
Outcome characteristics	(refer to Table 2)
Management characteristics	Initial management site and referrals for additional evaluation or therapy Up to 40 different therapeutic interventions

national data collection system (NDCS) to report their experiences.[3] This system consists of a large data base of prospectively collected data obtained during routine management of poison cases. PCCs provide consultation to the community and health care professionals regarding initial triage and subsequent management of patients exposed to poisonous agents; approximately 40% of these exposures involve pharmaceutical products. Data are routinely collected on an NDCS medical record form and later transferred to a data collection form which can be optically scanned and recorded on magnetic tape. The limitations of the NDCS, described in detail elsewhere,[4] include potential bias due to voluntary reporting and inability to collect detailed, clinical-trial-type information in a systematic manner. For example, information regarding drug dose and past medical history are not included in the NDCS data base (see Tables 1 and 2). Retrospective reviews of hospital records have described the frequency, type, and outcomes of overdose exposures for particular health care facilities,[5-9] intensive care units[10] and factors related to outcome for specific drugs.[11] Similar studies have been done using death certificates[12] and coroners' cases.[13] The major problem with retrospective studies is that certain information may be missing from the record or inadequately documented. Studies utilizing hospital records to identify cases are often limited to those cases managed at one institution; therefore the number of cases of a particular drug is usually small when compared to the NDCS data base. Drugs infrequently prescribed, especially those recently marketed, may not be detected at all. Reviews of death certificates have used larger populations but provide few clinical details and are restricted to only those cases with a fatal outcome. Case reports of drug overdose provide detailed clinical information but are limited to descriptions of either one or a small number of cases; the frequencies of various clinical findings are not available. None of the available sources of data can provide clinical-trial-type data, e.g., detailed clinical observations based on a structured protocol, along with the capability to monitor infrequently prescribed or newly marketed drugs.

Table 2. National Data Collection System Classification of Medical Outcome

No effect	The patient developed no symptoms as a result of the exposure.
Minor effect	The patient exhibited some symptoms as a result of the exposure but those symptoms were not life-threatening. The symptoms resolved rapidly, usually involved skin or mucous membrane manifestations and the patient returned to a preexposure state of well-being without residual disability or disfigurement. Some examples: mild gastrointestinal symptoms, drowsiness, skin irritation, or first-degree burn.
Moderate effect	The patient exhibited symptoms as a result of the exposure which were more pronounced, more prolonged, or more systemic in nature than minor symptoms. Usually some form of treatment was indicated. Symptoms were not life-threatening and the patient returned to a preexposure state of well-being with no residual disability or disfigurement. Some examples: a corneal abrasion, acid-base disturbance, high fever, disorientation, hypotension that rapidly responds to treatment, and isolated brief seizures that resolve spontaneously or readily respond to treatment.
Major effect	The patient exhibited some symptoms as a result of the exposure. The symptoms were life-threatening or resulted in residual disability or disfigurement.
Unknown, nontoxic exposure	The patient was lost to follow-up; however, in your estimation the exposure was likely to be nontoxic because the agent involved was nontoxic or the degree of the exposure (or route) was insignificant and unlikely to result in toxicity.
Unknown, potentially toxic exposure	The patient was lost to follow-up and in your estimation the exposure was significant and may have resulted in toxic manifestations.
Unrelated effect	The patient exhibited symptoms that were initially thought to be related to a toxic problem; however, the symptoms were ultimately diagnosed as not related to a toxic problem.
Death	The patient died, as a result of the exposure or a direct complication of the exposure, which was unlikely to have occurred had the toxic exposure not preceded the complication.

The objectives of our surveillance system are to:

1. identify cases at the time of exposure and follow them prospectively
2. collect detailed clinical data on each patient in a systematic manner
3. minimize bias in exposure assessment by determining the concentration of drug in the blood for each case
4. correlate dose (blood level) with clinical effects and outcome
5. characterize the drug's toxicity profile in a population of overdose cases

METHODS

Overview

Our plan to develop a surveillance system for drug overdoses started in April 1985 with a pilot study to evaluate the toxicity profile of ibuprofen. Ibuprofen is a nonsteroidal antiinflammatory agent and analgesic which changed in 1984 from prescription to over-the-counter status in the United States. This study utilized the Intermountain Regional Poison Control Center of Salt Lake City,

Utah to extend routine data collection efforts using the NDCS to include more detailed information regarding drug dose, patient outcome, and clinical course. Blood samples were obtained for determination of ibuprofen serum concentrations. The pilot study enlisted 42 of 43 hospital-based emergency departments and all 15 freestanding emergency centers in Utah. The next step was to expand these methods to include a drug overdose surveillance network (DOSNET) of other PCCs which utilize the NDCS. We have recently undertaken a multicenter study to evaluate the effects of phenolpropanolamine overdose. The Intermountain Regional Poison Control Center serves as the coordinating PCC for five other PCCs located in geographically distinct areas. Each PCC has a designated region, e.g., state or metropolitan boundaries, and the total population served by all six PCCs is approximately 16.5 million. Approval was obtained for both the pilot and DOSNET studies from the Institutional Review Board (IRB) at the University of Utah and by the IRBs at participating Utah health care facilities. Other PCCs in the DOSNET obtained IRB approval from their affiliated institutions and from participating health care facilities. Because this study is in progress, only a brief overview of the methods will be reported here.

Study

The pilot study included all patients with a history of accidental or intentional overdose of ibuprofen who were treated in a participating Utah health care facility and who provided a signed informed consent for obtaining blood samples. When the PCC was contacted first, cases were referred to a health care facility if the exposure was intentional or if the history indicated that greater than 100 mg/kg ibuprofen had been ingested. If the patient initially circumvented the PCC and went directly to a health care facility, participating facilities reported qualifying cases to the PCC when they presented. A finder's fee was paid to health care facility personnel for eligible cases. All study patients received standard care for their overdoses.

Data collection included a structured, study-specific data collection form to prompt the poison information specialist for certain information regarding possible toxicity. Specific assessments of the presence, time of onset, and relation to ibuprofen (judged by the poison information specialist) were made for gastrointestinal findings (nausea, vomiting, diarrhea, gastrointestinal pain); central nervous system findings (lethargy, stupor, coma, nystagmus, dizziness); cardiovascular findings (hypotension, bradycardia, tachycardia); dermal findings (rash, itching, hives, angioedema); respiratory findings (dyspnea, chest pain); and other findings such as tinnitus, headache, and loss of color. Also recorded were findings that occurred but were not included in the above assessment, preexisting medical conditions that could account for any of these findings, and laboratory data routinely collected during case management. Data were collected at 0, 1, 4, 8, 12 and 24 hours for hospitalized cases. If the patient was discharged after a short time in the emergency department, telephone follow-up continued at 8- to 12-hour intervals for the first 24 hours. Data collection continued every 24 hours until all symptoms resolved. Additionally, the NDCS data collection form was completed, as it is for all exposure cases reported to the PCC. The NDCS form was used to corroborate data on the study form.

Approximately 7 mL of whole blood was collected in a clot tube from eligible cases as soon as possible after arrival at the health care facilty. A second sample was obtained approximately two hours after the first. In Metropolitan Salt Lake City, health care facilities sent the whole blood to the PCC via a delivery service. The samples were centrifuged and the serum frozen in silanized tubes with Teflon* caps. Health care facilities outside metropolitan Salt Lake City centrifuged the whole blood, transferred the serum to silanized tubes and mailed the samples in preaddressed Styrofoam mailers. All samples were stored frozen and later analyzed by high pressure liquid chromatography at the Center for Human Toxicology, University of Utah.

DOSNET Study

The DOSNET study, presently in progress, expands the methods used in the pilot study to five other PCCs and two other sources of data collection. The health care personnel record objective clinical findings at designated time intervals on a study flow sheet and obtain an electrocardiogram in patients meeting specific criteria. The patients record specific subjective findings on a visual analog scale.

The Intermountain Regional Poison Control Center serves as the coordinator for five other PCCs and has the following responsibilities: liaison among the associate centers and the sponsor; distribution of protocols, data collection instruments, and other materials to the associate PCCs; collection of completed data files and blood samples on all patients and ECGs on cases meeting specific criteria; data entry, maintenance, and analysis; and preparation of the initial draft of the study report. Each associate PCC has a designated associate investigator responsible for on-site training, sample processing and shipment to the Center for Human Toxicology, and overall coordination of the study. Because of the amount and complexity of data collected for each case and our primary objectives for evaluating phenylpropanolamine, e.g., dose-response correlations, we are using only selected health care facilities. The selection of participating health care facilities is based on the ability of their emergency departments to conduct the study, the working relationships between them and the PCC, and their proximity to the PCC. Presently, an investigator is visiting each health care facility to oversee the data collection process.

---

*Registered trademark of E.I. du Pont de Nemours and Company, Inc., Wilmington, Delaware.

Table 3. Outcome of Exposure to Ibuprofen

Outcome*	N	%
No effect	12	14.1
Minor effect	64	75.3
Moderate effect†	5	5.9
Major effect‡	2	2.4
Unknown effect, potentially toxic	1	1.2
Death‡	1	1.2

*See Table 2 for descriptions of outcomes.
†Four of five cases had serum ibuprofen concentrations below 30 mg/L. One patient had an ibuprofen serum concentration of 616 and 252 mg/L at two and four hours, respectively (postingestion). This patient had a two-hour postingestion ETOH level of 95 mg/dL and a four-hour postingestion acetaminophen level of 27 mg/L. He arrived at the health care facility obtunded, was intubated, placed on room air (no ventilator), and extubated after lavage. Over the next six hours his sensorium improved, and he became alert and oriented.
‡Serum ibuprofen concentrations were below 35 mg/L for all three patients. Cause of death was listed on the death certificate as sepsis.

RESULTS

During the 18-month ibuprofen pilot study, 344 patients reported a potentially toxic exposure to ibuprofen, and 329 had complete NDCS records. Of these, 93 patients were treated in a participating health care facility and 89 provided an informed consent. The PCC referred 41 of these patients to a health care facility, and 48 were already in a health care facility. Blood samples were lost, broken, or hemolyzed and unusable on four patients (there were no consistent patterns regarding the cause of unusable samples). This report describes our findings for the remaining 85 patients, who differed on several variables, mostly relating to the severity of ingestion, from the 236 patients with complete records who were treated at home. The average reported amount of ibuprofen ingested was 7.7 times greater in the study group than those cases managed at home (9898 mg vs 1340 mg; $t = 5.6$; $df = 66$; $p < 0.001$) and the median amount was 10 times greater. Intentional exposures were more likely in the study group (67% vs 10%; chi-square = 111.7; $df = 1$; $p < 0.001$) as were the presence of co-ingestants (32% vs 5% with two or more ingestants; chi-square >40; $df = 1$; $p < 0.001$).

The medical outcomes (NDCS classification) of the study group are shown in Table 3. Of note, 76 of 85 patients (89.4%) had an outcome of either no effect or minor effect. Only one of the nine patients with a moderate or greater effect could be linked to ibuprofen based on toxic blood levels. Specific outcomes are shown in Table 4. Gastrointestinal symptoms were more frequently reported than other findings. This assessment was confounded by decontamination procedures, e.g., ipecac, lavage or activated charcoal, and co-ingestants that produce gastrointestinal symptoms, e.g., alcohol. Central nervous system effects comprised the next largest group. This assessment was also confounded by co-ingestants such as alcohol, benzodiazepines, and antidepressants that produce central nervous system depression.

The distribution of initial serum ibuprofen concentrations, i.e., those sam-

Table 4. Type of Symptoms Reported

Type of Symptom	Unrelated* N	Unrelated* %	Related* N	Related* %	Relation Unknown* N	Relation Unknown* %	Total N	Total %
Gastrointestinal	24	11.8	23	11.3	59	29.1	106	52.2
CNS†	17	8.4	11	5.4	32	15.8	60	29.6
CV‡	3	1.5	2	1.0	9	4.4	14	6.9
Dermal	0	—	0	—	1	0.5	1	0.5
Respiratory	2	1.0	0	—	4	2.0	6	3.0
Other	2	1.0	1	0.5	13	6.4	16	7.9
Total	48	23.6	37	18.2	118	58.1	203	100.0

Note: Multiple assessments were made for each category of symptoms, and some cases had more than one symptom per category.
*Assessment by poison information specialist.
†Central nervous system effects.
‡Cardiovascular effects.

ples drawn at the time of admission, were as follows: 1 of 85 (1.2%) was missing; 9 of 85 (10.6%) were negative; 29 of 85 (34.1%) were positive but <50 mg/L; 24 of 85 (28.2%) were between 50 and 100 mg/L; 11 of 85 (12.9%) were between 100 and 200 mg/L; and 11 of 85 (12.9%) were >200 mg/L. Because the time from exposure to initial presentation varied from case to case, we extrapolated the ibuprofen serum concentration versus time plot to time zero for all patients to estimate initial serum concentration with the same frame of reference for all cases. The relation between the estimated initial ibuprofen serum concentration, gastrointestinal and central nervous system findings, and outcome is shown in Table 5. We did a point by serial correlation (continuous variable with a dichotomous variable) of the estimated initial serum ibuprofen concentration of the 85 study patients (83 df) with the presence of any gastrointestinal findings ($r = -0.177$), the presence of any central nervous system findings ($r = 0.176$), the presence of co-ingestants ($r = 0.078$), and whether the patient had a bad outcome, i.e., moderate or worse ($r = 0.087$), and found poor correlations for each. We then tried to control for co-ingestants by correlating the estimated initial ibuprofen concentrations of those 36 study patients who reported ingesting ibuprofen alone (df = 34) with the presence any gastrointestinal findings ($r = -0.023$), the pres-

Table 5. Relation Between Estimated Initial Ibuprofen Serum Concentration at Time Zero, Symptoms, Co-Ingestants, and Outcome

Estimated Initial Serum Level Ibuprofen (mg/L)	N	% Patients with at least 1 GI Sx	% Patients with at least 1 CNS Sx	% Patients with Co-Ingestants	% Patients with Moderate or Worse Outcome
0	15	86.7	53.3	60.0	13.3
0, <10	10	80.0	30.0	40.0	20.0
> 10, <50	11	63.6	45.5	54.5	9.1
> 50, <100	9	100.0	55.6	55.6	22.2
> 100, <200	13	84.6	46.2	61.5	0.0
>200	27	70.4	70.4	66.7	3.7

Table 6. Relation Between Age, Estimated Initial Ibuprofen Serum Concentration at Time Zero, Co-ingestants, and Outcome

Age	N	% with Exposure > 100 mg/L	% Cases with Co-ingestants	% with Moderate or Worse Outcome
Infant < 2 yr	2	50.0	50.0	0.0
Child 2–12 yr.	8	0.0	12.5	0.0
Adolescent 13–17 yr	16	43.8	50.0	0.0
Adult >17 yr	59	50.9	67.8	13.6

ence of any central nervous system findings ($r = 0.055$), and whether the patient had a bad outcome ($r = 0.051$), and again found poor correlations. Fifty of 85 cases had a second serum ibuprofen concentration measured, which allowed calculation of drug clearance from serum. The relation between clearance and estimated initial serum concentration was evaluated. Patients with estimated serum concentrations at time zero >200 mg/L ($n = 24$) had a faster clearance rate than those with estimated concentrations ≤200 mg/L ($n = 26$). (−0.00723 vs −0.00461 mg/L/minute; $t = 3.74$; $p < 0.01$). Evaluation of other cutting points showed less significant differences.

The relation between age and estimated ibuprofen serum concentration at time zero, co-ingestants, and outcome is shown in Table 6. Adults (age >17 years) formed the largest age category, comprising 59 of 85 cases (69.4%), followed by adolescents (age 13 to 17 years), comprising 16 of 85 cases (18.8%). Thus nearly all (88.2%) of the study group was more than 12 years old and all cases with a moderate or worse outcome were more than 17 years old. Of the 10 patients who were less than 13 years old, only one had an estimated serum concentration at time zero which was greater than 100 mg/L and only two had co-ingestants present.

DISCUSSION

We attempted to develop a method for prospectively monitoring drug overdose patients that will have significant advantages over present methods. The pilot study demonstrated that a poison-control-center-based surveillance system for drug overdoses is workable and capable of providing more information than the NDCS. One significant advantage over other methods of overdose surveillance is that exposure assessment is made determining the actual amount of drug in the blood. Our analytical laboratory, the Center for Human Toxicology, is capable of developing drug assays if they are not commonly available. Based on our experience with the pilot study, we believe poison-control-center-based surveillance has the potential to be expanded and refined into a drug overdose surveillance network of PCCs which could serve a larger population base than Utah. The main problems encountered in the pilot study involved improper sample storage by health care facilities (e.g., freezing whole blood before separation, resulting in a hemolyzed sample) before delivery to our facility and evaluating the confounding variables. We developed more explicit protocols for sample processing and have made inclusion criteria more stringent for the DOSNET study. By eliminating subjects with a history of other ingestants, we can more economically deal with these confounders than by controlling for them in the analysis. The expenses associated with this type of study are directly related to the amount and detail of data collected. Thus the cost per case of the DOSNET study is higher than for the pilot study. Compared to other data sources for drug overdose surveillance, this method is more costly than the NDCS and, depending on the study, may be more expensive than retrospective studies. However, in most situations, it is the only method that can provide detailed descriptions of the clinical effects of drug overdose and dose-response correlations.

CONCLUSIONS

A poison-control-center-based drug overdose surveillance system was developed and used to evaluate the toxicity profile of ibuprofen overdose. Ibuprofen was shown to be relatively nontoxic in overdose, even at exposure levels up to 10 times the upper limit of the therapeutic range. The pilot study utilized health care facilities located in the poison control center's service area to aid in identifying eligible cases and to obtain blood samples. We were able to evaluate the correlation between dose (serum concentration) and toxicity, provide frequencies of various outcomes among cases of ibuprofen overdose treated in health care facilities, and provide information regarding drug clearance in overdose. This method appears promising for further development as a drug overdose surveillance network consisting of other poison control centers.

ACKNOWLEDGMENT

We are grateful to David C. Bradford for assistance with data analyses.

REFERENCES

1. Faich GA: *Postmarketing Surveillance of Prescription Drugs: Current Status*. Monograph from the editors of the Clinical Real Life Studies Program, Oct 1986, pp1–12.
2. Wardell WM, Tsianco MC, Anavekar SN, et al: Postmarketing surveillance of new drugs. I. Review of objectives and methodology. *J Clin Pharmacol* 1979;Feb-Mar:85–94.
3. Litovitz TL, Normann SA, Veltri JC: 1985 Annual report of the American

Association of Poison Control Centers National Data Collection System. *Am J Emerg Med* 1986;4:427–458.

4. Veltri JC, McElwee, NE, Schumacher MC: Interpretation and uses of data collected in poison control centers in the U.S. *Med Toxicol* 1987;2:389–397.
5. Fazen LE, Lovejoy FH, Crone RK: Acute poison in a children's hospital: A two-year experience. *Pediatrics* 1986;77:144–151.
6. Ianzito BM: Attempted suicide by drug ingestion. *Dis Nerv Syst* 1970;31:453–458.
7. Smith JP: Drug overdose: Changing concepts for modern drugs. *Southern Med J* 1986;79:1230–1232.
8. Strong JM: Changing trends in drug overdose over a six-year period. *Mil Med* 1984;148:17–20.
9. Whelton A, et al: Acute toxic drug ingestions at the Johns Hopkins Hospital – 1963 through 1970. *Johns Hopkins Med J* 1973;132:157–167.
10. Strom J, Thisted B, Krantz T, et al: Self-poisoning treated in an ICU: Drug pattern, acute mortality and short term survival. *Acta Anaesthesiol Scand* 1986;30:148–153.
11. Greenblatt DJ, Allen MD, Harmatz JS, et al: Overdosage with pentobarbital and secobarbital: Assessment of factors related to outcome. *J Clin Pharmacol* 1979:Nov-Dec;758–768.
12. Callaham M, Kassel D: Epidemiology of fatal tricyclic antidepressant ingestion: Implications for management. *Ann Emerg Med* 1985;14:1-9.
13. Finkle BS, McCloskey KL, Kiplinger GF, et al: A national assessment of propoxyphene in postmortem medicolegal investigation, 1972–1975. *J Foren Sci* 1981;21:706–742.

14. *Current Status of the Saskatchewan Prescription Drug Plan*

WINANNE DOWNEY

The government of Saskatchewan funds a health care system whereby each resident in the province, regardless of his or her ability to pay, is entitled to a broad range of health care services. The government pays for health care on behalf of each resident. Under some programs (e.g., hospital and medical care), the resident has little or no direct cost; for other programs (e.g., the prescription drug plan), the resident is responsible for a portion of the cost.

As a result of these programs, large data bases exist that contain information on outpatient prescription drug use, hospital separations, physician claim data, and cancer cases for a population of about a million people.

One feature that helps make these data bases so valuable for such things as pharmacoepidemiology is the unique identifier assigned to each individual and used by all data bases. Each eligible resident in Saskatchewan is assigned a "Health Services Number." This eight-digit number permits electronic linkage of an individual's records from various data bases. The first six digits of this number designate the family unit; the last two numbers identify the individual within the family unit. Although there are circumstances when an individual's health services number may change (e.g., individual turns 18, marries, divorces, etc.), the newly assigned number can be matched to the old number through a master registry.

The procedures for use of the data maintained by Saskatchewan Health require that a written protocol be submitted. This application for research data must then be approved by each agency whose data are required. For example, if a project requires information on outpatient prescription use and hospitalization, the Prescription Drug Plan and the Hospital Services Plan must each authorize the use of their data. Furthermore, any protocol that requires data from more than one health agency must be reviewed by a committee of Saskatchewan Health research personnel. This committee reviews requests primarily to ensure that confidentiality of user or provider will not be breached. The committee may wish to meet with the researcher to discuss the project; often, however, this is not necessary.

The Saskatchewan Prescription Drug Plan is one of the newest health programs in the system and has been in operation since September 1975. This program operates with a formulary that currently lists over 1700 drug products. These products are estimated to represent about 90% of the prescription drugs dispensed in Saskatchewan.

Up until July of 1987, the Drug Plan provided first-dollar coverage. Eligible residents paid a nominal prescription charge for any drug listed in the Saskatchewan Formulary, and the dispensing pharmacy submitted a claim to the Drug Plan for reimbursement of the balance of the prescription cost. Over 51.5 million prescription claims have been submitted by pharmacies since the Drug Plan began, and these claims form the Drug Plan's data base.

The information in the data base on these claims includes:

- the individual's unique eight-digit health services number
- the identification of the drug dispensed (brand, strength, form)
- quantity of drug dispensed
- date of dispensing
- prescriber identification
- cost information

In an attempt to curb the increasing costs of funding the Drug Plan, on July 1, 1987, the government changed the features of the program from first-dollar coverage to a deductible system. Under the new deductible system, residents are required to pay 100% of their total prescription costs to the pharmacy at time of purchase. Then, once their total costs exceed the deductible level, residents submit claims to the Drug Plan for reimbursement of 80% of the costs in excess of the deductible. (The annual deductible is $50 for a single senior aged 65 or over, $75 for a family with at least one spouse aged 65 or over, and $125 for all other families.)

There are several groups of people exempted from the program change. The two main groups are residents of special-care homes (licensed nursing homes, about 6000 people) and beneficiaries of the Saskatchewan Assistance Plan (social welfare recipients, about 50,000 people). For these residents, pharmacies continue to submit claims directly to the Drug Plan. Consequently, with the exception of identification of the prescriber, the data maintained on those beneficiaries are the same as under the former program.

The data compiled on the majority of the population, however, (i.e., those who submit their own claims) will be on those whose drug costs exceed the deductible and who submit claims for reimbursement; no information will be captured on the drug use of those who do not exceed the deductible and who do not send in their claims.

For those people who do submit claims, the data compiled will be on a *family unit* basis and will include:

- the family's six-digit health services number
- the same drug identification as under the old system (brand, strength, form)

- quantity dispensed
- date dispensed
- cost information

The main impact of these changes on the Drug Plan's data base, then, is that drug use data are not compiled by individual user, and information is not received on "low" drug users, i.e., those whose family drug costs do not exceed their particular deductible.

The limitations of these "new" data for such things as pharmacoepidemiology, postmarketing surveillance, drug use review, and so on are recognized by the Department of Health. Although the department will continue to examine ways to address these limitations, it is not likely that changes in the type of data captured will be made within the current year. In the meantime, however, Saskatchewan Health continues to be interested in enhancing the use of the existing data and working with researchers to achieve that goal.

The economic situation in Saskatchewan that prompted the government to change the Prescription Drug Plan has also necessitated a downsizing of staffing levels. Consequently, this has had an impact on the level of involvement we have been able to provide in this area. Sometimes work on projects takes longer than originally anticipated, or work is rescheduled, or review of and response to inquiries takes longer than optimum. Nevertheless, the Department of Health encourages interested researchers to use Saskatchewan as a resource for research, to submit proposals, and to persevere with us as we attempt to further develop the use of the data maintained by the province.

Effective 1 January 1989, changes were again made to the Drug Plan that restored the usefulness of the data for pharmacoepidemiology in that the data base will contain information comparable to that compiled prior to 1 July 1987. As well, Saskatchewan Health has established a Pharmacoepidemiology Unit to facilitate research using linked data.

15. *Early Experience with the COMPASS Data Base*

JEFFREY L. CARSON

INTRODUCTION

The Computerized On-line Medicaid Pharmaceutical Analysis and Surveillance System (COMPASS) is a data base composed of Medicaid billing data. COMPASS derives its data as a by-product of the Medicaid Management Information System, which is a computerized claims processing and management information program for this large health care system. Over the past 10 years, the Food and Drug Administration has funded the development of COMPASS as a potential data resource for conducting postmarketing drug surveillance studies. Software has been created to store, retrieve, and abstract that fraction of each patient's record that is useful for research. This chapter will briefly review the strengths and weaknesses of the COMPASS data base and describe several of the logistical issues related to performing epidemiologic studies. These comments are based upon five years of experience with the system.

ADVANTAGES OF COMPASS

- Large number of patients
- Relatively inexpensive
- Avoids logistic problems related to performing cohort studies
- No interviewer or recall bias

The principal advantage of COMPASS is the very large population available for study. There are currently 8.9 million patients from 10 states in the data base. To illustrate the large sample size available for study, we identified 88,000 patients during 1980 from two states who were exclusively dispensed one of seven nonsteroidal antiinflammatory drugs (NSAIDS).[1] There were approximately 36,000 patients dispensed ibuprofen, almost 15,000 patients dispensed sulindac, and 10,000 patients dispensed indomethacin. Similarly, there are very large numbers of patients with common diseases. Examples include upper respiratory tract infections, 1.4 million patients; abdominal pain, 700,000 patients; urinary tract infection, 700,000 patients; and pneumonia, diabetes, and asthma, between 150,000 and 500,000 patients.

The second advantage of COMPASS is that it is relatively inexpensive to use because the data are gathered as a by-product of a billing and claims process. Although using the system incurs considerable expense, it costs much less than using traditional epidemiological techniques.

Third, COMPASS has a significant advantage with regard to cohort studies. Cohort studies of adverse drug reactions identify individuals exposed to a drug and follow them forward in time looking for an adverse drug reaction (ADR). The principal disadvantage of this design is that it often requires a large number of patients. Logistically, this is very difficult and the process can be (and traditionally is) very expensive. Consider how difficult it would be to observe 88,000 patients for GI bleeding who were dispensed an NSAID. Since the COMPASS data set already exists, this is not a problem.

Similarly, COMPASS has significant advantages when performing case-control studies. In a case-control study of ADRs, a group of patients with a disease of interest (cases) and a similar group without the disease (controls) are identified and antecedent drug exposure is sought. One potential problem with this type of study is recall bias. This results from patients who developed the ADR remembering antecedent drug exposure better than patients who had not had an ADR. Since information on drug exposure is collected in COMPASS as a by-product of billing data, rather than by interview or medical record review, this is not a problem. A second potential difficulty with case-control studies is the selection of a unbiased control group. Once again, with COMPASS, controls can be chosen as a random sample from the entire healthy population.

DISADVANTAGES OF COMPASS

- Inpatient and over-the-counter drugs not available
- Some confounding variables not available, i.e., smoking, alcohol use
- Time lag before data is entered
- Uncertain generalization
- Uncertain validity of diagnosis data

There are several significant disadvantages that should be considered when using this data base. Information is not available on inpatient drugs or over-the-counter drugs. There is a time lag before data is entered into the system which may delay the study of newly marketed drugs. The generalizability of the results if uncertain, since this data base only includes indigent patients. This could be resolved with the inclusion of non-Medicaid patients. Because of the large sample sizes available, it is often easy to demonstrate statistically significant differences. One must always question, however, if a statistically significant difference is clinically/biologically important. A major limitation is that some important confounding variables are unavailable in the system, such as diet, parity, occupation, and smoking. If these variables are important for a given study, then it should not be performed using COMPASS.

A potentially serious problem is that there may be gaps in patients' eligibility. Thus, it is possible that the absence of a given diagnosis may actually represent an individual's having left the system. This is only a problem, however, in the unexposed or the healthy group because there is no indication that the individual is in the system. For an exposed individual or diseased patient, the drug prescription itself indicates that s/he is in the system. Several techniques have been used to solve this problem. (1) The first is an *admissibility screen* for all individuals. Before and after the study's selected time period, a claim for any medical service is sought. When found, the assumption is then made that the individual is in the system within that time period, and only data on those patients are analyzed. Of course, this is applied to both the cases and the controls in any study. This method has been found to have two problems. First, it creates a study with a sicker control population than normal because medical services are required for entry into the study. Second, the method significantly reduces the sample size available. In one study, this admissibility screen resulted in a reduction of approximately 50% of the sample size. Loss of this number of patients may represent a significant problem for some studies. (2) An alternative approach is to *focus on each prescription* rather than the entire study period. This procedure selects a study time period and looks back in time from the beginning of that period and forward beyond the time period for any claim of service. If a claim for medical service exists both before and after the time period, then the patient is assumed to be in the system during the time of interest. The same procedure is followed in the control patient during the identical time period. If the admission criteria are met for the case and the control, then this study period is examined. If the patient receives a second prescription, the procedure is followed for the second time period. If the admissibility criteria are met for the second prescription, both time periods are examined. If the admissibility criteria are not met for the second time period, then only the first time period is examined. Since more history is available for each study period to ascertain eligibility, there are many fewer patients lost, and this should reduce the bias toward obtaining a sicker population.

The final potential disadvantage of COMPASS is the validity of the diagnosis information in the data base. This is the crucial issue surrounding the future use of this or any other data base used for rigorous research. The Food and Drug Administration has sponsored a validation study of COMPASS which compared COMPASS data to its primary sources: hospitals, physicians, and pharmacy records.[2] Within the preestablished limits, birth date agreed in 94% of the records but could not be determined in 2.5%. Sex agreed with the medical record in 95% and could not be determined in 4%. The date that the drug was dispensed agreed in 97% of patients. However, data regarding medical services were much more questionable. There was no agreement in 28% of the diagnoses. Agreement to three digits of ICD-9-CM code was present in

41%. With less stringent criteria, such as broad diagnostic criteria, there was an additional 16% agreement (57% total). This would include the same body system or type of illness. Within the remaining 43% of patients, 12% of the records had no diagnosis given by the provider, and approximately 3% had multiple diagnoses. Clearly, this study raises important doubts about the validity of the diagnosis data in COMPASS.

This validation study, however, has serious methodologic problems. First, patients were sampled only from urban areas, i.e., Minneapolis and Detroit, and this sample may not be representative of the accuracy in the entire system. Second, only 55% of the physicians participated. Third, and most important, only the primary office records were examined. This is important because 50% of physicians in Michigan and Minnesota have second offices. If one searches for a diagnosis or medical services and does not check all the potential places in which patients may have been seen, it is unreasonable to conclude that the problem is with the data base. Fourth, claims were sampled, not patients. This could result in a patient with a diagnosis of diabetes mellitus on June 1 and a diagnosis of hypertension on June 15 being considered disagreements if the COMPASS data set shows opposite dates. In many situations, this would not be an important error. The FDA study was an investigation of disagreement, using medical records as the *gold* standard. This is not the best method to determine the validity of any system. Criteria should be developed, perhaps based upon the clinical presentation of a patient. This presentation can then be compared with both the providers' records and the COMPASS data base. This is especially important because there is a recent study which compared billing data to the primary records and concluded that the billing data were more accurate than the primary provider's record.[3] Finally, some minor differences resulted in disagreement. The 28% in which there was no agreement included such instances as one patient presenting with melena while the other source recorded the patient having an upper GI bleed with a duodenal ulcer. These diagnoses are very similar. It is not appropriate to consider them as complete disagreements.

Our experience suggests that the data may be sufficiently useful for research. The data has face validity when the profiles of patients are reviewed. The drug utilization program, which Health Information Design uses, has also suggested that the data are valid. This program sends thousands of patient-specific alerts to physicians and pharmacists warning these professionals that a drug is being used incorrectly. These alerts request that the practitioner verify the accuracy of the billing data and, if they agree with the basis of the alert, modify the patient's drug therapy regimen to minimize the risk of possible ADRs. Over 70% of these alerts gain appropriate response, and less than 1% of the responses indicated that the medical event was incorrect. In addition, several studies have been done that have replicated known associations. These include NSAIDS and upper GI bleeding (including dose-response and duration response).[4] NSAIDS, as a class, were demonstrated to be associated with hypersensitivity reactions, and zomepirac was found to be associated with the highest incidence of anaphylaxis among the NSAIDS.[5] Other associations found in COMPASS include oral contraceptives and gall bladder disease, oral contraceptives and thromboembolic disease, ticrynafen and liver disease, phenothiazine and liver disease, and procainamide and neutropenia.

It is also important to consider how an incorrect diagnosis, with its resulting misclassification bias, might affect the results of such a study. With misclassification bias, if the diagnosis inaccuracies are random, the relative risk estimate should tend toward unity. Therefore, positive studies may underestimate the rate of ADRs, but the associations are likely to be correct. Negative studies may not be interpretable in the face of these diagnostic inaccuracies.

The validation study raises very important concerns that must be addressed. Therefore, when using COMPASS or any other Medicaid data set, the investigator must build into each study validation tests. The best method to deal with uncertainty about the diagnosis data is to obtain primary records on a sample of patients. This may be possible in the near future.

CONCLUSIONS

In summary, COMPASS has great potential for providing a population-based, relatively inexpensive data base to conduct studies with very large sample sizes. The ultimate usefulness of this data base, however, lies with the documentation of its validity.

ACKNOWLEDGMENT

This work was supported in part from FDA Grant FD-4-000079-01.

REFERENCES

1. Carson JL, Strom BL, Morse ML, et al: The relative gastrointestinal toxicity of the nonsteroidal anti-inflammatory drugs. *Arch Intern Med* 1987; 147:1054–1059.
2. Lessler JT, Harris BDH: *Medicaid data as a source for post marketing surveillance information: Final report.* Research Triangle Park, NC, Research Triangle Institute, 1984.
3. Studney, DR, Hakstian AR: A comparison of medical records with billing diagnostic information associated with ambulatory medical care. *Am J Public Health* 1981;71:145–149.
4. Carson JL, Strom BL, Morse ML, et al: The association of nonsteroidal anti-inflammatory drugs and upper GI bleeding. *Arch Intern Med* 1987;147:85–88.
5. Strom BL, Carson JL, Morse ML, et al: The effect of indication on hypersensitivity reaction associated with zomepirac sodium and other non-steroidal anti-inflammatory drugs. *Arthritis Rheum* 1987;30:1142–1148.

16. *Postmarketing Surveillance in Tayside: A Further Assessment of Record Linkage Using Five Nonsteroidal Antiinflammatory Drugs*

PAUL H.G. BEARDON
SHEILA V. BROWN
DENIS G. MCDEVITT

INTRODUCTION

The need for comprehensive systems of postmarketing surveillance in the United Kingdom has been reinforced by the report of the adverse reactions working party.[1] The spontaneous reporting system (the yellow card system), although perhaps the most suitable method for detecting rare adverse effects[2], has several limitations. The most important of these is the degree of underreporting[2-5] due to the fact that only 16% of prescribers use the system.[3,4] Also, the system does not allow for the calculation of incidence rates, since only the number of prescriptions dispensed can be determined and not the number of persons receiving a prescription. The data are also uncontrolled, and allowance has to be made for biases, confounding factors, and the absence of formal controls for comparision. Reporting may also be delayed and incomplete.[6] Other methods of postmarketing surveillance have been considered and include monitored release, restricted release,[7,8] recorded release,[9] and *ad hoc* studies, but the cost of these may be too prohibitive to allow long-term follow-up. More recently, prescription event monitoring has been introduced[10] and the feasibility of computerized record linkage in Tayside assessed using cimetidine.[11-16] The role of record linkage in Tayside is being further assessed using nonsteroidal antiinflammatory drugs (NSAIDs) to determine whether adverse drug reactions (ADRs) can be detected and their rate calculated for various age groups and sex. NSAIDs were chosen, since they are widely prescribed (5% of all NHS prescriptions),[17] thus allowing the rapid accumulation of a large cohort over a relatively short time, and they are responsible for 25% of all ADRs reported on yellow cards to the Committee on the Safety of Medicines (CSM);[17] these adverse effects have also been well documented. It should thus be possible to compare the results obtained in this study to those from other studies.

RECORD LINKAGE IN TAYSIDE

All residents in the United Kingdom are required to register with a general medical practitioner, and in Tayside all residents so registered are allocated a unique patient identifier—the community health number (CHNo).[18] This is a 10-digit number where the first six figures indicate age (DDMMYY); the following three figures are sequentially allocated to persons with the same date of birth, with odd numbers representing males and even numbers females; and the final digit is a check digit based on the modulus-11 system.

The community health number is used on all hospital inpatient records, where diagnoses and deaths are coded according to the *International Classification of Diseases* (ninth revision)[19] and operations to the *Classification of Surgical Operations* of the Office of Population Censuses and Surveys.[20] The principal diagnosis, up to five secondary diagnoses, and two surgical operations may be recorded on the form SMR1[21] and subsequently stored on the health board computer. Other data routinely collected and computerized include maternal discharge diagnoses (form SMR2), neonatal discharge diagnoses (form SMR11), child development records, and psychiatric discharge diagnoses (form SMR4). Mortality records are also stored on the health board computer. Tayside was chosen as an ideal area for record linkage studies, since hospital morbidity and mortality data are readily available on computer and the population of approximately 400,000, although not large enough to detect rare adverse events, is sufficient to demonstrate the feasibility of record linkage.

In Scotland, all community prescriptions dispensed by pharmacists are sent, on a monthly basis, to the Prescription Pricing Division in Edinburgh to enable pharmacists to be reimbursed under the National Health Service scheme for the cost of the prescription. After one year, the minimum time that these prescriptions are held, they are sent to the Medicines Evaluation and Monitoring Group. Here prescriptions for the drugs being studied, in this case NSAIDs, are extracted. Five drugs were examined: Osmosin, indomethacin, naproxen, piroxicam, and ibuprofen. No attempt was made to differentiate between formulations (except Osmosin) or amount of drug consumed. The community health numbers were then traced for each name appearing on the prescriptions from a master index and keyed into the health board computer. A control group was selected by matching age (within five years), sex, and

Table 1. Use of Nonsteroidal Antiinflammatory Drugs in Tayside, by Gender

	Males	Females	Total
Osmosin	389	772	1,161
Indomethacin	2,182	2,973	5,155
Naproxen	2,867	5,323	8,184
Piroxicam	1,428	2,999	4,427
Ibuprofen	2,398	4,634	7,032
Total	9,258	16,701	25,959

general practitioner through the computer. The system ensures that drug takers do not appear in the control group.

During a selected time period, the morbidity of the drug takers and controls was retrieved from the computer and compared.

The relative risk for the drug takers was then determined using the Mantel-Haenszel (MH) method[22] and the attributable or excess rate calculated from the difference in event rates (per thousand persons) between the groups; the 95% confidence intervals were also determined.[23]

MORBIDITY PATTERNS

During this study, 25,959 persons received one or more prescriptions for one of the five NSAIDs. In all, there were 16,701 females and 9258 males (ratio 1:8; female-to-male ratio for Tayside = 1:1). Females were thus more likely to receive a prescription for NSAIDs than males. The most frequently prescribed drug was naproxen, followed by ibuprofen, indomethacin, and piroxicam. In all cases, more females received one or more prescriptions compared to males (Table 1). Osmosin was withdrawn from the market during the prescription collection period.

Table 2 shows the number of hospital discharges among NSAID takers and controls. Clearly the NSAID takers enter hospitals more frequently than controls, with female NSAID takers having a higher admission rate than males. Among controls there was no difference in admission rates between males and females.

Table 3 shows the overall morbidity profile of NSAID takers and controls,

Table 2. Hospital Discharges Among Nonsteroidal Antiinflammatory Drug Takers and Controls, per 1000 Persons

	NSAID Takers	Controls	Difference (95% CI)
Persons with one or more discharges	366	256	110 ± 8
Male	355	262	93 ± 8
Female	372	252	120 ± 8
Difference	17	10	27
95% CI	± 12	± 12	± 8

Table 3. Morbidity Profile of Nonsteroidal Antiinflammatory Drug Takers and Controls, per 1000 Persons

Disease Category (ICD code)*	NSAID Takers	Controls	Excess†
Musculoskeletal (710–739)	159	33	126 ± 5
Blood and blood forming system (280–289)	18	8	10 ± 2
Skin and subcutaneous tissue (680–709)	31	21	10 ± 3
Infections (001–139)	11	6	5 ± 2
Digestive system (520–579)	112	77	35 ± 5
Endocrine disorders (240–279)	34	21	13 ± 3
Symptoms, signs, and ill-defined conditions (780–799)	102	71	31 ± 5
Genitourinary system (580–629)	80	59	21 ± 4
Nervous system and sense organs (320–389)	61	47	13 ± 4
Circulatory system (390–459)	215	172	47 ± 7
Respiratory system (460–519)	72	59	13 ± 4
Mental disorders (290–319)	18	18	0

*Discharge diagnoses.
†Includes 95% confidence interval.

and in all cases, except for mental disorders, NSAID takers exhibited a higher morbidity than controls. These differences are statistically significant. In some cases, this was expected, since the drugs are used to treat the disease; for instance, we would expect higher morbidity among NSAID takers in diseases of the musculoskeletal system, since these drugs are used to treat symptoms of these diseases. Similarly, among endocrine disorders the higher morbidity among NSAID takers is due to the treatment of gout.

Of particular concern are adverse effects concerning the gastrointestinal system. Table 4 shows the number of events (ICD 520–579: diseases of the digestive system; and 787: symptoms involving the digestive system) occurring among NSAID takers and controls for both males and females. Among male NSAID takers the attributable or excess risk was 23 per 1000, and among female NSAID takers 47 per 1000. These figures represent relative risks of 1.28 and 1.67, respectively, and are statistically significant. Table 5 shows the event

Table 4. Gastrointestinal Events (ICD 520–579 & 787) Among Males and Females, per 1000 Persons

	Male (n = 9268)	Female (n = 16,701)	Attributable Risk (95% CI)
NSAID takers	114	127	13 ± 8
Controls	91	80	11 ± 7
Attributable risk	23	47	24 ± 4
95% CI	± 9	± 7	
Relative risk	1.28	1.67	2.16*
95% CI	1.16–1.41	1.55–1.79	1.85–2.52

*Relative excess risk between male and female NSAID takers (Mantel-Haenszel method[22]).

Table 5. Gastrointestinal Events (ICD 520–579 and 787), per 1000 Persons, by Age

	-49	50–59	60–69	70–79	80–99
Number	7926	4693	5702	5370	2268
NSAID takers	57	86	120	182	286
Controls	37	62	91	126	175
Attributable risk	20	24	29	56	111
95% CI	±7	±11	±11	±14	±24

Note: Relative risk (Mantel-Haenszel method[22]) 1.54 (1.45–1.63).

Table 6. Gastrointestinal Events (ICD 520–579 and 787), per 1000 Females, by Age

	-49	50–59	60–69	70–79	80–99
Number	4598	2940	3667	3734	1762
NSAID takers	60	79	109	185	295
Controls	35	53	85	107	178
Attributable risk	25	26	24	78	117
95% CI	±9	±13	±14	±16	±28

Note: Relative risk (Mantel-Haenszel method[22]) 1.70 (1.58–1.83).

rates with respect to age. As can be seen, the number of events increases among both NSAID takers and controls with increasing age. At the lower age groups, the difference in event rates between NSAID takers and controls is similar (about 20 per 1000), but this difference increases after the 70–79 age band and is even greater in the 80–99 age band. This effect is more noticeable in females (Table 6) than males (Table 7). It is also possible to compare the relative excess risk between male and female NSAID takers. In this case, this relative excess risk for females compared to males was 2.16 (95% confidence interval 1.85 to 2.52). In other words, females were twice as likely to develop an NSAID-associated gastrointestinal event than males.

LIMITATIONS

Since there is no comprehensive prescribing data base, only the drugs of interest can be studied, and this imposes limitations upon the interpretation of the results. In this case, only five NSAIDs were examined, and it is not known what other drugs were being taken by the NSAID takers or controls. It is also

Table 7. Gastrointestinal Events (ICD 520–579 and 787), per 1000 Males, by Age

	-49	50–59	60–69	70–79	80–99
Number	3328	1753	2035	1636	506
NSAID	52	99	138	178	257
Controls	40	79	100	171	168
Attributable risk	12	20	38	7	89
95% CI	±10	±19	±20	±26	±50

Note: Relative risk (Mantel-Haenszel method[22]) 1.29 (1.17–1.42).

not known whether controls were taking any of the other NSAIDs (approximately 17 at the time of the study), thus it is possible that the number of gastrointestinal events occurring among controls is high. Similarly, the drug histories immediately prior to the prescription collection period are not known, and this would also limit interpretation of the results.

Patient identification also presents problems. Since only 92% of the prescriptions could be allocated a community health number, the remaining unidentified persons receiving prescriptions could appear in the control group because they cannot be excluded.

These problems may be minimized by establishing a prescribing data base where all prescriptions issued in Tayside are stored on a computer together with the patient identifier. To reduce errors in patient identification, this identifier should appear on the prescription. This approach has been investigated using embossed plastic cards carrying patient details.[24] With the advent of a computerized pricing system currently being developed at the Prescription Pricing Division in Edinburgh, it may be possible to develop a prescribing data base incorporating patient details.

SUMMARY

This study shows that among NSAID takers there was an increased degree of morbidity compared to controls. NSAIDs were also associated with a higher rate of gastrointestinal events, which increased in the elderly, particularly females.

Despite the current limitations, record linkage in Tayside is a useful means of postmarketing surveillance, and the ability to detect drug-associated events has been demonstrated. The results are similar to those obtained in other studies, and both the relative and attributable risks can be calculated. Control subjects can be readily identified, allowing the background morbidity rate to be determined. The establishment of a comprehensive prescribing data base would greatly enhance the interpretation of results as well as allow stricter inclusion or exclusion criteria to be applied to both test subjects and controls.

The current study has demonstrated the ability of record linkage in Tayside to detect differences in gastrointestinal event rates between NSAID takers and controls (nontakers).

ACKNOWLEDGMENTS

We gratefully acknowledge the assistance of the Tayside Health Board Computer Consortium for keying-in prescription data, and in particular to P. McInstry and P. Tovey, for retrieving morbidity data. We are indebted to the University of Dundee computing department, in particular D. McDonald, for developing analysis programs. We also thank the Prescription Pricing Division

(Scotland) for providing prescriptions and the clerical staff of MEMO for painstakingly processing the prescriptions. This study was supported by grants form the The Department of Health and Social Security and the Scottish Home and Health Department.

REFERENCES

1. Committee on Safety of Medicines: *Adverse Reactions Working Party Report,* London, Department of Health and Social Security, 1984, part 2.
2. Inman WHW: Post-marketing surveillance of adverse drug reactions in general practice. 1: Search for new methods. *Br Med J* 1981;282: 1131–1132.
3. Speirs CJ, Griffin JP, Weber JCP, et al: Demography of the UK adverse reactions register of spontaneous reports. *Health Trends* 1984;16:49–52.
4. Griffin JP, Weber JCP: Voluntary systems of adverse reaction reporting—part 1. *Adverse Drug Reactions and Acute Poisoning Reviews* 1985;4:213–230.
5. Lumley CE, Walker SR, Hall GC, et al: The under-reporting of adverse drug reactions seen in General Practice. *Pharmaceutic Med* 1986;1:205–212.
6. Mann RD: The yellow card data: The nature and scale of the adverse drug reactions problem, in Mann RD (ed): *Adverse Drug Reactions: The Scale and Nature of the Problem.* Cranforth, Lancashire, United Kingdom, Parthenon Publishing, 1987, pp 5–66.
7. Lawson DH, Henry DA: Monitoring adverse reactions to new drugs: "Restricted release" or "Monitored release"? *Br Med J* 1977;1:691–692.
8. Harcus AW, Ward AE, Smith DW: Methodology of monitored release of a new preparation: buprenorphine. *Br Med J* 1979;2:163–165.
9. Dollery CT, Rawlins MD: Monitoring adverse reactions to drugs. *Br Med J* 1977;1:96–97.
10. Inman WHW: Postmarketing surveillance of adverse drug reactions in general practice. II: Prescription Event Monitoring at the University of Southampton. *Br Med J* 1981;282:1216–1217.
11. Crombie IK, Brown SV, Hamley JG: Postmarketing surveillance by record linkage in Tayside. *Journal of Epidemiology and Community Health* 1984;38(3):226–231.
12. Crombie IK: The role of record linkage in post-marketing drug surveillance. *Br J Clin Pharmac* 1986;22:77S-82S.
13. Crombie IK: Dundee record linkage study, in Walker SR, Goldberg A (eds): *Monitoring for Adverse Drug Reactions.* Lancaster, England, MTP Press, 1984, pp 81–87.
14. Beardon PHG, Brown SV, McDevitt DG: Post-marketing surveillance by record linkage in Tayside: Follow-up morbidity study of cimetidine. *Acta Pharmacologica et Toxicologica* 1986;59(suppl. V):157.
15. McDevitt DG, Beardon PHG, Brown SV: Mortality amongst cimetidine takers: A long-term follow-up study using cimetidine. *Acta Pharmacologica et Toxicologica* 1986;59(suppl V):157.
16. McDevitt DG, Beardon PHG, Brown SV: Record linkage in Tayside: An

assessment of present development, in Mann RD (ed): *Adverse Drug Reactions: The Scale and Nature of the Problem*. Carnforth, Lancashire, United Kingdom, Parthenon Publishing, 1987, pp 107–114.

17. Anon: Non-steroidal anti-inflammatory drugs and serious gastro-intestinal reactions-1. *Br Med J* 1986;292:614.
18. Angus J, Cameron L, Finlayson CF, et al: *The Tayside Master Patient Index*. Dundee, Tayside Health Board, 1978.
19. *International Classification of Diseases*, rev 9. London, World Health Organization, HMSO, 1977, vol 1.
20. *Classification of Surgical Operations*, rev 3. London, Office of Population Censuses and Surveys, 1975.
21. Heasman MA: Scottish hospital in-patient statistics—sources and uses. *Health Bull* (Edin) 1968:26;10–18.
22. Mantel N, Haenszel W: Statistical aspects of the analysis of data from retrospective studies of disease. *Journal of the National Cancer Institute* 1959;22(4):719–748.
23. Wonnacott TH, Wonnacott RJ: *Introductory Statistics*, ed 3. New York, John Wiley and Sons, 1977, p 227.
24. Marshall D, Crombie IK, Beardon PHG, et al: The use of plastic identification cards and hand imprinters in general practice. *Health Bull* (Edin) 1986;44(6):374–379.

SECTION FOUR

Drugs, Populations, and Outcomes: Specific Studies

Introduction

Section Four presents an array of individual studies dealing with specific drugs, populations, and outcomes.

Nonsteroidal antiinflammatory drugs (NSAIDs) are widely marketed in the United States. Drs. Strom and Carson investigated the relative incidence of clinically apparent upper gastrointestinal bleeding by analyzing data from the Computerized On-Line Medicaid Pharmaceutical and Surveillance System (COMPASS). The COMPASS data base is an important resource for Medicaid claims data. This study shows how a historical cohort study can be carefully conducted using these records.

The impact of NSAID use on general GI upset in the elderly was examined by Bigelow and Collins, using Wisconsin Medicaid billing data. The study provides an interesting methodological approach to discerning GI upset by including patients identified by appropriate ICD codes or those receiving histamine antagonists and antacids presumably not prescribed prophylactically.

Dr. David Henry et al. investigated the relationship of NSAIDs and peptic ulcer death in Australia. They present the results of a case-control study. Cases were defined as all patients who died from ulcer complications in Newcastle hospitals between 1980 and 1986. Controls were chosen from peptic ulcer survivors.

Whenever a pharmacoepidemiologic study identifies an apparent drug effect, the investigator must consider whether the effect is due to the underlying condition being treated or the drug (confounding by indication). Dr. Tennis et al. use the Saskatchewan Health automated data files to investigate a possible increased risk of neoplasia with rheumatoid arthritis. Potential confounders considered are disease-modifying drugs (DMARDs), sex, and age.

Acyclovir was marketed in oral formulation in January 1985 for the treatment and suppression of genital herpes. Because of the high exposure potential among women of reproductive age, the manufacturer developed a program to study the drug. Dr. Andrews et al. describe the program, the Acyclovir in Pregnancy Registry, and the joint industry, government, and private sector advisory committee that was established.

Recombinant DNA technology has enabled the production of synthetic human growth hormones, one of which was developed to eliminate the transmission of Creutzfeldt-Jakob disease through pituitary-derived human growth hormone. Dr. Bernad reports on the safety of this synthetic growth hormone.

Without question, the AIDS epidemic has received more publicity and generated more concern by the general public than any other recent public health issue. In March 1987, Retrovir became the first drug approved in the United

States for the treatment of HIV infection. Drs. Joseph and Creagh-Kirk briefly review the epidemiology of AIDS, the innovative open-label trial that was conducted jointly by the Burroughs Wellcome Company and the National Institutes of Health, and describe the Retrovir postmarketing surveillance program.

It has been reported that blacks and whites are prescribed psychotropic medications differently. Dr. Batey et al. investigate this question through a retrospective study of black and white patients admitted to a Southern state mental health facility. Medical charts were reviewed and patients interviewed for sociodemographic data, psychological variables, and medications prescribed during hospitalization. Outpatient drug exposure was determined from medication history completed by the patient during the hospitalization.

Though the elderly utilize a disproportionately high percentage of health care resources, premarketing drug studies generally exclude them because of their multiple diseases and concurrent use of "nonstudy" medications. Dr. Stewart et al. have collected longitudinal information on drug use and health in ambulatory elderly subjects, using the Dunedin health screening program in Florida. Data are presented on frequency of drug use, therapeutic indications, hematological and biochemical test results, and symptoms.

Dr. Chrischilles et al. report on an interesting examination of the impact of psychotropic drug use on mortality in nursing home patients. The investigation was part of the Iowa 65+ Rural Health Study, which is a prospective study of all persons aged 65 years and older residing in two rural Iowa counties. Participants in this survey were residents of one of 11 chronic care facilities.

The last chapter in this section provides an example of research in the important area of measuring the economic impact of drugs. Dr. Eisenberg et al. present an interesting nested case-control study conducted at six Philadelphia hospitals that investigated the cost of nephrotoxicity associated with aminoglycosides.

17. *Nonsteroidal Antiinflammatory Drugs and Upper Gastrointestinal Bleeding*

BRIAN L. STROM
JEFFREY L. CARSON

INTRODUCTION

A number of new nonsteroidal antiinflammatory drugs (NSAIDs) have been marketed in the recent past. The major motivation for the use of these drugs is the known gastrointestinal toxicity of aspirin. From premarketing studies it was known that these drugs, as well, could cause subclinical gastrointestinal bleeding, but there were no controlled studies of the association between NSAIDs and clinically apparent upper gastrointestinal (UGI) bleeding. There also was no information on the relative incidence of UGI bleeding associated with the use of different NSAIDs. This pair of studies was undertaken to address these questions, as well as to test the validity of a new computerized data base for postmarketing drug surveillance.[1,2]

METHODS

Data Source

COMPASS – the Computerized On-line Medicaid Pharmaceutical Analysis and Surveillance System – is a data base composed of Medicaid claims data. Its characteristics, advantages, and disadvantages have been described elsewhere.[3] Data are now available from 11 Medicaid states, totaling over 8 million individuals.

Adapted from: (1) Carson JL, Strom BL, Soper KA, et al: The association of nonsteroidal anti-inflammatory drugs with upper gastrointestinal tract bleeding. *Arch Int Med* 1987;147(1):85-88. (2) Carson JL, Strom BL, Morse ML, et al: The relative gastrointestinal toxicity of the nonsteroidal anti-inflammatory drugs. *Arch Int Med* 1987;147(6):1054-1059.

At the time of these studies, data were available from only the states of Michigan and Minnesota, including 1.2 million patients. Data available for each patient included age; sex; state; inpatient and outpatient diagnoses, recorded using the ninth revision of the *International Classification of Diseases, Clinical Modification* (ICD9-CM)[4]; and outpatient drugs dispensed. Data are now available on race, procedures, and deaths, but were not available at the time these studies were performed. Data on over-the-counter drugs were only available if the drugs were prescribed. During this study, Medicaid regulations in these states generally permitted the dispensing of up to a 30-day supply of a drug at one time, but never more than a 90-day supply at one time.

Design

A retrospective (historical) cohort study was performed. After excluding patients known to have been prescribed aspirin, generally part of combination cold preparations or combination analgesics, there were a total of 100,124 patients exposed to NSAIDs.

For the first part of this study, to ensure that patients included in the study were eligible for Medicaid benefits throughout the study period, an admissibility screen was applied. First, patients were included only if they were exposed to an NSAID between March through August 1980. Second, patients who did not have a claim for some medical service both before March 1980 and after August 1980 were excluded. Exposed patients with a diagnosis of UGI bleeding earlier in 1980 were also excluded. This resulted in 47,136 exposed patients for the study. For each patient exposed to NSAIDs, an unexposed patient was then selected from the same state, who met the same admissibility screen, did not have prior UGI bleeding, and was matched to the exposed subject by sex and age (within 10-year age strata). Matched unexposed patients could be found for 44,634 (95%) of these exposed patients.

For the second part of the study, the entire subset of 100,124 patients was subdivided into mutually exclusive cohorts of patients exposed to one and only one of the seven NSAIDs available; 12,074 patients were thereby excluded.

Analysis

For the first part of this study, the days at risk associated with an NSAID prescription were defined as the 30 days after each prescription was dispensed or until the next NSAID prescription. For unexposed patients, the identical days at risk were used as for the matched exposed patients. Follow-up for each patient ended after a diagnosis of upper GI bleeding during a day at risk or at the end of the observation. The rate of UGI bleeding during a day at risk was compared between the NSAID-exposed and the unexposed groups, and relative risks with 95% confidence intervals were calculated.[5] Similar univariate analyses were performed to determine whether each potential confounding variable was associated with UGI bleeding. The association between NSAIDs and UGI bleeding was then reevaluated using stratification to control for sex, age (as a continuous variable), and each other potential confounder, one at a time.[6] Finally, logistic regression was used to evaluate the effects of NSAIDs on UGI bleeding, adjusting for the joint effects of all the potential confounders.[6]

For the second part of the study, days at risk were calculated as above. A chi-square test was performed to test whether the overall differences observed among the seven drugs were statistically significant. Then pairwise comparisons of each NSAID to ibuprofen were made. Ibuprofen was chosen as a reference drug because it had the largest number of users and so provided the most stable baseline for comparisons. Potential confounding variables were again controlled using logistic regression to control for age, sex, state, and each of the confounding variables separately.

In order to examine duration- and dose-response relationships, a subsampled cohort study was performed. Cases were all subjects with a diagnosis of UGI bleeding during a day at risk. Controls were selected at random from the remaining exposed patients who did not develop UGI bleeding, with two controls per case. In order to examine duration-response, the cases were divided into categories according to the number of prescriptions they received until their diagnosis of UGI bleeding occurred. The observed proportion of days at risk in each category for the cases was compared to the expected proportion of days at risk in each category estimated from the control group. Average daily dose was then calculated as the number of pills dispensed, multiplied by the dose per pill, divided by the number of days between each prescription. These were compared to the maximum recommended daily dose provided in the 1981 *Physicians Desk Reference*.[7] Patients were divided into categories of low, medium, or high average daily dose, with cutoffs for each category selected to result in nearly equal numbers of subjects in each category. The dose-response relationship was then evaluated using the Armitage chi-square test.[8]

RESULTS

Of the 47,136 exposed individuals, 155 developed UGI bleeding within 30 days after each prescription (see Table 1). Of the 44,634 unexposed individuals, 96 developed UGI bleeding. The unadjusted relative risk for developing UGI bleeding in patients exposed to an NSAID was 1.5 (95% confidence interval 1.2–2.0) (Table 1).

Univariate analyses were performed to determine if each potential confounding variable was associated with UGI bleeding (see Table 2). The factors related to UGI bleeding were age (older subjects more than younger subjects, $p < 0.001$), sex, state, alcohol-related diagnoses, anticoagulants, and preexisting abdominal conditions. Use of antacids/H_2 blockers and corticosteroids were not associated with UGI bleeding, although both occurred infre-

Table 1. Association of Exposure to Nonsteroidal Antiinflammatory Drugs with Upper Gastrointestinal Tract Bleeding

	Exposed Patients	Unexposed Patients
No. of patients	47,136	44,634
Patients with upper gastrointestinal tract bleeding	155	96
Rate of upper gastrointestinal tract bleeding per 10,000 persons	33	22
Rate of upper gastrointestinal bleeding per 10,000 person-months*	12.7	8.3
Unadjusted relative risk (95% confidence interval)	1.5 (1.2–2.0)	
Adjusted relative risk† (95% confidence interval	1.5 (1.1–1.9)	

Source: Carson JL, et al.[1]

*The number of person-months was estimated from the cohort of 47,136 exposed patients who passed the eligibility screen. This calculation assumed one month of follow-up (up to a maximum of six months) for each prescription, using the average number of prescriptions per patient.

†Adjusted for all potential confounding variables by logistic regression.[6]

quently. The indication for NSAID use also was not associated with UGI bleeding. Inclusion of each of these variables with NSAIDs, state, age, and sex in a logistic regression model did not result in substantive changes in these estimates.

The risk of UGI bleeding rose with higher doses of NSAIDs, indicating a linear dose-response relationship (see Figure 1). The duration-response analysis revealed a steadily increasing risk for the first through fourth exposures, followed by a steadily decreasing risk, statistically compatible with a quadratic model ($p < 0.001$) (see Figure 2).

A highly significant difference was seen among the rates of the UGI bleeding associated with the use of the different NSAIDs ($p < 0.001$) (see Tables 3 and 4). Interdrug comparisons revealed that only sulindac had an elevated risk when compared with ibuprofen. These results were similar when restricted to patients hospitalized for UGI bleeding. When the average daily dose of sulindac was divided by its maximum recommended dose,[7] it was notably higher than that of the other drugs (sulindac 93%, ibuprofen 71%, fenoprofen 71%, phenylbutazone 65%, naproxen 63%, tolmetin 51%, and indomethacin 49%). The distribution of indications differed among the NSAIDs ($p < 0.001$), with indomethacin and phenylbutazone used preferentially for crystal arthropathy and ibuprofen used preferentially for dysmenorrhea. Using logistic regression to adjust for age, sex, state, and each of the potential confounding variables did not change these relationships.

Examination of the number of prescriptions dispensed for each drug revealed that, on average, more prescriptions were dispensed for sulindac (3.98) and fewer prescriptions were dispensed for phenylbutazone (1.52) than for the other NSAIDs (3.0 to 3.4). The number of prescriptions was an important predictor of UGI bleeding ($p = 0.02$). However, the association between

Table 2. Potential Confounding Variables Evaluated for Their Association with Upper Gastrointestinal Tract Bleeding

Variable	Patients with Variable	Patients with UGI Tract Bleeding	Unadjusted Relative Risk (95% Confidence Interval) *	Adjusted Relative Risk (95% Confidence Interval) †
Sex	15,878	55	1.3 (1.0–1.8)	1.3 (1.0–1.8)
State (Michigan vs Minnesota)	73,062	230	2.8 (1.8–4.4)	3.1 (2.0–4.9)
Alcohol-related diagnoses	1,025	12	4.5 (2.5–8.0)	5.0 (2.5–8.1)
Use of anticoagulants	1,298	9	2.6 (1.3–5.1)	2.8 (1.4–5.6)
Preexisting abdominal conditions	3,873	18	1.8 (1.1–2.8)	1.5 (0.9–2.5)
Antacids/cimetidine	2,560	8	1.1 (0.6–2.3)	1.1 (0.6–2.3)
Corticosteroids	4,265	16	1.4 (0.8–2.3)	1.4 (0.8–2.2)

Source: Carson JL, et al.[1]

* Haldane method.[5]

† Adjusted for exposure to nosteroidal antiinflammatory drugs, age (as a continuous variable), and all other variables in the table by logistic regression.[6]

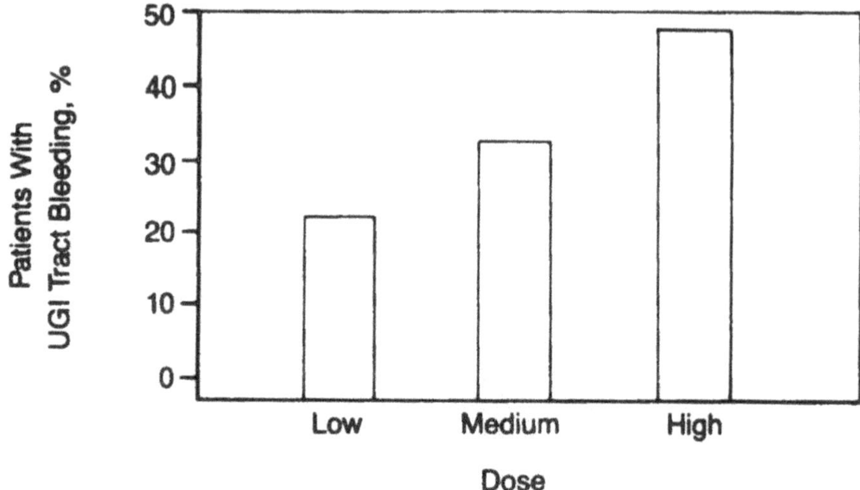

Figure 1. Dose-response relationship between the average daily dose and the risk of UGI bleeding.

the number of prescriptions and UGI tract bleeding was similar for each of the study drugs ($p = 0.94$), and after controlling for the number of prescriptions by logistic regression, differences in the rate of UGI bleeding among users of the drug persisted, although they became less dramatic ($p = 0.075$).

An interaction was observed between use of NSAIDs and the presence of an alcohol-related diagnosis ($p = 0.017$), with the differences among the NSAIDs becoming exaggerated in patients who had alcohol-related diagnoses (see Table 5).

The possibility of selection bias was explored in several ways. First, prior cimetidine and/or antacid use was controlled for as described above. Second, preexisting abdominal conditions were controlled for as described above. In both cases, although the variables were themselves associated with UGI tract bleeding, adjusting for them did not change our results. Third, because many physicians may believe that indomethacin and phenylbutazone are more toxic to the gastrointestinal tract than the newer NSAIDs, these two drugs were excluded. However, differences persisted among the five newer NSAIDs ($p = 0.003$). Fourth, we evaluated 1981 Medilink data for the proportion of new prescriptions for each drug which were due to a change in therapy from some other NSAID. Tolmetin, naproxen, and ibuprofen replaced other NSAIDs more frequently than sulindac (10.4%, 6.5%, 4.2%, and 3.6%, respectively). Phenylbutazone, indomethacin, and fenoprofen replaced other NSAIDs slightly less frequently than sulindac (3.1%, 3.1%, 3.0%, and 3.6%, respectively). Most changes were for perceived lack of efficacy rather than for adverse reactions (average 69%).

Lastly, because it was not an *a priori* hypothesis that sulindac would be

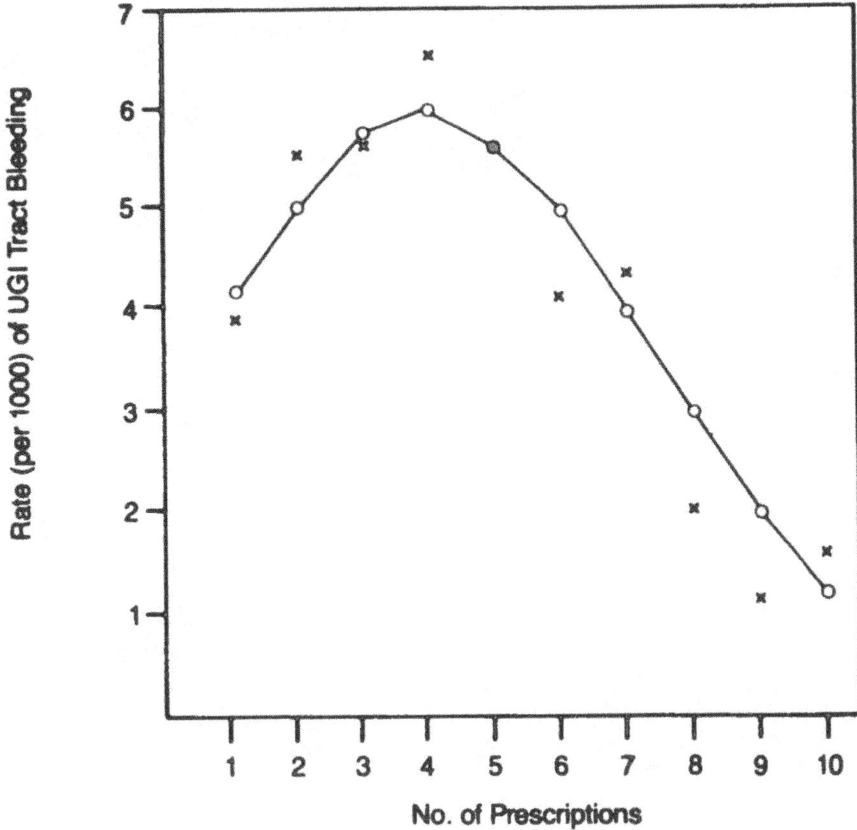

Figure 2. Duration-response relationship between the number of NSAID prescriptions and the risk of UGI bleeding.

associated with a higher rate of UGI bleeding than the other six NSAIDs, this was tested again by repeating the study, investigating patients exposed to one and only one NSAID in Michigan in 1982 (Tables 4 and 6). The rate of UGI bleeding remained different among users of the nine NSAIDs ($p = 0.046$). Sulindac users once again were associated with the highest incidence of UGI bleeding, and compared to all of the other drugs, sulindac was statistically different (one-sided $p = 0.004$). Notably, sulindac remained the only drug that was different from ibuprofen ($p = 0.022$). When only the original seven drugs were considered, a significant difference among the drugs persisted ($p = 0.0049$). Fenoprofen and tolmetin exchanged positions from the 1980 to the 1982 data, but in both data sets the apparent differences between these two drugs were compatible with chance. To test the possibility that in 1980 physicians had given their highest risk patients the most recently marketed NSAID, i.e., sulindac, the rates of UGI bleeding among users of the two newest NSAIDs in 1982 (piroxicam and zomepirac) were compared with those of the

Table 3. Risk of Upper Gastrointestinal Tract Bleeding Associated with the Use of Each Nonsteroidal Antiinflammatory Drug: 1980 Data

	Number of Patients					Incidence of UGI
Drug	**UGI Tract Bleeding**	**UGI Tract Bleeding Resulting in Hospitalization**	**No UGI Tract Bleeding**	**Total**	**Overall Incidence of UGI Tract Bleeding (per 1000 Exposed Patients)** *	**Bleeding Resulting in Hospitalization (per 1000 Exposed Patients)** *
Sulindac	76	35	14,351	14,427	5.3	2.4
Tolmetin	20	9	4,626	4,646	4.3	1.9
Naproxen	32	11	8,478	8,510	3.8	1.3
Ibuprofen	112	32	35,918	36,030	3.1	0.9
Indomethacin	30	10	10,323	10,353	2.9	1.0
Fenoprofen	9	4	4,286	4,295	2.1	0.9
Phenylbutazone	19	9	9,770	9,789	1.9	0.9

Source: Carson JL, et al.[2]

* $p < 0.001$ not adjusted for confounding variables.

Table 4. Interdrug Comparisons of Risk of Upper Gastrointestinal Tract Bleeding

Drug	1980 Unadjusted Relative Risk (95% Confidence Interval) *	1980 Unadjusted Relative Risk (95% Confidence Interval) * for Hospitalized Patients †	1980 Adjusted Relative Risk (95% Confidence Interval) ‡	1982 Unadjusted Relative Risk (95% Confidence Interval) ‡
Sulindac	1.7 (1.3–2.3)	2.7 (1.7–4.4)	1.4 (1.1–1.9)	1.8 (1.1–2.9)
Tolmetin	1.4 (0.9–2.2)	2.2 (1.0–4.6)	1.4 (0.9–2.3)	1.0 (0.5–2.1)
Naproxen	1.2 (0.8–1.8)	1.5 (0.7–2.9)	1.2 (0.8–1.7)	1.1 (0.7–1.7)
Ibuprofen	1.0 (reference)	1.0 (reference)	1.0 (reference)	1.0 (reference)
Indomethacin	0.9 (0.6–1.4)	1.1 (0.5–2.2)	1.0 (0.6–1.4)	1.0 (0.5–1.9)
Fenoprofen	0.7 (0.3–1.3)	1.0 (0.4–3.0)	0.7 (0.3–1.3)	1.6 (0.9–2.7)
Phenylbutazone	0.6 (0.4–1.0)	1.0 (0.5–2.2)	1.4 (0.9–2.3)	0.2 (0.0–1.3)

Source: Carson JL, et al.[2]

* Comparisons of each drug with ibuprofen calculated by the Haldane method.[5]

† Upper GI tract bleeding in outpatients was excluded.

‡ Adjusted for the number of prescriptions for each drug in the entire 12-month time period using logistic regression.[6]

Table 5. Alcohol-Drug Interaction

	Patients with Alcohol-Related Diagnoses				
	UGI Tract Bleeding	No UGI Tract Bleeding	Total	Incidence (per 1000)	Overall Incidence (per 1000)
Sulindac	6	230	236	25.4	5.3
Tolmetin	4	70	74	54.1	4.3
Naproxen	2	131	133	15.0	3.8
Ibuprofen	3	788	791	3.8	3.1
Indomethacin	0	203	203	0.0	2.9
Fenoprofen	0	84	84	0.0	2.1
Phenylbutazone	1	176	177	5.7	1.9

Source: Carson JL, et al.[2]

Note: $p<0.001$ for the association between alcohol-related diagnoses and upper gastrointestinal (UGI) tract bleeding; $p=0.017$ for alcohol-nonsteroidal antiinflammatory drug interaction, using logistic regression.[6]

older drugs. Compared to the seven older drugs, there was no difference in the rate of bleeding among users of piroxicam (relative risk 1.0, 95% confidence intervals 0.4–2.5) or zomepirac (relative risk 0.8, 95% confidence intervals 0.5–1.2).

DISCUSSION

Our results confirm that NSAIDs as a class are associated with UGI bleeding, but the magnitude of risk associated with their use is reassuringly small. However, these data reveal that there are significant differences in the rates of UGI bleeding associated with the use of the different NSAIDs. Sulindac users had the highest incidence of UGI bleeding, and sulindac was the only drug associated with a rate of UGI bleeding statistically different from ibuprofen.

Table 6. Risk of Upper Gastrointestinal Tract Bleeding: 1982 Data

	Number of Patients			1982 Incidence (per 1000 Exposed Patients)	1980 Incidence (per 1000 Exposed Patients)
Drug	UGI Tract Bleeding	No UGI Tract Bleeding	Total		
Sulindac	24	4,752	4,776	5.0	5.3
Fenoprofen	15	3,390	3,405	4.4	2.1
Naproxen	30	9,697	9,727	3.1	3.8
Piroxicam	5	1,718	1,723	2.9	—
Ibuprofen	63	22,174	22,237	2.8	3.1
Indomethacin	11	3,900	3,911	2.8	2.9
Tolmetin	8	2,858	2,866	2.8	4.3
Zomepirac	29	12,700	12,729	2.3	—
Phenylbutazone	1	1,998	1,999	0.5	1.9

Source: Carson JL, et al.[2]

Note: $p=0.046$ for overall rate of UGI tract bleeding in 1982 data; $p=0.049$ for overall rate of UGI tract bleeding, including only drugs from the 1980 analysis (i.e., excluding piroxicam and zomepirac); $p=0.004$ (one-sided) for sulindac vs other drugs.

This was confirmed in a separate data set in 1982. This association was even stronger when the analysis was restricted to hospitalized patients. A synergistic effect was found between the presence of alcohol-related diagnoses and the risk of UGI bleeding associated with the use of each drug.

There are several potential confounding variables that must be considered. We controlled for state, age, sex, indication, use of anticoagulants, use of corticosteroids, use of cimetidine and/or antacids, the presence of other conditions previously associated with UGI bleeding, and the average number of prescriptions for each drug. However, we could not control for family history, smoking, blood type, and aspirin use. Over-the-counter ibuprofen was unavailable at the time of this study. The first three variables are probably unrelated to the use of NSAIDs and so should not result in significant confounding. The use of aspirin could be, however, and was not accurately measured in the study, as aspirin is available over-the-counter and is inexpensive, and COMPASS includes only information on prescribed drugs. Although we excluded the considerable number of patients who were prescribed aspirin, it is likely that some patients who were not excluded were taking the drug. It is possible that use of aspirin was different in the group of NSAID users compared to the nonusers. If users of NSAIDs were more likely to be using aspirin, then the real risk from NSAIDs might be even smaller. If users of NSAIDs were less likely to be using aspirin, then the real risk from NSAIDs might be larger. It seems unlikely that aspirin use is distributed unequally among the seven NSAIDs, unless perhaps sulindac was perceived as less effective and thereby more often supplemented by aspirin.

Similarly, our ability to control for alcohol use was limited. Our patients with alcohol-related diagnoses are likely to be heavy alcohol users, although some heavy alcohol users would be excluded from this group. Any misclassification of alcohol use here is unidirectional, however. This would mask an interaction between alcohol-related diagnoses and the use of NSAIDs, rather than create one.

A major potential problem when using claims data is data validity. In particular, when this study was conducted, unlike now, we were unable to obtain copies of primary medical records. A previous report of ours discusses this issue in detail, concluding that the diagnosis data in this data set appear to be sufficiently valid to be useful.[3] In addition, there are a number of findings in this study which would be expected clinically and were observed, suggesting that the data are valid. Included are the relative utilization rates of the different NSAIDs, including the preferential use of ibuprofen for dysmenorrhea and indomethacin and phenylbutazone for crystal arthopathy, and the association of UGI bleeding with elevated age, male sex, residence in the more urban states, preexisting abdominal conditions, anticoagulants, use of cimetidine and/or antacids, and alcohol-related diagnoses. In addition, the average daily dose[9] and the incidence of UGI bleeding[10] were similar to that found in previous studies, and dose-response and duration-response relationships were seen. Lastly, when the analysis was restricted to subjects admitted to the hospital with discharge diagnoses of UGI bleeding, diagnoses much less subject to problems of validity, the differences among the NSAIDs were increased, rather than eliminated.

Another potential limitation is that these conclusions are derived from a Medicaid population only. Although there are no obvious reasons to believe that these findings cannot be generalized to other populations, this must be considered.

In conclusion, our data confirmed that NSAIDs are associated with UGI bleeding, although the magnitude of the risk is relatively small. Differences were apparent among the different NSAIDs in the risk of UGI bleeding associated with their use. Specifically, sulindac was associated with a higher risk than the other drugs, a finding which was reproduced in a separate 1982 data set. The reason for this could be some unique property of the drug. Alternatively, if sulindac were perceived as less effective, this could result in physician use of a higher average daily dose, as observed, or more frequent use of concomitant aspirin. Either of these could create a higher risk of UGI bleeding. Nevertheless, these results should be confirmed from other sources before they can be considered proven.

ACKNOWLEDGMENT

This study was supported by Cooperative Agreement FD-U-00079 from the U.S. Food and Drug Administration and grants from The Henry J. Kaiser Family Foundation, The Andrew W. Mellon Foundation, and The Rockefeller Foundation.

REFERENCES

1. Carson JL, Strom BL, Soper KA, et al: The association of nonsteroidal anti-inflammatory drugs with upper gastrointestinal bleeding. *Arch Intern Med* 1987;147:85–88.
2. Carson JL, Strom BL, Morse ML, et al: The relative gastrointestinal toxicity of the nonsteroidal anti-inflammatory drugs. *Arch Intern Med* 1987; 147:1054–1059.
3. Strom BL, Carson JL, Morse ML, et al: The Computerized On-line Medicaid Pharmaceutical Analysis and Surveillance System: A new resource for postmarketing drug surveillance. *Clin Pharmacol Ther* 1985;38:359–364.
4. *International Classification of Diseases, Clinical Modification* (ICD-9-CM). Ann Arbor, Michigan Commission on Professional and Hospital Activities, 1980.
5. Everitt BS: *The Analysis of Contingency Tables*. New York, John Wiley & Sons Inc, 1977.

6. Kleinbaum DG, Kupper LL, Morgenstern H: *Epidemiology Research: Principles and Quantitative Methods*. New York, Van Nostrand Reinhold Co, 1982.
7. *Physicians' Desk Reference*, ed 35. Oradell, NJ, Medical Economics Co, 1981.
8. Armitage P: Tests for linear trends in proportions and frequencies. *Biometrics* 1955;42:375–386.
9. Baum C, Kennedy DL, Forbes MB: Utilization of non-steroidal anti-inflammatory drugs. *Arthritis Rheum* 1985;28:686–692.
10. Cutler JA, Mendeloff AI: Upper gastrointestinal bleeding: Nature and magnitude of the problem in the US. *Dig Dis Sci* 1981;26(Suppl):90–96.

18. *Impact of Nonsteroidal Antiinflammatory Agents on General Gastrointestinal Upset in an Elderly Population*

WAYNE BIGELOW
TED COLLINS

INTRODUCTION

Numerous studies have evaluated the effect of nonsteroidal antiinflammatory drugs (NSAIDs) on acute gastrointestinal (GI) problems, specifically, upper GI bleeding and the incidence of esophageal and duodenal ulcers.[1-3] To date, these studies have shown that, controlling for age, sex, concomitant drug use and other prior conditions (e.g., smoking and alcohol consumption), NSAID users are more at risk of acute GI problems than other persons.

But, although these studies investigated the impact of NSAID use on acute GI problems, none investigated the association between NSAIDs and generalized GI distress. Additionally, no studies specifically evaluated the impact of NSAIDs on general GI distress in an elderly population. An evaluation of the effect of NSAIDs on general GI distress among an elderly population is particularly germane, since the elderly are already subject to a complex spectrum of health problems, sometimes aggravated by drug regimens consisting of multiple drug classes and agents.

The current study provides preliminary estimates of the impact of NSAIDs on the risk of general GI upset among Wisconsin Medicaid recipients aged 65 and older for the period April 1984 to March 1987. General GI distress was measured using both diagnostic codes indicative of GI upset (Appendix 1) and the use of histamine antagonists and antacids as indicators or markers of general GI distress. These preliminary figures estimate the impact of NSAIDs on several levels:

- for patients receiving long- vs short-acting NSAIDs
- for patients receiving full, therapeutic, and low doses of NSAIDs
- for institutionalized and noninstitutionalized elderly
- for five specific NSAIDs

PATIENT SELECTION

Wisconsin Medicaid billing data for the period April 1, 1984, to March 31, 1987, were used to estimate the impact of NSAID use on general GI upset among the elderly. All persons aged 65 or older receiving services for which a bill was received by Medicaid were initially included in the analysis. For the entire period, a total of 102,739 elderly Medicaid recipients received services.

The population was then reduced by eliminating patients with a history of GI upset. To determine whether patients had a prior history of GI upset, diagnostic codes indicative of GI upset and bills submitted for histamine antagonists or antacids during the first 90 days of observation for each patient were used (Appendix 2). Patients with evidence of GI upset during the first 90 days were excluded from analyses. Additionally, patients with fewer than 90 days' worth of bills submitted were excluded from the analysis, since these patients were deemed not to have a sufficient observation period to determine a prior history of GI upset.

Patients with a diagnostic code indicative of alcohol abuse at any point during the period of observation were also eliminated. Finally, a subset of diagnostic codes indicative of GI difficulties, but not presumed to be causally linked to NSAID use, was used to exclude patients from the analysis if these codes were evidenced at any point during the observation period. Since these conditions may be, and often are, related to our outcome measure, it was necessary to control for them in the analysis. Observation ended when any evidence of GI upset was found for a specific patient.

OUTCOME MEASURES

A dichotomous outcome measure was created based on (1) the presence of a subset of diagnostic codes indicative of GI upset that can be presumed to be attributable to NSAID use, and (2) bills submitted for histamine antagonists and antacids. The use of these two types of drugs as markers or indicators of GI upset is reasonable insofar as physicians often prescribe them to alleviate GI distress. However, physicians often prescribe these drugs prophylactically at the same time that NSAIDs are prescribed in order to alleviate anticipated GI upset. To control for the use of these agents as prophylaxis, patients whose prescriptions for histamine antagonists or antacids started on the same day or the day after the initiation of NSAID drug therapy were excluded from the analysis.

The presence of either the diagnostic codes or the drug indicators of general

Table 1. Nonsteroidal Antiinflammatory Drugs Included in the Study

NSAID	Action	Maximum Recommended Daily Dose
aspirin	short	5400 mg
piroxicam	long	20 mg
ibuprofen	short	2400 mg
sulindac	long	400 mg
naproxen	long	1250 mg
indomethacin	short	200 mg
diflunisal	short	1500 mg
ketoprofen	short	300 mg
phenylbutazone	short	600 mg
tolmetin	short	2000 mg
meclofenamate	short	400 mg
fenoprofen	short	3200 mg

GI distress had to occur within 30 days of the end of an NSAID prescription in order for GI distress to be attributed to NSAID use.

Independent variables were (1) sex; (2) age group (75–84 or 85 and older); (3) institutionalization status; and (4) use of corticosteroids or anticoagulants.

NSAID USE

Two types of measures were constructed for evaluating the impact of NSAIDs on general GI upset. The first was based on the use of long-acting vs short-acting NSAIDs in a given month, as well as on a mix of long- and short-acting NSAIDs. A *long-acting* NSAID is one for which the half-life is approximately 12 or more hours, as defined in the *Physicians' Desk Reference*. The second measure was determined by the dose level of the drug. *Dose* was computed as the quantity of a given NSAID divided by the number of days of supply and multiplied by the milligrams per unit. The dose was then transformed into a percentage of the *maximum recommended daily dose* (RDD), as defined in the *Physicians' Desk Reference*.

The 12 NSAIDs included in the study are shown in Table 1. NSAID therapy was coded as full dose (100% of the maximum RDD); therapeutic dose (34–99% of the maximum RDD); or low dose (≤33% of the maximum RDD) for each month of observation.

MONTH OF OBSERVATION

Since the period of time a specific recipient could be "observed" was variable (from 4 to 37 months), and since patients who exhibited GI upset were deleted from further observation, selection bias might occur if the length of observation was not controlled. If patients with no GI upset during earlier months of observation were less likely to ever experience GI upset, not controlling for the length of observation would negatively bias our estimates. As such, we added a

Table 2. Distribution of Patients and Patient-Months over Major Variables

	Recipients	
	Number (N=77,905)	%*
Sex		
Male	22,251	28.56
Female	55,654	71.44
Age		
65–74	29,660	38.07
75–84	33,278	42.72
85 and older	24,461	31.40
Institutionalized	40,598	52.11
Noninstitutionalized	56,094	72.00
Corticosteroid use	3,925	5.04
Anticoagulant use	3,137	4.03
NSAID Therapy		
Low Dose	1,656	2.13
Therapeutic Dose	5,591	7.18
Full Dose	11,524	14.79
GI upset	15,472	19.86

Note: Total number of patient-months = 1,684,994; average number of months per patient = 21.63.

*Numbers sum to greater than 100% due to that recipients could be in more than one "status" of a given variable over the three-year observation period.

variable equal to the number of months (measured as 30-day periods) that a specific patient was observed.

STATISTICAL METHOD

For each patient-month (30-day period), one observation record was created. Each record contained information on the independent variables and outcome measures described above. These records were grouped or aggregated over all patients. Logistic regression was then used to estimate the effect of NSAID use on the likelihood of general GI upset.

RESULTS

Table 2 presents the distribution of patients and patient-months over relevant variables after excluding those patients who (1) evidenced a history of GI upset or alcohol abuse, (2) were missing demographic information, (3) were prescribed histamine antagonists or antacids as prophylaxis, or (4) evidenced diagnostic codes for conditions linked to our outcome measure but not presumed to be attributable to NSAID use. After these exclusions, a total of

Table 3. Effects of Long-, Short-, and Mixed Long/Short-Acting Nonsteroidal Antiinflammatory Drug Therapy on General Gastrointestinal Upset

Variable/Category	Adjusted Logit Coefficient (Relative Risk)
Female	0.0187 (1.01)
Aged 75 to 84	0.0264 * (1.03)
Aged 85 or older	0.0230 (1.02)
Noninstitutionalized	−0.4432 ** (0.64)
Use of corticosteroids and/or anticoagulants	0.5348 ** (1.71)
Month of observation	0.0022 ** (1.00)
Short-acting NSAID use only	0.3698 ** (1.45)
Long- and short-acting NSAID use	0.6045 ** (1.83)
Long-acting NSAID use only	0.3871 ** (1.47)

* $p < 0.01$.
** $p < 0.001$.

77,905 patients remained. As would be expected in an elderly Medicaid population, females predominated, comprising 71% of this population. During the observation period, 56,094, or 72% of the population, were not institutionalized, and 52% were institutionalized at some point. Additionally, 5% of patients received corticosteroids and 4% received anticoagulants at some point while receiving services during the period. Thus, about 24% of our population entered a nursing home during the observation period after having been in a noninstitutionalized setting, or, left a nursing home to enter such a setting. Since elderly Medicaid recipients often enter a nursing home for short periods after a hospital stay and are highly at risk to enter nursing homes at any point, this is not surprising.

For the NSAIDs and general GI upset measures, almost 20% of the population received NSAIDs, and 20% (15,742) had indications of general GI upset at some point.

DOSE LEVEL AND SHORT- VS LONG-ACTING NSAIDs

Tables 3 and 4 present the logit coefficients and the converted relative risk estimates for general GI upset in the population for two models estimating GI upset. The first model (Table 3) estimates the likelihood of GI upset with NSAID use categorized by long- vs short- vs long- and short-acting. The second model (Table 4) provides estimates categorizing NSAID use by full-, therapeutic-, and low-dose levels.

Table 4. Effects of Low-, Therapeutic-, and Full-Dose Nonsteroidal Antiinflammatory Drug Therapy on General Gastrointestinal Upset

Variable/Category	Adjusted Logit Coefficient (Relative Risk)
Female	0.0175 (1.01)
Aged 75 to 84	0.0264* (1.03)
Aged 85 or older	0.0218 (1.02)
Noninstitutionalized	−0.4435** (0.64)
Use of corticosteroids and/or anticoagulants	0.5324** (1.70)
Month of observation	0.0022 (1.00)
Low-dose NSAID use	0.1596** (1.17)
Therapeutic-dose NSAID use	0.3897** (1.48)
Full-dose NSAID use	0.4272** (1.53)

* $p < 0.01$.
** $p < 0.001$.

For both models, the age coefficients indicate minor, generally insignificant, effects of increasing age on GI upset. The same is true for sex. As expected, the use of corticosteroids and/or anticoagulants has a large and significant impact, increasing the likelihood of GI upset by almost 70%. There is a large and significant negative coefficent associated with being noninstitutionalized, those persons being 36% less likely to experience GI upset than the institutionalized.

In Tables 3 and 4, the parameters for NSAID use are all positive and significant. In Table 3, which contains the coefficients for the model with long-acting vs short-acting NSAIDs, it is seen that mixed use of NSAIDs (long- and short-acting during the same 30-day period) had the largest impact, increasing the risk by 83% in comparison to patients not receiving any NSAIDs. Patients receiving only long-acting NSAIDs were 47% more likely to experience general GI upset than those not receiving any NSAIDs, and those only on short-acting NSAIDs experienced a 45% greater chance. We had expected long-acting NSAIDs to evidence the greatest positive impact on GI upset, and so the finding that mixed use was associated with a larger likelihood was rather surprising.

Table 4 shows the coefficients for the model with NSAID use broken down by full, therapeutic, and low doses. As expected, there was a positive effect on the likelihood of general GI upset. Patients on low doses of NSAIDs were at 17% increased risk of GI upset compared to the population not receiving NSAIDs; patients on therapeutic doses had a 48% higher rate of GI upset; and those on full doses had a 53% higher likelihood of GI upset.

Table 5. Interaction Effects of Dose and Long/Short-Acting NSAIDs on General Gastro-intestinal Upset

Variable/Category	Adjusted Logit Coefficient (Relative Risk)
Low dose —short-acting use only	0.1514** (1.16)
Low dose —short- and long-acting use	na
Low dose —long-acting use only	0.5233* (1.69)
Therapeutic dose —short-acting use only	0.3913** (1.48)
Therapeutic dose —long- and short-acting use	0.7073** (2.21)
Therapeutic dose —long-acting use only	0.3342** (1.40)
Full dose —short-acting use only	0.4329** (1.54)
Full dose —long- and short-acting use	0.5970** (1.82)
Full dose —long-acting use only	0.3979** (1.49)

Note: na = insufficient cases to estimate parameters.
* $p<0.01$.
** $p<0.001$.

Since higher dosage levels of NSAIDs were positively related to GI upset, the finding that mixed use of long- and short-acting NSAIDs had the largest impact on general GI upset might simply be the result of mixed use being associated with higher dosage levels. To investigate this possibility, we estimated the effects of long-acting, short-acting, and mixed NSAID use within dose levels. Table 5 presents the coefficients only for the NSAID variables, taken from the full model containing the same parameters as those described for Tables 3 and 4. Even within dose levels, the use of short- and long-acting NSAIDs during the same month was associated with a higher risk of GI upset than the use of short- or long-acting NSAIDs alone. Therefore, we could not conclude that the relation between short- and long-acting NSAIDs and GI upset was linked to the dose levels associated with the half-life of a specific NSAID.

DIFFERENCES BETWEEN THE INSTITUTIONALIZED AND NONINSTITUTIONALIZED ELDERLY

Part of the goal of this preliminary research was to determine if the impact of NSAID use differed between institutionalized and noninstitutionalized elderly populations. Table 6 presents the coefficients and converted relative risk estimates for the model containing long-acting versus short-acting NSAID use for the two populations.

Table 6. Effects of Long-, Short-, and Mixed Long/Short-Acting NSAID Therapy on General Gastrointestinal Upset, by Institutional Status

Variable/Category	Adjusted Logit Coefficient (Relative Risk)[a] Institutionalized	Non – Institutionalized
Female	0.0214 (1.02)	– 0.0059 (0.99)
Aged 75 to 84	0.0754** (1.08)	– 0.0160 (0.99)
Aged 85 or older	0.0756** (1.08)	– 0.0832** (0.92)
Use of corticosteroids and/or anticoagulants	0.5100* (1.67)	0.5549** (1.74)
Month of observation	0.0009 (1.00)	0.0045** (1.00)
Short-acting NSAID use only	0.1570** (1.17)	0.4912** (1.63)
Long- and short-acting NSAID use	0.4659** (1.59)	0.6843** (1.98)
Long-acting NSAID use only	0.3342** (1.40)	0.4169** (1.52)

[a] Relative risk ratio converted from logit coefficient is in parentheses.
* $p < 0.01$.
** $p < 0.001$.

Some differences could be noted for the two populations. Increasing age appeared to be positively related to GI upset for the Wisconsin institutionalized elderly, but negatively related for the noninstitutionalized elderly. For both populations, the use of short- and long-acting NSAIDs in the same period was associated with a higher risk of GI upset than either used separately. However, for the institutionalized elderly, the use of only long-acting NSAIDs had a higher risk associated with GI upset than did short-acting NSAID use only (1.40 versus 1.17). Conversely, among the noninstitutionalized elderly, this association was not present. The relative risk associated with short-acting NSAID use among the noninstitutionalized elderly was 1.63, while the relative risk of long-acting NSAID use was only 1.52.

DIFFERENCES BETWEEN SPECIFIC NSAID AGENTS

Estimates for the impact of five specific NSAID agents, derived from the full model, are shown in Table 7. The five NSAID agents included in the analysis were naproxen, sulindac, piroxicam, ibuprofen, and all long-acting NSAIDs combined. Adjusted logit coefficients and the 95% confidence intervals for these NSAIDs are presented. The goal for this component of the preliminary research was to determine if specific NSAID agents were more highly related to increased GI upset than others. The relative impact of the five NSAID agents was similar, with piroxicam increasing the likelihood of GI

Table 7. Adjusted Effects of Specific NSAIDs on General Gastrointestinal Upset

Variable/Category	Adjusted Logit Coefficient	95% Confidence Interval for Relative Risk	
ibuprofen	0.3753**	1.38	1.53
piroxicam	0.4024**	1.40	1.60
sulindac	0.3944**	1.38	1.60
naproxen	0.3589**	1.35	1.52
all long-acting NSAIDs	0.3871**	1.41	1.53

** $p < 0.001$.

upset by the largest amount (between 40% and 60%), and naproxen increasing the likelihood by the smallest amount (between 35% and 52%). However, considering the confidence intervals associated with the five NSAIDs, the overlap was extensive, indicating that there was little difference in the impact of the five agents on general GI upset among elderly Medicaid recipients. The lack of differences revealed in the Table 7 may be partially due to the lack of a dose measure in the models. In the future, we intend to add such measures to the model.

CONCLUSIONS

As anticipated, institutionalized elderly Medicaid recipients were more at risk of GI upset than were the noninstitutionalized elderly. Much of the research investigating the impact of NSAID use on acute GI problems to date has utilized Medicaid data, and differences between these two groups of elderly have not been controlled for. Our preliminary estimates suggested that this patient dimension should be adjusted for in future research, and Medicaid billing data contains the necessary information to do so.

Unlike some reports, our analysis found very few significant or substantive impacts of either age or sex on GI upset. This may have been due to the more selective nature of our population or the more general nature of our outcome measure in comparison to other research.

Our preliminary findings also indicated that NSAID use was positively related to general GI upset among the elderly. Also, this risk generally appeared to be positively related to dose levels. However, there did not appear to be any specific pattern of effect associated with long- vs short-acting NSAID use for the elderly population as a whole. Finally, there were remarkably few differences in the impact of five different NSAID agents on general GI upset, although this may be due to the lack of a dose measure in our models.

Future research will attempt to explicate the relation between the diagnostic code and drug indicators in our models to more fully determine whether it is appropriate to use drug indicators to identify GI upset. Additionally, we intend to further examine the impact specific NSAIDs have on general GI upset among the elderly, including controls for dose level. Insofar as we can determine specific combinations of drugs and/or doses and their relation to negative outcomes among the elderly, the value of research utilizing Medicaid billing data may have significant quality-of-care and financial impacts.

REFERENCES

1. Bartle W, Gupta A, and Lazor J: Non-steroidal anti-inflammatory drugs and gastro-intestinal bleeding. *Arch Intern Med* 1986;146:2365–2367.
2. Carson JL, Strom BL, Soper KA, et al: The association of nonsteroidal anti-inflammatory drugs and gastro-intestinal bleeding. *Arch Intern Med* 1987;147:85–88.
3. Collier DStJ: NSAIDs and peptic ulcer perforation. *Gut* 1985;26:359–363.

APPENDIX 1.

Criteria Used in Determining the Presence of GI Upset

Drug Therapy Criteria

Histamine antagonist drug therapy
Antacid drug therapy

Diagnostic Criteria

530.0	Diseases of the esophagus
531.0	Gastric ulcer
532.0	Duodenal ulcer
533.0	Peptic ulcer, site unspecified
534.0	Gastrojejunal ulcer
535	Gastritis and duodenitis
536.8	Dyspepsia and other specified disorders of function of stomach
536.9	Unspecified functional disorder of stomach
537.8	Other specified disorders of stomach and duodenum
537.9	Unspecified disorders of stomach and duodenum
578	Gastrointestinal hemorrhage
787.1	Heartburn
787.2	Dysphagia
787.3	Flatulence
789	Abdominal pain

APPENDIX 2.

Criteria to Be Used in Excluding Patients from Analysis if They Occur Within the First Three Months of a Patient's Initial Recipiency

Drug Therapy Criteria

Histamine antagonist drug therapy
Antacid drug therapy

Diagnostic Criteria

150	Malignant neoplasm—esophagus
151	Malignant neoplasm—stomach
152	Malignant neoplasm—small intestine, including duodenum
197.4	Secondary malignant neoplasm—small intestine, including duodenum
197.8	Secondary malignant neoplasm—other digestive organs
291.0	Benign neoplasm—esophagus
211.1	Benign neoplasm—stomach
211.2	Benign neoplasm—duodenum, jejunum, and ileum
230.1	Carcinoma in situ—esophagus
230.2	Carcinoma in situ—stomach
230.7	Carcinoma in situ—colon
230.9	Carcinoma in situ—other and unspecified digestive organs
239.0	Unspecified neoplasm—digestive system
251.5	Abnormality of secretion of gastrin
306.4	Physiological malfunction—mental factors: gastrointestinal
456.0	Esophageal varices in diseases classified elsewhere
456.1	Esophageal varices without mention of bleeding
456.2	Esophageal varices in diseases classified elsewhere
530.0	Diseases of the esophagus
531.0	Gastric ulcer
532.0	Duodenal ulcer
533.0	Peptic ulcer, site unspecified
534.0	Gastrojejunal ulcer
535	Gastritis and duodenitis
536.8	Dyspepsia and other specified disorders of function of stomach
536.9	Unspecified functional disorder of stomach
537.8	Other specified disorders of stomach and duodenum
537.9	Unspecified disorders of stomach and duodenum
555	Regional enteritis
558	Other noninfectious gastroenteritis and colitis
564.8	Other specified functional disorders of intestine
564.9	Unspecified functional disorders of intestine
569.8	Other specified disorders of intestine
569.9	Unspecified disorder of intestine

578	Gastrointestinal hemorrhage
750.3	Tracheoesophageal fistula
750.4	Other specified anomalies of esophagus
750.5	Congenital hypertrophic pyloric stenosis
750.6	Congenital hiatus hernia
750.7	Other specified anomalies of stomach
750.8	Other specified anomalies of upper alimentary tract
750.9	Unspecified anomaly of upper alimentary tract
787.1	Heartburn
787.2	Dysphagia
787.3	Flatulence
787.9	Other symptoms involving digestive system
788	Symptoms involving urinary system
789	Abdominal pain
866.22	Injury to esophagus, without open wound
863.1	Injury to GI tract, stomach, without open wound
863.2	Injury to GI tract, stomach, with open wound
863.3	Injury to GI tract, small intestine

19. *NSAIDs as a Cause of Morbidity and Mortality from Peptic Ulcer Complications in New South Wales*

DAVID A. HENRY
PAMELA R. HALL
ANNE JOHNSTON
ANNETTE DOBSON

INTRODUCTION

While few would doubt that there is a relation between use of nonsteroidal antiinflammatory drugs (NSAIDs) and peptic ulcer and its complications, the association was, until recently, inadequately studied. In the last three years epidemiological investigations, including case control and prospective record linkage studies, have produced a wide range of estimates of the relative risks of upper gastrointestinal hemorrhage (UGIH) and ulcer perforation associated with use of NSAIDs.[2-6] The highest estimates of risk have come from the United Kingdom, where a controversy has arisen over the number of deaths from ulcer complications which can be attributed to the use of NSAIDs. Estimates have ranged from 200 to over 3000 deaths annually.[5-6] The figures supporting the higher estimate were published by Armstrong and Blower, and recalculation of their data reveals that the odds ratio for use of NSAIDs by patients who died from ulcer complications compared with those who survived was 3.4.[6] Although these authors did not set out specifically to compare patients who died with those who survived peptic ulcer complications and thus did not control for factors that might confound the relation between use of NSAIDs and mortality, their data raise the possibility that NSAIDs are associ-

Note: Part of this work has been published previously.[1] The relevant sections have been included in this manuscript with the knowledge and approval of the editor of the *British Medical Journal*.

ated with an increased case fatality rate. If this was confirmed, it would be important, as estimates of attributable mortality which have been calculated from morbidity studies, making the assumption of a "normal" case fatality rate, would need to be revised. An increased case fatality rate might be due to a direct effect of the drugs on bleeding time or renal function but would more likely be due to confounding, particularly by chronic diseases that were more common in users of NSAIDs and worsened their prognosis after an episode of hemorrhage or perforation.

The present study was set up to test the hypothesis that NSAIDs are associated with an increased case fatality rate from peptic ulcer complications. The roles of aspirin and corticosteroids were also examined.

SUBJECTS AND METHODS

The study was approved by the Hunter Regional Research Ethics Committee. Records of all separations from public and private hospitals in the Greater Newcastle area in New South Wales are held by the Hunter Health Statistics Unit. Information that can be accessed includes hospital unit record numbers, demographic data, mode of separation from hospital (discharged, died, transferred, etc.) and up to five separate diagnoses.

Cases were defined as all patients who had died from ulcer complications in Newcastle hospitals between January 1980 and June 1986, and they were identified by examination of the original hospital records of all patients who died in-hospital and whose separation diagnoses included any diagnostic code for peptic ulcer (ICD-9-CM 531.0–531.9; 532.0–532.9; 533.0–533.9). The clinical notes were reviewed by a research nurse and a gastroenterologist, and only those patients who had died during the hospital stay and whose primary reason for admission to the hospital was considered to be a complication of a peptic ulcer (hemorrhage or perforation or both) were included in the study as cases. Patients who had developed peptic ulcer complications while in the hospital for other reasons were excluded.

Controls were drawn randomly from the records of all subjects who had been admitted to the hospital with a primary diagnosis of complicated peptic ulcer but who had survived and been discharged back to the community. As with the study cases, original records were examined by a research nurse and a gastroenterologist in order to validate the diagnoses. Two controls were matched individually to each case for age (to within five years), sex, date of separation from hospital (to within two years), site of ulcer (gastric or duodenal), and nature of complication (hemorrhage or perforation). Information on use of all drugs taken during the week prior to admission to hospital was obtained from the hospital records. Generally this information was recorded by the admitting intern or resident medical officer or was included in the referral letter from the family practitioner. No attempt was made to calculate dose or to determine drug use prior to one week before admission. Our experi-

Table 1. Drug Use, by Cases and Controls

	Cases (n = 80)	Controls (n = 160)	Unadjusted Odds Ratio*	Adjusted Odds Ratio*	P
NSAIDs	31(39%)	59(37%)	1.1(0.6, 2.1)	1.1(0.5, 2.1)	0.88
Aspirin	19(24%)	34(21%)	1.2(0.6, 2.4)	1.2(0.6, 2.6)	0.58
Corticosteroids	7(9%)	4(3%)	4.2(0.9,25.6)	6.0(0.7,50.9)	0.10

*95% CI.

ence is that medical staff who are responsible for patients with acute complications of peptic ulcer take detailed histories of previous use of aspirin and NSAIDs, presumably because they regard these drugs as important etiological factors. In a separate study of incident cases of peptic ulcer hemorrhage or perforation admitted to Newcastle during 1986 and 1987, we determined prior drug use by structured interview, cross-checked with family practitioner's prescribing records, and determined that the use of NSAIDs within the previous week (taking no account of dose) was in 97% agreement with the information recorded in the hospital notes.

In addition to drug use, information was collected from hospital records on previous history of peptic ulcer and other diseases, diagnoses present on admission to hospital, and new diagnoses made during the hospital stay. Account was also taken of the patient's social circumstances, the history of alcohol and tobacco usage, the presence of shock on admission, the quantity of blood transfused on the first day and during the entire admission, and the degree of renal failure present on admission.

Unadjusted odds ratios for previous use of NSAIDs, aspirin, and corticosteroids were calculated for matched triplets using the methods of Miettinen, and adjustments were made by conditional logistic regression.[7,8] After inspection of the univariate analyses the covariates that were included in the logistic regression model were (1) prior use of digoxin; (2) prior use of anti-ulcer drugs; (3) the presence of hypertension, cerebrovascular disease, chronic airways disease or chronic liver disease; (4) a history of previous uncomplicated peptic ulcer; (5) a history of living in care; (6) a total transfusion requirement of more than 6 units of blood; and (7) a serum creatinine level greater than 0.12 mmol/L.

RESULTS

During the six years of the study, 1003 patients were admitted to the study hospitals with a primary diagnosis of ulcer perforation or hemorrhage. On the basis of the case note review, 81 patients were judged to have died as a result of peptic ulcer complications during their hospital stay. Eighty of these were successfully matched for all variables.

Crude and adjusted odds ratios for recent use of the drugs of interest are given in Table 1. For each class of drugs, adjustment made little or no differ-

Table 2. Use of Individual Drugs, by Cases and Controls

	Cases (%)	Controls (%)
Indomethacin	32	37
Naproxen	32	30
Ibuprofen	18	6
Sulindac	9	7
Diflunisal	6	6
Diclofenac	3	6
Phenylbutazone	0	7

Note: 31 cases and 59 controls used NSAIDs. Each figure is the usage of an individual drug expressed as a percent of total usage of NSAIDs by that group of subjects.

ence to the relative risk estimates. With NSAIDs and aspirin there was no evidence that they were associated with any increase in case fatality rate.

The use of individual drugs by cases and controls is given in Table 2. There was no evidence that any particular agent was associated with a worse prognosis than the others. The numbers were small and any differences between drugs were likely to have occurred by chance.

Because there was no difference between cases and controls in their use of NSAIDs, they were combined in order to compare the usage of the drugs by particular subgroups of patients. As can be seen in Table 3, a higher proportion of women than men took NSAIDs. Usage by patients with duodenal ulcer was almost as high as those with gastric ulcer, and prevalence of NSAID use appeared to be unrelated to the nature of the ulcer complication. As expected, users on average were older than nonusers: mean 73.4 (range 51 to 90) years versus 65.8 (39 to 88) years.

In contrast, corticosteroids seemed to be associated with a reduced survival following hemorrhage or perforation, although the confidence interval for the estimated relative risk was wide and statistical significance was not achieved (Table 1). Examination of the clinical notes of the seven patients taking corticosteroids who died after developing ulcer complications revealed that four died as a result of sepsis, which included three cases of staphylococcal septicemia, of whom two were related to infection of intravenous cannulation sites.

DISCUSSION

This study provides no evidence that use of NSAIDs or aspirin is associated with an increased case fatality rate from bleeding or perforated peptic ulcer. The odds ratios for both classes of drugs were close to unity and were unchanged after adjustment. This suggests that users of the drugs were not "sicker" than nonusers, at least in terms of a higher prevalence of diseases that appeared, in this study, to be associated with a worse prognosis (notably, cerebrovascular disease and chronic liver disease).

As the study did not include a control group without ulcers, it is not possible to estimate directly the relative risk of users of NSAIDs developing peptic ulcer complications. However, the prevalence of the use of NSAIDs was 37% to

Table 3. Use of NSAIDs, by Subgroups

	n	NSAID Users
Men	169	50 (30%)
Women	71	40 (56%)
Duodenal ulcers	110	39 (35%)
Gastric ulcers	130	51 (39%)
Ulcer hemorrhage	166	64 (39%)
Ulcer perforation	74	26 (35%)

Note: For these analyses, cases and controls have been combined.

39%, which is considerably higher than would be expected in the normal population. As part of a 1983 survey of the prevalence of risk factors for coronary heart disease in the Hunter Region of New South Wales, 18% of over 1200 inhabitants aged 50 to 64 years selected from the electoral roll were found to be using NSAIDs. This is higher than the levels of community use recorded in other countries. If this is representative of community use during the period of this study, the levels of use by the cases and controls are compatible with a relative risk for peptic ulcer complications of between 2 and 3. The data indicate that patients with gastric and duodenal ulcers had a similar prevalence of use of NSAIDs, which, in contrast to previous work,[9] supports an elevated relative risk for development of ulcers in both sites. Our data give an estimated population-attributable fraction of between 20% and 30% for ulcer complications in the Newcastle area, which is similar to the figures given in an individually matched case control study conducted in the United Kingdom.[5] As there is no suggestion of an increase in case fatality rate, this study supports the lower of the two estimates of attributable mortality from the United Kingdom.[5] In the state of New South Wales during 1984 there were 1443 cases of ulcer complications in subjects over the age of 60 which resulted in 132 deaths. The data presented here predict that the morbidity and mortality attributable to NSAIDs in New South Wales comprises 300 to 400 cases and 25 to 40 deaths annually.

In contrast to NSAIDs and aspirin, the case fatality rate from peptic ulcer complications appears to be elevated by use of corticosteroids. Although the numbers were small and statistical significance was not achieved, the relative risk was high and the frequency of severe sepsis as a cause of death supported a causal association. Furthermore, adjustment for possible confounders did not reduce the estimated relative risk, although some of the diseases which were indications for corticosteroids were not common enough to be included in the logistic regression analysis. The occurrence of two cases of fatal staphylococcal septicemia arising from an infected intravenous cannulation site indicates the significance of these findings for patients being treated for peptic ulcer complications while on corticosteroids. Clearly this is a group that merits special attention.

CONCLUSION

Our data suggest that the intrinsic toxicity of NSAIDs and aspirin is not very high. NSAIDs may be associated with a doubling or trebling of the risk of ulcer hemorrhage or perforation, but there is no increase in case fatality rate. However, these drugs are very widely used in New South Wales and, as a result, account for 20% to 30% of all cases and deaths from ulcer complications. In comparison, corticosteroids are uncommonly used but their intrinsic toxicity is high, because they appear to be associated with an increased case fatality rate, with, in particular, an increased risk of serious sepsis as a cause of death among corticosteroid users who develop peptic ulcer complications.

REFERENCES

1. Henry DA, Johnston A, Dobson A, et al: Fatal peptic ulcer complications and the use of non-steroidal anti-inflammatory drugs, aspirin and corticosteroids. *Br Med J* 1987;295:1227–1229.
2. Carson JL, Strom BL, Soper KA, et al: The association of nonsteroidal anti-inflammatory drugs with upper gastrointestinal tract bleeding. *Arch Intern Med* 1987;147:85–88.
3. Jick SS, Perera DR, Walker AM, et al: Non-steroidal anti-inflammatory drugs and hospital admission for perforated peptic ulcer. *Lancet* 1987;2:380–382.
4. Bartle WR, Gupta AK, Lazor J: Nonsteroidal anti-inflammatory drugs and gastrointestinal bleeding. A case-control study. *Arch Intern Med* 1986;146:2365–2367.
5. Somerville K, Faulkner G, Langman M: Non-steroidal anti-inflammatory drugs and bleeding peptic ulcers. *Lancet* 1986;1:462–464.
6. Armstrong CP, Blower AL: Non-steroidal anti-inflammatory drugs and life threatening complications of peptic ulceration. *Gut* 1987;28:527–532.
7. Miettinen OS: Estimation of relative risk of individually matched series. *Biometrics* 1970;26:75–86.
8. Breslow NE, Day NE: *Statistical Methods in Cancer Research: The Analysis of Case-Control Studies.* Lyon, World Health Organization, 1980, pp 73–161.
9. Duggan JM, Dobson AJ, Johnson H, et al: Peptic ulcer and nonsteroidal anti-inflammatory agents. *Gut* 1986;27:929–933.

20. *The Relationship Between Rheumatoid Arthritis and Risk of Cancer, Controlling for the Effect of Drugs, in Hospitalized Patients of Saskatchewan, Canada*

PATRICIA TENNIS
ELIZABETH B. ANDREWS
HUGH H. TILSON

INTRODUCTION

Confounding by indication, or the lack of separation of the effect of a drug from the effect of the underlying condition for which the drug is prescribed, can confuse the interpretation of pharmacoepidemiologic studies. This issue has arisen when examining the effect of certain second-line drugs which are used in the treatment of severe rheumatoid arthritis. The second-line drugs include the corticosteroids (predominantly prednisone) and disease-modifying drugs (DMARDs) which consist of general rheumatoid suppressive drugs (penicillamine, gold, chloroquine) and immunosuppressive drugs (azathioprine and methotrexate). It has been suggested that DMARD use may increase risk of neoplasia,[1] especially of the lymphoproliferative type. However, it has also been suggested that the condition of rheumatoid arthritis, which involves a number of abnormalities of the immune system, may itself produce elevated risk of neoplasia.

A number of large prospective epidemiologic studies have compared the risk of neoplasia in the general population with the risk in subjects with rheumatoid arthritis (RA) in an effort to determine if RA is related to elevated risk of neoplasia.[2-4] In none of these studies was drug use controlled for; thus, it is still unclear how much of the observed risks was related to drug use or the underlying condition of rheumatoid arthritis.

The objective of this study is to determine whether there is increased risk of neoplasia associated with rheumatoid arthritis. Therefore, rheumatoid arthritis is considered to be the exposure, neoplasia is the outcome, and the potential confounders which are to be assessed are DMARD use, sex, and age.

The Saskatchewan Health automated data files provide a unique opportunity to address this question. A large number of patients could be identified in the Saskatchewan Hospital Services Plan file, thus allowing a prospective cohort design. By linking with other files through the health registration number, cancer outcomes were identified on the Cancer Foundation data file, drug exposures were identified on the Prescription Drug Plan file, and length of follow-up, i.e. eligibility in the plan, was identified on the Health Information Registration File.

METHODS

The basic rationale of the study involves the comparison of cancer incidence between a cohort of rheumatoid arthritis patients and two sets of controls: general controls and osteoarthritis controls. The osteoarthritis (OA) controls are expected to contain misdiagnosed rheumatoid arthritis (RA) patients and are thus expected to act as an intermediate set of controls. The general controls (CN) consist of hospitalized patients with discharge diagnoses other than RA, OA, and cancer. The three study groups were chosen from the Saskatchewan Hospital Services Plan file on the basis of their discharge diagnoses. All study subjects were chosen from hospitalizations with a discharge date during the period January 1, 1978 to Dec 31, 1980. The RA group was defined as anyone discharged from the hospital with a primary or secondary diagnosis of RA either during or prior to the enrollment period, and the osteoarthritis group was defined as those patients having a primary or secondary discharge of OA prior to or during the enrollment period. Both the OA and CN groups were matched to the RA group by date of enrollment and sex and age (5-yr age groups) at first discharge of the enrollment period. The study was designed to have a 6:1 ratio of CN to RA and a 2:1 ratio of OA to RA, but a ratio of 1.5:1 OA to RA was actually obtained.

Exclusions

Those dying at enrollment were excluded in order to obtain follow-up data on all subjects. In order to rule out people who were in the hospital because of early symptoms of undiagnosed cancer, anyone having a diagnosis of cancer up to one year after enrollment was excluded. In addition, those under the age of 30 were excluded in order to eliminate people with juvenile RA. In order to reduce the probability of misclassification of exposure, discharge diagnoses of other rheumatic diseases were used to exclude people from all three study groups. Such diagnoses might indicate incorrect diagnoses of what is truly RA in the CN and OA groups, and in the RA group they might indicate diagnoses that are incorrectly identified as RA.

Outcomes

Because of the high mortality and relatively short follow-up time per RA patient,[5-10] we adjusted outcome rates for follow-up time. For each subject follow-up started at one year after the first hospitalization during the enrollment period, and ended at whichever of the following came first: the first diagnosis date of cancer, date of death, date of last registration, or January 1, 1987, the last date for which data were available. Age-specific incidences were calculated by dividing number of cases for each 5-yr age group by the total amount of follow-up time for that age group. Then a directly age-adjusted incidence rate was calculated for each sex and study group by adjusting to the age distribution of the female RA group.

Several cancer outcomes were used. Total cancers were all neoplasms, excluding skin cancers, reproductive female cancers (largely cervical cancer), male reproductive cancers (largely prostate cancer), and *in situ* cancers. Incidence rates were calculated separately for each of the following: (1) the female reproductive cancers, (2) male reproductive cancers, (3) skin cancer, and (4) lymphoma, leukemia, and myeloma, which form a subset of total cancers, but were singled out because of past reported associations with RA.

Exposure

Because prednisone use was commonly linked with DMARD use, prednisone and DMARDs were combined into a single DMARD exposure category. Exposure was categorically defined as ever or never having any prescription for any of the included drugs. However, because of latency periods required for neoplasias, a neoplasia was attributed to drug exposure only if the exposure occurred at least one year prior to the diagnosis of the neoplasia. Therefore, DMARD-exposed subjects included those with any prescriptions in the DMARD category up to one year prior to the end of the follow-up period.

Data Quality Control and Validity

In an effort to minimize errors that occur in any large data base, a number of logical checks were performed, and consequently, exclusions of subjects and deletions of records were made:

- Deletion of duplicate hospitalizations (1090/110,000 records)
- Deletion of duplicate drug prescriptions (15,515/620,000 records)
- Exclusion of subjects if hospital file birthdate and registration file birthdate were different by more than 2.5 yr (387 subjects)
- Exclusion of subjects if inactivity date listed in registration file was earlier than enrollment date (seven subjects)
- Deletion of hospitalizations with the incorrect sex (110/110,000 records)
- If hospitalizations overlapped, then the length of the shorter hospitalization was subtracted from the length of the longer hospitalization (5000/110,000 hospitalizations)

Table 1. Comparison of Characteristics of Each Study Group, by Sex

	Females			Males		
	CN	OA	RA	CN	OA	RA
N	4720	1256	892	1906	597	343
Percentage of cohort	71.2	67.8	72.2	28.8	32.2	27.8
Mean age (yr)	63.4	69.3	64.9	62.4	65.6	62.9
Mean no. of hospitalizations in 3 yr prior to enrollment	1.7	3.0	2.7	1.8	2.5	2.7
Median length (days) of hospitalizations in 3 yr prior to enrollment	7	9	10	7	9	10

Note: CN = general controls; OA = osteoarthritis patients; RA = rheumatoid arthritis patients.

In addition, hospital charts for 150 subjects from each study group are being abstracted in order to determine the amount of misclassification of RA exposure. A pilot study of the abstract form showed that of 40 people discharged from the hospital with a diagnosis of RA made by a rheumatologist, 95% met the American Rheumatism Association criteria for RA.[11]

RESULTS

After making all exclusions and deletions from the original 13,333 subjects enrolled, 9714 subjects contributed follow-up time to the study (Table 1). The three study groups were fairly comparable, although there were some slight differences. As expected, each group was predominantly female. The OA group had a higher frequency of males and was slightly older than the RA and CN groups. With respect to hospitalization history (mean number of hospitalizations and median duration of hospitalizations during the three years prior to enrollment), the OA and RA were more comparable to each other than the CN group, and they tended to spend more time in the hospital than the CN group.

Table 2 describes the percentage of each study group, by sex, receiving prescriptions for drugs commonly used in the treatment of RA. NSAID prescriptions were comparable in the RA and OA groups and were more common in these two groups than in the CN group. DMARD prescriptions were most common in the RA group, and the diversity of these drugs was much greater in the RA group. The OA and CN groups were predominantly prescribed prednisone, whereas the RA group was most commonly prescribed prednisone, but received the other disease-modifying drugs chloroquine, penicillamine, gold, methotrexate, and azathioprine, as well. The difference in composition of these drugs within each group should be kept in mind when comparing different study groups.

Table 2. Prescriptions for Drugs Commonly Used to Treat Rheumatoid Arthritis: Percentage of Each Study Group, by Sex, Ever Receiving Such a Prescription

	Females			Males		
	CN	OA	RA	CN	OA	RA
N	4720	1256	892	1906	597	343
NSAIDs	77.5	95.6	97.6	66.6	92.8	95.6
Any DMARDs	16.3	22.2	66.5	14.9	18.6	66.3
chloroquine	0.9	1.0	16.4	0.6	1.0	13.7
penicillamine	0.1	0.1	30.0	0.2	0.3	29.4
gold	0.3	0.5	27.2	0	0.3	25.4
methotrexate	0	0	2.5	0	0	0.6
azathioprine	0.04	0.1	7.5	0.1	0.2	9.3
prednisone	15.2	21.3	48.0	14.5	17.1	50.2
Corticosteroids other than prednisone	5.0	12.3	14.8	4.5	8.5	17.8

Note: CN = general controls; OA = osteoarthritis patients; RA = rheumatoid arthritis patients.

In Figure 1, the age-adjusted incidences of total cancer are plotted by sex and by study groups. For females, the RA group clearly does not have an elevated incidence of cancer compared to the other two groups. The males, on the other hand, have somewhat greater incidence of cancer in the RA group when compared with the CN or the OA group. If the RA group is limited to those who have seen a rheumatologist (thus excluding people more likely to be

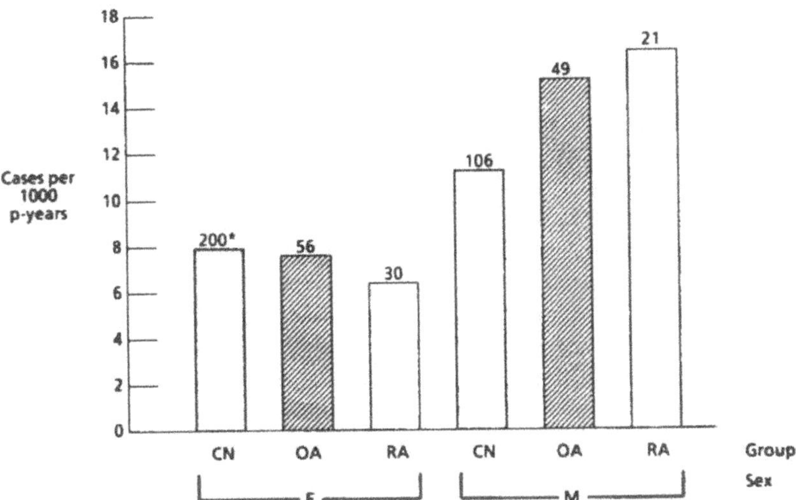

* Number of cases.

Figure 1. Age-adjusted incidence of total cancer, excluding reproductive cancers, skin cancers, and *in situ* cancers, by group and by sex.

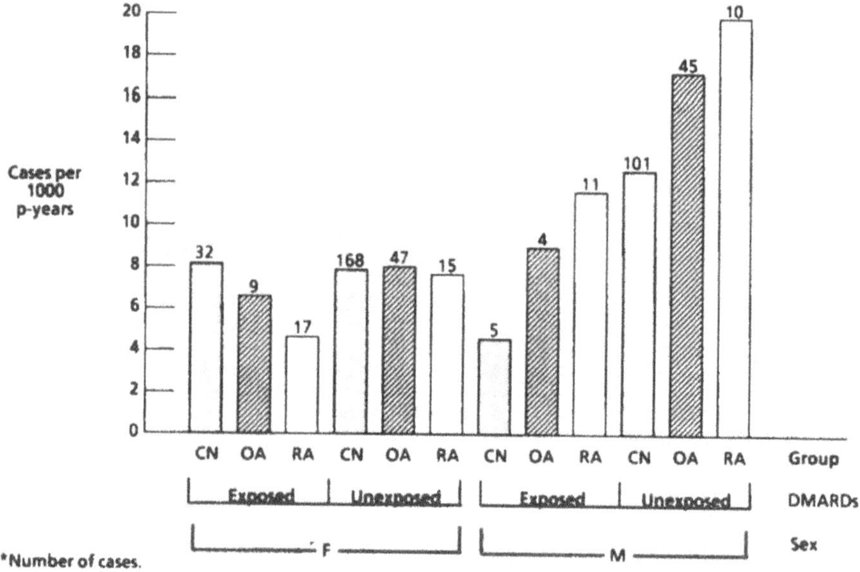

Figure 2. Age-adjusted incidence of total cancer, by group, sex, and DMARD exposure.

misdiagnosed as RA), the cancer incidence pattern is accentuated with an even lower incidence (4.95 cases/1000 p-yrs) for the female RAs and a higher incidence (20.4 cases/1000 p-yrs) for the male RAs. In Figure 2, the incidence of total cancer is shown by sex, group, and DMARD exposure. For the females, whether exposed or unexposed, the RA group does not have elevated incidence of cancer. However, for the males, whether exposed or unexposed, the RA group has the highest incidence of cancer. In addition, within each study group, the males exposed to second-line drugs tend to have lower incidence of cancer than the males unexposed, whereas the exposed women tend to have incidences similar to the unexposed.

A multivariate model (Cox Proportional Hazards Model) was used to adjust for age and sex and to estimate the effects of the RA and second-line drug use on a number of neoplastic outcomes (Table 3). When sex and age were the only other variables included in the model, the hazard ratios for RA were not significantly different from 1.0 for any of the outcomes, when compared with either the CN or the OA group. When DMARD exposure was added to the model, adjusting for DMARD use, RA still did not show a significant association with any of the outcomes examined (Table 4). However, the coefficient for DMARD use, controlling for study group, age, and sex, revealed a significant and negative association of total cancer with DMARD use. This unexpected result suggests questions regarding the comparability of DMARD category across the three study groups. Thus, an approach that does not involve all DMARD and RA exposure categories was considered more appropriate.

Table 3. Effect of Rheumatoid Arthritis, Controlling for Age and Sex: Hazard Ratios from Cox Proportional Hazards Model

	Hazard Ratios for RA	
Cancer Outcomes	**Compared with CN**	**Compared with OA**
Total cancer	0.91	0.83
Lymphoma, leukemia, and myeloma	1.12	0.68
Female reproductive	1.0	1.38
Male reproductive	1.53	1.03
Skin	0.95	0.68

Note: CN = general controls; OA = osteoarthritis patients.

Table 4. Effects of Rheumatoid Arthritis and Disease-Modifying Drugs, Controlling for Age and Sex: Hazard Ratios from Cox Proportional Hazards Model

	Compared with CN		Compared with OA	
Cancer Outcomes	**RA**	**DMARDs**	**RA**	**DMARDs**
Total cancer	1.04	0.76*	1.0	0.63†
Lymphoma, leukemia, and myeloma	1.08	1.07	0.52	1.68
Female reproductive	1.35	0.47	2.03	0.36
Male reproductive	1.71	0.77	0.93	0.89
Skin	1.08	0.76	0.72	0.88

Note: CN = general controls; OA = osteoarthritis patients; RA = rheumatoid arthritis patients; DMARDs = patients taking disease-modifying drugs (general rheumatoid suppressive drugs and immunosuppressive drugs).

* $p = 0.057$.

† $p = 0.025$.

The effect of RA on risk of neoplasia may be better assessed by limiting analysis to subjects who were never exposed to DMARDs. In this situation, comparison of cancer incidence across the groups will not be confounded by differing DMARD composition. When multivariate analysis is used to control for the effects of age and sex (Table 5), none of the cancer outcomes was associated with RA.

The effect of DMARDs on risk of neoplasia can be assessed by limiting the

Table 5. Effect of Rheumatoid Arthritis in Patients Unexposed to Disease-Modifying Drugs, Controlling for Age and Sex: Hazard Ratios from Cox Proportional Hazards Model

	Compared with CN		Compared with OA	
Cancer Outcomes	**No. Cases**	**Hazard Ratio**	**No. Cases**	**Hazard Ratio**
Total cancer	292	1.08	115	0.93
Lymphoma, leukemia, and myeloma	31	0.43	13	0.33
Female reproductive	33	1.58	10	2.45
Male reproductive	32	1.75	16	1.18
Skin	116	0.98	52	0.72

Note: $p > 0.10$ for all.

CN = general controls; OA = osteoarthritis patients.

analysis to the RA group and comparing the DMARD-exposed patients to the DMARD-unexposed. When controlling for age and sex through multivariate modeling, except for one outcome, all the hazard ratios for DMARD use are under 1.0 and are not statistically different from 1.0. The exception is lymphoma, leukemia, and myeloma with a hazard ratio of 3.4. Because of the small number of cases (seven cases), however, the 95% confidence limits for this hazard ratio range from 0.4 to 29. Because these are the cancers reported to be associated with DMARD use and with RA, this is an interesting finding; however, it is unclear whether it is a chance finding.

DISCUSSION

The objective of this retrospective cohort study was to determine if, after controlling for the effect of DMARD use, people with rheumatoid arthritis are at increased risk of neoplasia. Out of 13,333 hospitalized RA, OA, and CN patients in Saskatchewan, 9714 met the stringent inclusion criteria and contributed follow-up time to the study. When specific cancer incidences in the RA group were compared to the CN or the OA groups, there was no significant elevation of cancer in the RA group. When DMARD exposure across the three groups was controlled for, by using a multivariate model or by eliminating DMARD users, there was no significant increase in any neoplastic outcomes for the RA group compared with either the CN or OA groups.

Although there was no statistically significant increase in cancer associated with RA, the across-group pattern of total cancer incidence in the male RAs was consistent with the hypothesis of cancer associated with RA. That is, the lowest incidence occurred in the CN group and the highest incidence occurred in the RA group, even when stratified by DMARD use. This observation is consistent with other studies which have observed excess neoplasias or mortality from neoplasia in male RA subjects but not female RA subjects.[1,12] If risk of cancer were related to severity of RA and males had more severe RA than females, it is possible that a relation between cancer and RA would be most readily detected in men. However, the data on drug use and hospitalizations do not support the hypothesis that males have more severe RA than women, and the smaller numbers of men in this study make it difficult to differentiate chance findings from real associations.

Surprisingly, DMARD use was associated with significantly decreased total cancer when the study group was controlled in a multivariate model. However, in the RA group the DMARD exposure involved use of prednisone and DMARDs, while in the OA and CN groups DMARD exposure involved use of prednisone predominantly. The coefficient in the model represents the average effect of DMARD use across all three study groups. In the next phase of this study it will be important to separate steroid use from the DMARD category.

Within the RA group, DMARD use was not associated with a significant increase in any of the neoplasias. However, the estimated hazard ratio for

Table 6. Comparison of Variables Available to Check for Misclassification of Rheumatoid Arthritis: Percentage of Each Study Group, by Sex, Who Are Known to Have Received Health Care from a Rheumatologist

	Females			Males		
	CN	OA	RA	CN	OA	RA
Percentage ever hospitalized by rheumatologist	0.9	4.5	54.8	1.1	3.8	51.6
Percentage ever receiving prescription by rheumatologist	2.4	6.5	50.6	1.6	4.4	48.1
Percentage ever hospitalized or receiving prescription by rheumatologist	3.0	8.9	61.4	2.6	6.5	58.0

Note: CN = general controls; OA = osteoarthritis patients; RA = rheumatoid arthritis patients.

lymphoma, leukemia, and myeloma was somewhat elevated for DMARD use. Because of the low numbers of cases of these neoplasias it is unclear whether this is a chance finding. In addition, the combination of outcomes into one category and the combination of drugs into one category may mask a true association between a single drug and a specific neoplasia; however, the small number of RA subjects exposed to any one drug would make such an analysis uninterpretable. Because the focus of the current study was to measure the effect of RA, not the effect of a specific drug, numbers of subjects exposed to specific drugs was small. Nevertheless, the apparent success of this methodology suggests the feasibility of developing a still larger study of drug effects within this population.

Despite the measures used to control for RA and DMARD use, confounding by indication could still exist if risk for lymphoma, leukemia, and myeloma is directly related to severity of RA, and severity of RA is related to DMARD use. Unfortunately, it was not possible in this study to identify a group with RA severity similar to the DMARD group but not exposed to DMARDs.

As with any automated data set, other confounders not controlled because of lack of information may mask true associations; however, there is no reason to believe that important life-style factors would be differentially distributed over the three study groups. Nevertheless, these are hospitalized patients, and potentially confounding drugs not controlled in the analysis could be differentially distributed across the three groups.

An overall picture of the validity of exposure classification can be obtained by examining the frequency of health care by a rheumatologist within each group (Table 6). If we assume that those in the RA group who have been hospitalized by a rheumatologist or who have drugs prescribed by a rheumatologist have been correctly diagnosed, then we can estimate that the maximum amount of misclassification in this group is 40%; however, it is most certain that not all RAs who do not receive care from a rheumatologist are misdiagnosed. The 3% of the CN group who receive care by a rheumatologist suggests that there could be a small amount of misclassification of RA into this group. Completion of the ongoing hospital chart abstractions of a 10% subsample of this cohort will give a better estimate of the amount of misclassification in the RA group. As a check of the validity of the results reported here, analyses can be repeated including only RA subjects who receive care from a rheumatologist and excluding CN subjects who receive care from a rheumatologist. Numbers will be reduced, but the likelihood of less misclassification of exposure would make such an analysis desirable.

Although one must use caution in using an automated data set for purposes other that those for which it was developed, this data set has been very useful in addressing the question at hand. A relatively large sample size remained after stringent exclusion criteria were applied, it was completed in less than one year, it was relatively inexpensive for the sample size, and although it may have its own set of biases, it is unbiased relative to *a priori* knowledge of the study question. Such a data set can be a powerful tool if used with discretion.

ACKNOWLEDGMENTS

We would like to thank Saskatchewan Health for permission to use their data. In addition, we would like to acknowledge the very helpful advice of Dr. Claire Bombardier, Dr. Don Mitchell, and Dr. Barbara Hulka in the design of various aspects of this study.

REFERENCES

1. Hazleman BL, DeSilva, M: The comparative incidence of malignant disease in rheumatoid arthritis exposed to different treatment regimens. *Ann Rheum Dis* 1982;41(Suppl):12–17.
2. Isomaki HA, Hakulinen T, Joutsenlahti U: Excess risk of lymphomas, leukemia, and myeloma in patients with rheumatoid arthritis. *J Chron Dis* 1978;31:691–696.
3. Prior P, Symmons DPM, Hawkins CH, et al: Cancer morbidity in rheumatoid arthritis. *Ann Rheum Dis* 1984;43:128–131.
4. Katusic S, Beard CM, Kurland LT, et al: Occurrence of malignant neoplasms in the Rochester, Minnesota, rheumatoid arthritis cohort. *Am J Med* 1985;78(Suppl 1A):50–55.
5. Monson RR, Hall AP: Mortality among arthritics. *J Chron Dis* 1976;29:459–467.
6. Koota K, Isomaki H, Mutru O: Death rate and causes of death in RA patients during a period of five years. *Scand J Rheumatology* 1977;6:241–244.
7. Lewis P, Hazleman BL, Hanka R, et al: Cause of death in patients with rheumatoid arthritis with particular reference to azathioprine. *Ann Rheum Dis* 1980;39:457–461.
8. Allenbeck P, Ahlbom A, Allander E: Increased mortality among persons with rheumatoid arthritis, but where RA does not appear on death certificates. *Scan J Rheum* 1981;10:301–306.

9. Vandenbroucke JP, Hazevot HA, Cats A: Survival and cause of death in rheumatoid arthritis: A 25-year prospective follow-up. *J Rheum* 1984;11:158–161.
10. Mitchell DM, Spitz PW, Young DY, et al: Survival, prognosis, and causes of death in rheumatoid arthritis. *Arthritis Rheum* 1986;29:706–714.
11. *Primer on the Rheumatic Diseases*, ed 8. Rodnan GP, Schumacher HR (eds): Atlanta, GA, Arthritis Foundation, 1983.
12. Speerstra F, Boerbooms AM TH, Van De Putte LBA, et al: Side-effects of azathioprine treatment in rheumatoid arthritis: Analysis of 10 years of experience. *Ann Rheum Dis* 1982;41(Suppl):37–39.

21. *Collaborative Study of the Effects of Acyclovir in Pregnancy*

ELIZABETH B. ANDREWS
HUGH H. TILSON
JOSÉ F. CORDERO
E. RUSSELL ALEXANDER
KATHERINE M. STONE
SEVGI O. ARAL
MICHAEL ROSENBERG
BARRY HURN
L. GRAY DAVIS

INTRODUCTION

The epidemiologic, postapproval study of the reproductive effects of any drug poses numerous methodologic and practical challenges. While no ideal method has been found to identify a small increase in reproductive risks associated with any new drug, and specifically with acyclovir as a new product, a variety of mechanisms has been assembled to assure that a large increase in the risk of birth defects could be detected quickly using methods that minimize potential biases. This effort required the professional and institutional collaboration of Centers for Disease Control, the American Social Health Association, Teratology Information Resources, and the international network of Wellcome companies. A case-registration approach is described to illustrate this collaboration.

BACKGROUND

Acyclovir, marketed as Zovirax, is a nucleoside analog for antiviral chemotherapy specific for the herpes simplex virus (HSV). It was first marketed in oral formulation in the United States in January of 1985, indicated for the treatment and suppression of genital herpes. Three factors prompted decisions to evaluate the safety of acyclovir when used during pregnancy despite the lack of evidence of any substantial problems from preclinical reproductive and genetic toxicity tests.[1,2] First was the theoretic teratogenic potential of any new chemical entity and the historic precedent of other less specific antivirals that have caused genetic damage.[3] Second was the likelihood of unintentional exposures during pregnancy, since the treatment population includes significant numbers of sexually active women of childbearing age. Experience in large health maintenance organizations demonstrates that women between 15 and 45 years of age receive at least 40% of new prescriptions for oral acyclovir (Burroughs Wellcome Co., unpublished data). Third was the opportunity afforded by the decision to examine the overall safety experience with the drug, once in general use in a population large enough to detect the occurrence of relatively rare adverse outcomes, given the low expected rates of exposure.

METHODOLOGIC ISSUES

Primarily because of the high exposure potential among women of reproductive age, a program of perinatal monitoring was undertaken as a component of Wellcome's extensive general safety monitoring program for acyclovir, which includes observational epidemiologic studies in large health maintenance organizations. Several methodologic issues arose, however, that were specific to the study of reproductive outcomes.

One of the most challenging problems facing this project was the need for a sample size large enough to permit the study of rare events. Detection of any but an extremely large increase in the risk of specific birth defects would require the observation of immensely large numbers of pregnancies because of the low frequency of birth defects and the low rates of exposure. It is estimated that 6 out of 1000 women 15–44 years of age in the United States take oral acyclovir each year (Burroughs Wellcome Co., unpublished data). Use of data bases from any single large health maintenance organization, a traditional resource for drug safety monitoring, would be insufficient to address the teratogenicity question. For example, it was estimated that fewer than 20 live births over a three-year period would be exposed to acyclovir at Group Health Cooperative of Puget Sound, with 360,000 plan members. Moreover, the low exposure rate also lowered expectations about the feasibility of a case-control study of birth defects.

Figure 1 further illustrates the sample size problem: monitoring of approximately 1600 live births following first trimester acyclovir use would be required to detect a fivefold increase in the risk of specific defects that occur as frequently as 1 per 1000 live births; 250 would be required to detect a 20-fold increase.

Large systems for monitoring birth defects, another traditional resource, are unable to discover an increase in the population rate of specific defects associated with new exposures unless the exposure rate is high and the magnitude of the increase is great. Such programs include the Metropolitan Atlanta program

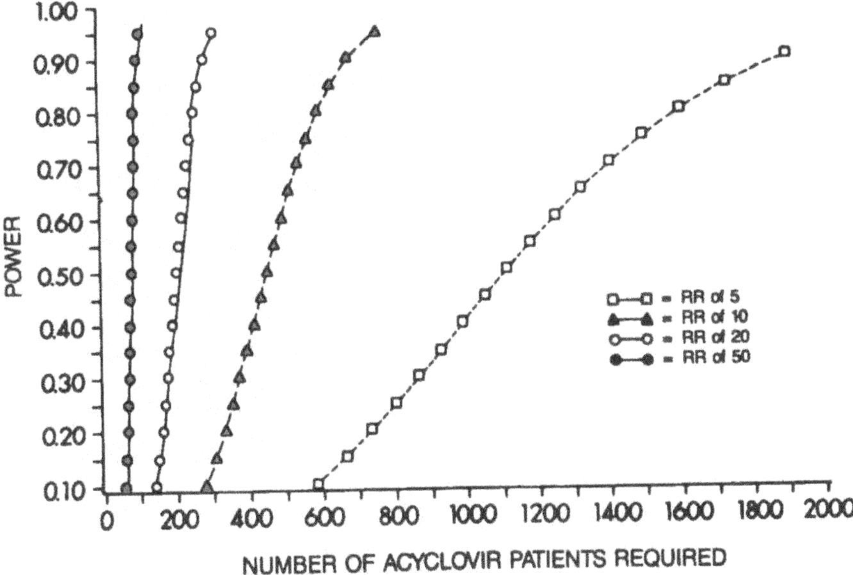

Figure 1. Power curves for a one-sided test. Assumes 0.1% of population comparison group will have specific defects.

that monitors 25,000 births and the nationwide Birth Defects Monitoring Program that monitors 1 million births annually.[4] This limitation was demonstrated in a recent examination of this methodology through the example of valproic acid, which increases 20-fold the risk of spina bifida (which normally occurs in 1 of 1000 live births). One million births in the population would need to be monitored in order to detect an increase in the population rate of spina bifida attributable to valproic acid, given that the exposure rate of valproic acid was 3 per 1000 pregnancies and that valproic acid-associated cases of spina bifida would represent only a small proportion of total cases. (It should be noted that this association was originally detected through a birth defects surveillance program that reviews approximately 80,000 birth defects per year.) Such programs alone would only detect abnormalities associated with acyclovir use if the exposure rate were greater than anticipated and the effect on rates of abnormalities extremely high.

The second problem in assessing potential reproductive risks of acyclovir is the difficulty of discriminating between the effects of acyclovir and the effects of HSV in the absence of an untreated HSV comparison group. Reported adverse reproductive effects associated with HSV include spontaneous abortion; fetal infection that could affect the skin, eye, central nervous system, and general growth and development of the fetus; and neonatal herpes.[6] Because most of this evidence is based on individual case reports and small studies of women with primary herpes during pregnancy, the magnitude of the increase among persons similar to the acyclovir-treated population (with primary and recurrent herpes) has not been estimated. There are not sufficient data to determine if an association exists between HSV and birth defects. An association between HSV and adverse reproductive outcomes could create a spurious association between acyclovir and adverse outcomes when studied in the absence of baseline HSV risk data. Therefore, in addition to needing a large sample size, data on the risks associated with herpes are needed to fully assess the potential risk of acyclovir.

A third methodologic problem is the potential for bias in voluntary retrospective reporting of reproductive outcomes. Through these systems, such as adverse drug experience reporting systems, physicians generally report abnormal rather than normal outcomes. Moreover, even abnormal outcomes are generally underreported. A voluntary registry of exposures to isotretinoin, a known human teratogen, demonstrated a significant difference in rates of abnormalities among pregnancies reported prospectively (during early pregnancy), and those reported retrospectively (after abnormalities could have been detected). Among infants and fetuses monitored in that program, 5 of 28 (17.9%) prospective cases and 16 of 19 (84.2%) retrospective cases involved abnormalities.[7] Additionally, even with prospective reporting of exposures, selective reporting of pregnancy outcomes is possible if follow-up is incomplete.

OVERALL STUDY PLAN

The overall plan for studying the safety of acyclovir took these methodologic problems into consideration in establishing objectives. For example, given the estimated exposure rate of oral acyclovir, it would be possible to detect only a large increase in the risk of specific birth defects. The following objectives were established: (1) to identify as many exposed pregnancies as possible and as quickly as possible, (2) to document the risks of birth defects associated with herpes itself, and (3) to minimize the biases associated with ascertainment of outcomes. A multiplicity of approaches was taken to attempt to meet these objectives.

Among the approaches were record-linkage general safety studies in at least two health maintenance organizations. These data bases provided the ability to detect exposed pregnancies and identify their outcomes efficiently. Additionally, other outcomes that might also be related to an increase in birth defects were studied.[8] Spontaneous abortions, which occur more frequently than birth defects, could be assessed in a population where pregnancies are detected early and reflected in the data bases. Because spontaneous abortions are more frequent, fewer exposed pregnancies need to be studied. Additionally, women with genital herpes and no exposure to acyclovir could be studied to begin documenting the rates of abnormal outcomes associated with herpes itself.

THE ACYCLOVIR IN PREGNANCY REGISTRY

The principal effort to address the safety-in-pregnancy question was through the Acyclovir in Pregnancy Registry, a case-registration study established by Burroughs Wellcome Co. in January 1985. Through the registry, exposed pregnancies reported through a network of organizations are enrolled and followed to gather information on acyclovir exposure, potentially confounding factors, and pregnancy outcome.

An advisory group was assembled which includes representatives from the Division of Sexually Transmitted Diseases and Division of Birth Defects and Developmental Disabilities of the Centers for Disease Control (CDC) and the American Social Health Association (ASHA). The advisory committee actively guides the study and encourages referrals in a manner sensitive to public policy concerns. In guiding the study, the committee oversees methods and materials, and reviews all data prior to the general release of any summary information. In the event of an adverse pregnancy outcome, they assist in case investigation.

The committee plays an active role in stimulating reporting. In this sensitive public policy area, the registry needs to maximize the study size by encouraging exposure reporting. Further, an important function of the registry is to provide clinicians with data to assist in patient care decisions. However, the need to disseminate information must be balanced by caution about possible misinterpretations of the study. Possible misperceptions range from the impression that the drug has been demonstrated to be safe in pregnancy and its use is thereby encouraged in the absence of controlled studies, to the impression that a known teratogenic risk exists, and even motivates the study, when such risk has not been demonstrated. The committee has therefore recommended that distribution of registry information be restricted to selected medical professions, such as obstetricians and gynecologists who might be treating patients who have been or are likely to be exposed during pregnancy.

An additional method of increasing the number of exposures reported to the registry was a referral mechanism established through the advisory committee. Any call received by the Centers for Disease Control or American Social Health Association is referred to the registry. Additionally, all teratology information services are routinely sent information and encouraged to refer exposures to the registry.

INTERIM PROGRESS

Despite the efforts to disseminate information widely to physicians most likely to detect exposures, the progress of the registry in recruiting reports and tracking outcomes has been only moderate. Figure 2 shows the number of reports made to the registry by month. The average number of reports has increased from 4 per month in the first year, to 6 per month in 1986, to 8 per

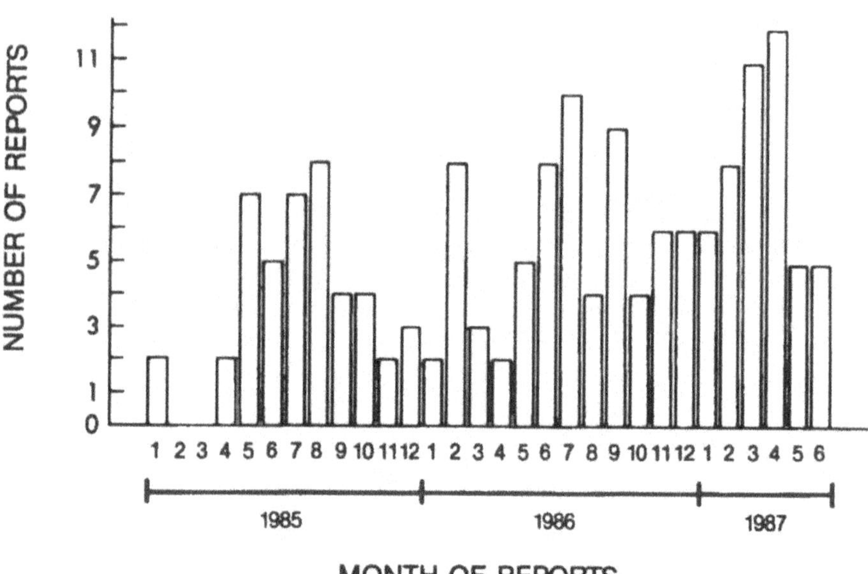

Figure 2. Frequency of reports, by month, January 1, 1985–June 30, 1987.

month in the first six months of 1987. A small increase was seen after an announcement of the registry appeared in March 1987.[9] The 151 reported exposures represent only a fraction of the 2000–3500 prenatal exposures which are estimated to have occurred in the United States, based on exposure rates and U.S. birth rates.[5]

While the U.S. registry is accumulating exposure reports at a moderate pace, an additional source of reports was made available through collaboration with the Wellcome Foundation in London. The medical directors of all Wellcome companies worldwide are encouraged to maintain an active case registration and follow-up system as in the United States and instructed to report all known cases to the Wellcome Foundation, where they are assembled and transmitted to Wellcome in the United States for inclusion in the registry. Through June 30, 1987, an additional 115 cases were reported from 15 other countries.

To minimize potential biases of voluntary case reporting, reports were separated by timing of the report relative to the outcome of pregnancy. Rates of abnormal outcomes were calculated only from cases enrolled prospectively (prior to pregnancy outcome). All reports, prospective and retrospective, were reviewed for patterns of abnormalities.

An additional potential source of reporting bias is selective loss to follow-up. In anticipation of a high rate of patients lost to follow-up, a protocol was established to schedule multiple and prompt reminder letters and telephone calls to the reporting physicians. A microcomputer-assisted tracking file has

Table 1. Acyclovir in Pregnancy Registry: Follow-up Status of Prospectively Monitored U.S. Patients by Trimester of Exposure, January 1, 1985–June 30, 1987

Trimester of Exposure	Outcomes Known	Reports Not Due	Lost to Follow-up	Status Unknown	Total
First	42	36	9	26	113
Second	1	6	0	3	10
Third	8	1	0	5	14
Unkown	0	7	3	4	14
Total	51	50	12	38	151

been maintained to trigger the mailing of data forms at the estimated date of delivery.

Despite efforts to track each case and conduct rigorous follow-up, the rate of confirmed follow-up has been approximately 50%. As shown in Table 1, of the 151 reports through June 30, 1987, 33% were not eligible for follow-up since the patients had not yet delivered. Of the remaining cases, outcomes were known for 50.5%. An additional 11.9% had been identified by the reporting physician as "lost to follow-up," and 37.6% were eligible for follow-up (the patient's estimated delivery date had passed), but no information on the outcome had been provided.

Data are summarized in a semiannual report to participating physicians. The most recent report shows that, among outcomes of 42 prospective reports of first trimester exposure in the U.S. registry, no infants with abnormalities have been reported. While the sample size remained small, individual patient experience was also summarized in graphical form, as shown in Figure 3 for three example cases. Dose and indication for acyclovir therapy, timing of

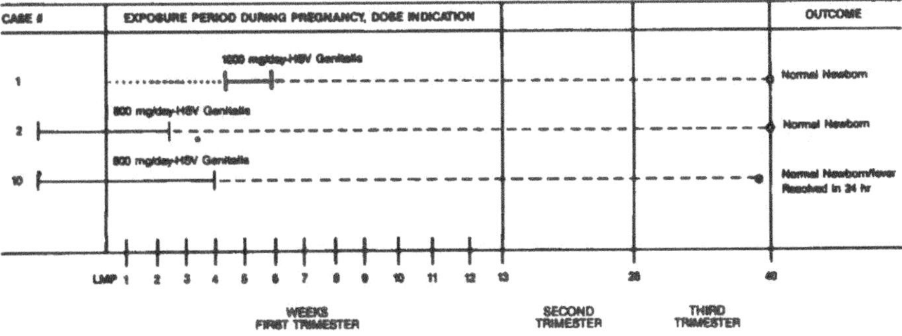

Figure 3. Outcomes among prospectively monitored patients, January 1, 1985–June 30, 1987, example of data.

exposure, and outcome were displayed for each case, enabling clinicians to make direct comparison between their patients and the registry experience.

COMMENT

This collaborative observational study registers and follows all reported pregnancies occurring among women taking acyclovir. Over a 30-month period in the United States, 151 such pregnancies were registered; 113 involved first trimester exposures, of which 42 were monitored to term. The number of first trimester exposures reported to date is too small to justify many conclusions about the safety of acyclovir, and the registry will therefore continue to enroll and follow new cases.

Conclusions based on a sample of this size are limited to the power to detect only major increases in the risks of specific birth defects, for example, a relative risk of 100 over specific defects which occur at a rate of 1 per 1000 live births in the general population. By comparison, a similar registry examining pregnancy outcomes following exposure to isotretinoin, a known strong teratogen, documented an increase in overall birth defects and an increase in selected birth defects with only 36 exposed pregnancies. Despite limitations in this study, there is no indication that acyclovir is associated with such a strong teratogenic effect.

It is possible that reporting of outcomes has been selective, and that the unreported outcomes differ from reported outcomes. Whether any bias actually exists in the current data is unknown. It would be anticipated, however, that the direction of bias would be toward underreporting normal rather than abnormal outcomes.

While no single study can adequately address the teratogenicity question, and even multiple approaches are insufficient to detect small increases in risk, the current approach to acyclovir should enable early detection of any major safety problems. Moreover, the methods used and the collaborative process are an improvement over conventional methods of ascertaining teratogenicity risk from observational data. Through a network of organizations and individuals interested in the safety of drugs during pregnancy, reporting of exposures is encouraged, and thereby the sample size is increased. At the current rate of reporting, it is estimated that 500 first trimester exposures will be monitored through the first five years of experience with oral acyclovir. This would enable the detection of a relative risk of 15 for individual birth defects occurring at a rate of 1 per 1000 live births, and a relative risk of 2 for total defects occurring at a rate of 3 per 100 live births, comparing the registry experience with existing population-based congenital defects registries. In addition, biases inherent in voluntary reporting systems with incomplete follow-up are minimized by the reliance on prospective reports. While even these reports are subject to biases, such biases are significantly less than those in spontaneous, retrospective outcome reporting systems. Additionally, the appropriate comparison group for this study is constituted of pregnancies among women with genital herpes, which are being studied in a companion project.

Moreover, the case-registration approach is substantially strengthened through the collaborative efforts of the Acyclovir in Pregnancy Registry Advisory Committee in three ways. First, there is significantly greater case ascertainment using a network of collaborating institutions. Second, the advisory panel process provides an impartial examination of all registry data. Third, this process provides a mechanism for public policy deliberations and information dissemination.

Finally, the success of such a study depends on the participation of practicing physicians who notify the registry of exposures and provide follow-up information postpartum. The assistance of all reporting physicians is greatly appreciated.

REFERENCES

1. Clive D, Turner NT, Hozier J, et al: Preclinical toxicology studies with acyclovir: Genetic toxicity tests. *Fundam Appl Toxicol* 1983;3:587–602.
2. Moore HL, Szczech GM, Rodwell DE, et al: Preclinical toxicology studies with acyclovir: Teratologic, reproductive and neonatal tests. *Fundam Appl Toxicol* 1983;3:560–568.
3. Briggs GG, Freeman RK, Yaffe SJ: *Drugs in Pregnancy and Lactation*, ed. 2. Baltimore, Williams and Wilkins, 1986, pp 10, 218, 469–470.
4. Edmonds LD, Layde PM, James LM, et al: Cogenital malformation surveillance: Two American systems. *Int J Epidemiol* 1981;10:247–252.
5. Khoury MJ, Holtzman NA: On the ability of birth defects monitoring to detect new teratogens. *Am J Epidemiol* 1987;126:136–143.
6. Guinan ME, Wolinsky SM, Reichman RC: Epidemiology of genital herpes simplex virus infection. *Epidemiol Rev* 1985;7:127–146.
7. Lammer EJ, Chen DT, et al: Retinoic acid embryopathy. *New Eng J Med* 1985;313:837–841.
8. Kline J, Stein Z, Strobino B, et al: Surveillance of spontaneous abortions: Power in environmental monitoring. *Am J Epidemiol* 1977;106:345–350.
9. Acyclovir use during pregnancy charted in national registry. *American College of Obstetricians and Gynecologists Newsletter* 1987;31(3):8–9.

22. *Creutzfeldt-Jakob Disease, Human Growth Hormone, and Its Replacement with Synthetic Growth Hormone*

PETER G. BERNAD

Recently, recombinant DNA technology has enabled the production of human hormones. One such synthetic hormone is a genetically engineered growth hormone for children with congenital or otherwise short stature or life-threatening hypoglycemia, infrequently encountered after birth or in early infancy. Development of the synthetic material has been accelerated most recently in reaction to reports of possible iatrogenic transmission of Creutzfeldt-Jakob disease (CJD).[1] Seven recipients of human pituitary-derived growth hormone (hGH) died of CJD.[1-9] No new cases are known since December 1986. All seven persons died before the age of 40. Recognizing the rarity of CJD, such an association of human growth hormone ingestion and severe neurologic disease has been understandably frightening and of great concern to the medical community. The seven patients had all received their last dose of human growth hormone by the early 1970s. Some authorities have suggested that the similar batches of hGH prepared in the same laboratory (for one New Zealand and three American patients) were contaminated with a CJD agent.[10] It is interesting to note that no such association has been found in any of the European countries producing hGH, that is, in Hungary, Switzerland, Sweden, or in Israel and Japan. The laboratory extraction process and preparation of hGH have undergone significant technological changes, primarily in the 1970s, thus significantly decreasing the likelihood of transmitting CJD.[11]

What is Creutzfeldt-Jakob disease? Two German neurologists first described the clinical features and studied the pathological findings in the condition that bears their names approximately 67 years ago.[12,13] The condition is best characterized as a form of dementia which is frequently very rapid and occasionally subacute, rarely lasting longer than one year. The condition affects both males and females, and the usual onset is after the age of 45. I am not aware of well-described pathologically proven cases of CJD before age 35 except for those seven already mentioned, who had received pituitary-derived human growth hormone therapy. Clinically, the patients present most often with abnormalities in higher cortical functioning: frequent memory lapses, confusion, difficulties with concentration, poor judgment, and decreased attention span. They may go on to have clumsiness, ataxia, and myoclonus. Motor function then deteriorates and patients may end up being institutionalized prior to death. Laboratory tests rule out other treatable causes of dementia.[14] The electroencephalogram shows generalized periodic discharges in a complex consisting of a single wave, usually triphasic in configuration, lasting from 100 to 600 milliseconds (average 360) with an amplitude of about 100 microvolts. This is usually followed by a burst of rhythmical discharge at 3 to 7 hertz or, alternately, a period of flattening for about one second. Periodicity ranging from 0.5 to 4 seconds is seen late in the evolution of the disease. Routine studies such as CT scanning of the brain and magnetic resonance imaging of the brain tend to be normal. Cerebrospinal fluid analysis is not helpful except to rule out other causes of dementing illness. Pathologically, there is a marked spongiform vacuolation of the cortical grey matter as well as astrocytosis and cerebellar atrophy. Similar findings have been noted in other diseases such as kuru, identified in the natural environment in Papua, New Guinea.[15] Kuru has been associated in the past with cannibalism but has become rare since the elimination of such human activity. Scrapie, another condition that is similar, is seen in sheep and goats, and has been seen in Iceland. The other condition that is reminiscent of CJD is transmissible mink encephalopathy. These conditions together have been regarded as forms of "spongiform encephalopathies," or slow transmissible viral diseases.

The recognition that CJD may be transmitted was a medical breakthrough of Nobel Prize dimensions. Initially in reviewing the epidemiology of CJD, clusters of cases were occasionally observed in families and some in marital partners.[16] It was in the late 1960s, after kuru had been transmitted to chimpanzees, that CJD was reported in a chimpanzee after intracerebral and intravenous inoculation with brain material from a patient who had died with CJD.[17] Transmission from chimpanzee to chimpanzee with an incubation period of 12 to 14 months was then demonstrated.[18] Transmission to small primates has also occurred.[19] The finding that iatrogenic transmission of CJD was a possibility was noted first in 1974.[20] This occurred in a female patient who had received a corneal transplant from another patient who had died of CJD. Eighteen months after the transplant, the patient showed signs of CJD and died within eight months. The second report of iatrogenic transmission of CJD occurred three years after that, when there were two cases in patients who had undergone neurosurgical excision of epileptic foci.[21] In both of those cases, the same electrodes were used for deep cortical electroencephalography of brain structures. Apparently they were the same electrodes that had been used in a patient who had unknowingly died from CJD. This occurred in spite of conventional sterilization of the electrodes, which were treated with 70%

ethanol followed by 48-hour exposure to formaldehyde vapor. It has since been recognized that the CJD agent is highly resistant to heat, formaldehyde, and even ionizing radiation. The CJD infectious particle, similar to the scrapie agent, prion, is viral-like but has not as yet been completely characterized.[22] Rod-shaped structures which have been found to cross-react immunologically with scrapie protein have been found in CJD-affected brains.[23] An advisory group had indicated that tissues for transplant should not be harvested from patients who died with dementia and that the pituitary glands from such patients should not be used for the manufacture of hormone preparations.[24] Unfortunately, techniques such as gel filtration and ion exchange chromatography were not available in the 1960s and the 1970s, so that older preparations, coming frequently from single laboratories, may not have been as pure as those using more modern techniques of preparation. Screening techniques may have been less strict in the elimination of pituitaries from suspect cases. Since the middle of the 1980s, with the advent of recombinant DNA technology, synthetic human growth hormone has become available from various pharmaceutical laboratories around the world. Unfortunately, the newer synthetic growth hormone has not been without some medical complications and adverse side effects.

The actual incidence of adverse drug reaction to any new medication is difficult to estimate. One approach to ADR assessment is spontaneous physician and pharmaceutical company reporting to the Spontaneous Reporting System (SRS), Division of Drug and Biological Product Experience (DDBPE) of the Food and Drug Administration. During the first three months of marketing (February to May 1986) Genentech's protropin (met-hGH), 57 adverse reactions were reported to the Food and Drug Administration.[25] These 57 reactions occurred in 22 patients. There were four deaths of patients who were on protropin, and at least two of them were on protropin only. A brief summary of the deaths and the analysis of the adverse reactions follow:

1. A seven-year-old boy with hypopituitarism, hypoglycemia, and seizures since birth developed a flu-like syndrome. This was characterized by fever, vomiting, and diarrhea. The patient's course was complicated by prolonged seizures that resulted in cardiac arrest, coma, and death.
2. A nine-year-old girl had a craniopharyngioma and hypopituitarism. She was on full replacement therapy with protropin. The tumor recurred. She was treated surgically and had cranial irradiation vasculitis.
3. An eight-month-old girl with floppiness at birth, central diabetes insipidus, and growth hormone deficiency had a history of frequent respiratory arrests and episodes of apnea and bradycardia. The patient also had episodes of severe hypoglycemia. She had a cardiorespiratory arrest and required prolonged respiratory therapy prior to death.
4. A 10-year-old boy with growth hormone deficiency, presumably secondary to an intracranial tumor, died suddenly with no immediately preceding symptoms. He had previously undergone surgery, irradiation, and

chemotherapy. Preliminary autopsy results showed a ruptured cerebral aneurysm. This patient was on no other medications except protropin.

The following is a list of other adverse reactions associated with protropin: (1) Addisonian crisis seen in five occurrences; (2) convulsions seen in five occurrences; (3) vomiting seen in four occurrences; (4) hypoglycemia seen in three occurrences; (5) somnolence seen in three occurrences; (6) hypotension seen in two occurrences; (7) a rash seen in two occurrences; (8) somnolence and stupor seen in two occurrences; and (9) tremor seen in one occurrence.

A number of theories may be proposed to explain the relation between this new synthetic growth hormone and the medical adverse reactions described above. An allergic response to met-hGH seems plausible. Other explanations include lack of or inadequate euglycemic effect of the synthetic material. Lack of antiinsulin or procortisol effect or lack of full biological activity are other possible explanations.

These and the rest of the 57 adverse reactions reported in a three-month period of utilization of this synthetic drug should be of some concern to clinicians. I have not become aware of any similar adverse reactions with the use of natural hGH during the 25 or more years of its clinical use, even though only recently a great deal of appropriate concern has been raised about the association of natural hGH therapy in the 1950s and 1960s with iatrogenic CJD. These adverse reactions are of concern to treating physicians and to the medical community at large. Although protropin has been associated with each of the reactions in the 22 patients, including the four deaths, a causal relationship remains to be established. All adverse reactions to any new drugs should be carefully scrutinized to reach accurate conclusions rather than those based on a variation of the old ecologic fallacy, which would lead to spurious associations.

Other potential medical problems have been reported with synthetic GH, using both the natural sequence synthetic materials from Eli Lilly & Company and the methionyl growth hormone from Genentech, Inc. These problems include risk of hypoglycemia, with alternate-day synthetic GH injections.[26] Fasting hypoglycemia developed in three growth hormone-deficient children after the start of treatment with synthetic GH. This activity, which occurred 36 to 60 hours after each injection, may have been due to insulinoid effects of endogenous somatomedins after weaning of insulin antagonism induced by growth hormone. In this particular study, daily growth hormone injections were recommended to maintain normal plasma glucose levels in young children requiring growth hormone replacement. The knowledge concerning human growth hormone, both synthetic and pituitary-derived, has increased so that potential medical and neurological adverse effects may be eliminated in the not too distant future. The synthetically produced, genetically engineered replacement growth hormones have their own share of medical problems as seen above. Immunogenicity may be a problem, partly because synthetic growth hormones contain an extra methionyl residue as an amino acid terminal. This amino acid has been the starting point from which the *Escherichia coli*, used for the manufacture of GH, makes the protein chain. Traces of *E. coli* antigens are also present in the preparation. It is hoped that future preparations of synthetic GH will not have this extra amino acid as in natural-sequence synthetic GH, and that pure monoclonal proteins will be made. Whatever the drawbacks or problems associated with any synthetic material, it is reasonable to expect that this material does not have the potential to transmit CJD. Further research is still necessary to develop the ideal growth hormone replacement for symptomatic patients.

REFERENCES

1. Koch TK, Berg BO, De Armand SD, et al: Creutzfeldt-Jacob disease in a young adult with idiopathic hypopituitarism and possible relationship to administration of cadaver human growth hormone. *N Engl J Med* 1985;313:731–733.
2. Cibbs CJ Jr, Joy A, Heffner R, et al: Clinical and pathological features and laboratory confirmation of Creutzfeldt-Jakob disease in a recipient of pituitary-derived human growth hormone. *N Engl J Med* 1985;313:734–738.
3. Powell-Jackson J, Weller RO, Kennedy P, et al: Creutzfeldt-Jakob disease after administration of human growth hormone. *Lancet* 1985;ii:244–246.
4. Tintner R, Brown P, Hedley-Whyte T, et al: Neuropathologic verification of Creutzfeldt-Jakob in the exhumed American recipient of human pituitary growth hormone: Epidemiologic and pathogenetic implications. *Neurology* 1986;36:932–936.
5. Croxson M, Brown P, Synek B, et al: A new case of Creutzfeldt-Jakob disease associated with human growth hormone therapy in New Zealand. *Neurology* 1988;38:1128–1130.
6. Marzewski DJ, Towfighi J, Harrington MG, et al: Creutzfeldt-Jakob disease following pituitary-derived human growth therapy: A new American case. *Neurology* 1988;38:1133–1134.
7. New MI, Brown P, Teneck JW, et al: Preclinical Creutzfeldt-Jakob disease discovered at autopsy in a human growth hormone recipient. *Neurology* 1988;38:1133–1134.
8. Hintz R, MacGillivray JA, Tintner R: Fatal degenerative neurologic disease in patients who received pituitary derived human growth hormone. *MMWR* 1985;34:359–366.
9. Brown P, Gajdusek CD, Gibbs CJ, et al: A potential epidemic of Creutzfeldt-Jacob disease from human growth hormone therapy. *New Engl J Med* 1985;313:728–731.
10. Brown P: The decline and fall of Creutzfeldt-Jakob disease associated with human growth hormone therapy. *Neurology* 1988;38:1135–1137.
11. Chapman GE, Renwick AGC, Livesey JH: The isolation of human pituitary hormones from frozen glands. *J Clin Endocrinol Metabol* 1981;53:1008–1013.

12. Creutzfeldt HG: Uber eine eigenartige herdformige Erkrankung des Zentralnervensystems. *Ztschr f d ges neurol u Psychiat*, Berlin, 1920;57:1–18.
13. Jakob A: Uber eigenartige Erkrankungen des Zentralnervensystems mit bemerkens-werten anatomischen Befunde. (Spastiscke Pseudosklerose-Encephalomyelopathie mit disseminierten Degenerationsherden). *Ztschr f d ges neurol u Psychiat*, Berl Orig, 1921;64:147–228.
14. Klass WD, Daly DD (eds): *Current Practice of Clinical Electroencephalography*. New York, Raven Press, 1980.
15. Prusiner SB, Hadlow WJ (eds): Epidemiology and ecology of kuru, in *Slow Transmissible Diseases of the Nervous System*. New York, Academic Press, 1979, vol 1.
16. Matthews WB: Epidemiology of Creutzfeldt-Jakob disease in England and Wales. *J Neurol Neurosurg Psychiatry* 1975;38:210–213.
17. Gibbs CJ, Gajdusek DC, Asher DM, et al: Creutzfeldt-Jakob disease (spongiform encephalopathy) transmission to the chimpanzee. *Science* 1968;161:388–389.
18. Gibbs CJ, Gajdusek DC: Infection as the etiology of spongiform encephalopathy (Creutzfeldt-Jakob disease). *Science* 1969;165:1023–1025.
19. Zlotnick I, Grant DP, Dayan, et al: Transmission of Creutzfeldt-Jakob disease from man to squirrel monkey. *Lancet* 1974;ii:435–438.
20. Duffy P, Wolf J, Collins G, et al: Possible person to person transmission of Creutzfeldt-Jakob disease. *New Engl J Med* 1974;290:692.
21. Bernoulli C, Siegfried J, Baumgartner G, et al: Danger of accidental person to person transmission of Creutzfeldt-Jakob disease by surgery. *Lancet* 1077;i:478–479.
22. Prusiner SB: Prions: Novel infectious pathogens. *Adv Virus Res* 1984;29:1–56.
23. Bockman JM, Kingsbury DT, McKinley MP, et al: Creutzfeldt-Jakob disease prion proteins in human brains. *New Engl J Med* 1985;312:73–78.
24. *Report of the Advisory Group on the Management of Patients with Spongiform Encephalopathy (Creutzfeldt-Jakob Disease [CJD])*. Department of Health and Social Security Circular DA (84) 16, 1981.
25. FDA Report, 1986.
26. Press M, Notarfrancesco A: Risk of hypoglycemia with alternate-day growth hormone injection. *Lancet* 1987;i:1002–1004.

23. *Retrovir: The Challenge of Postmarketing Surveillance*

MICHAEL C. JOSEPH
TERRI CREAGH-KIRK

INTRODUCTION

This chapter covers the wide spectrum of the social, political, regulatory, and medical aspects of the AIDS epidemic and shows the uniqueness of Retrovir® development, testing, and surveillance—with an emphasis on public health and regulatory issues. We will provide a quick recap of AIDS followed by a review of the clinical trials, then describe the innovative, open-label trial, i.e., the treatment IND (investigational new drug), or compassionate release study, and briefly discuss the immediate postapproval period and the post-marketing surveillance projects.

ACQUIRED IMMUNODEFICIENCY SYNDROME

Since the first cases of AIDS were reported in 1981, a coordinated response has been mounted by the public and private sectors. The recognition of the geometric increases in incidence (Figure 1), the high mortality rates, and the associated health-care costs combined to accelerate drug development and clinical research efforts.

The disease spread rapidly among the homosexual population, and gradual reports of cases among hemophiliacs and intravenous drug abusers narrowed the search for an etiology toward an infectious agent transmittable sexually or by blood or other body products. The etiologic agent, the human immunodeficiency virus, or HIV, was identified in 1983, and screening tests were developed to protect the blood supply for transfusions by mid-1985. Despite the recent increase in cumulative incidence to more than 40,000 AIDS cases in the United States, the general proportions by risk group remain the same. It was estimated in the August 14, 1987 *Morbidity and Mortality Weekly Report*[1] that 6000 to 8000 additional cases, or roughly 15–20% of the accumulated total,

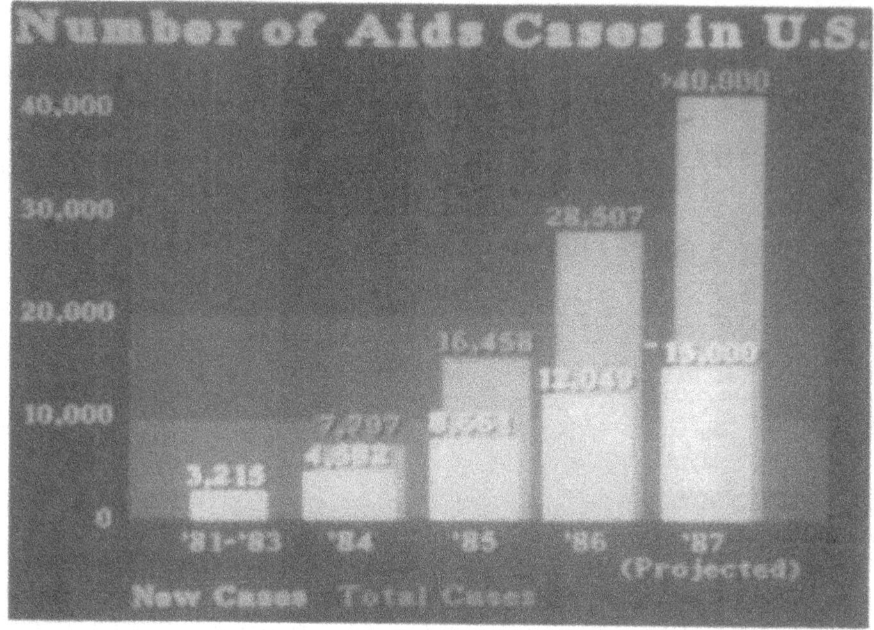

Figure 1. Number of AIDS cases in the United States. (Reported by state and territorial epidemiologists to the AIDS Program, Center for Infectious Diseases, Centers for Disease Control.)

had been diagnosed already and would be reported to the Centers for Disease Control by December 1987.

The magnitude of the AIDS problem is graphically displayed in the two iceberg plots in Figure 2, representing 1987 and projections to 1991. The 1991 estimates were derived by CDC in 1986 by combining various assumptions of HIV prevalence, viral transmission rates, conversion rates from the asymptomatic carrier state, and survival models based on existing cohorts of homosexual males. The two significant parameters in these estimates are the cumulative increases in all three categories of HIV infection by a factor of 9 or 10, and the conversion of at least one-third of asymptomatic HIV carriers (as of 1987) to clinical AIDS (by 1991) if present trends continue. The Surgeon General estimates that by 1991, 270,000 cases and 179,000 deaths will have occurred in the first decade of experience with AIDS, with 145,000 AIDS patients needing help and supportive services at an annual cost of between $8 and $16 billion.

CLINICAL TRIALS

In February 1985, Retrovir was first shown to be effective against HIV.

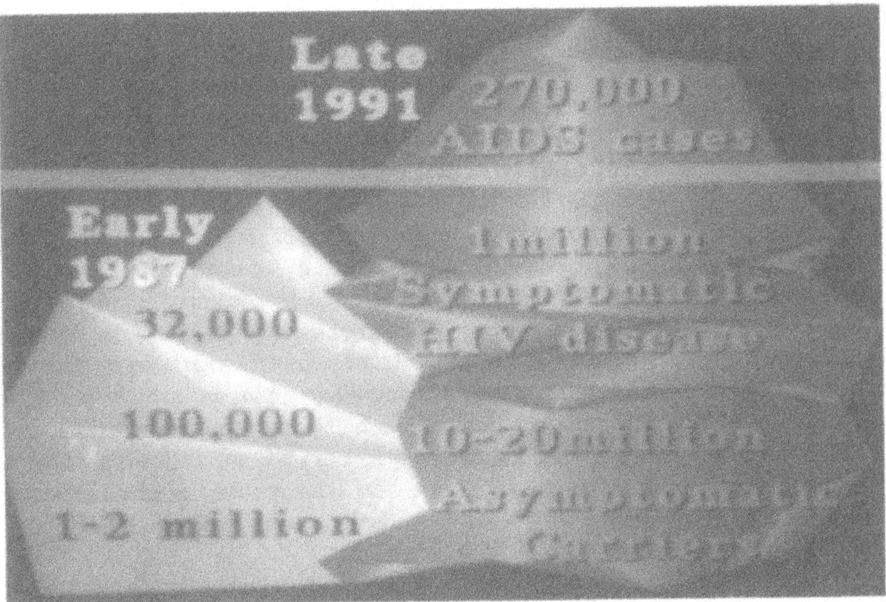

Figure 2. Projected number of AIDS cases in 1991 compared with 1987. (Reported by state and territorial epidemiologists to the AIDS Program, Center for Infectious Diseases, Centers for Disease Control.)

February '85—Activity in human retrovirus (HIV)
April '85—Pre-IND meeting with FDA. Project group formed
June '85—IV IND submitted 6/14/85; approved 6/21/85
July '85—First patient dosed
November '85—Capsule IND (approved in 1/2 day)
December '85—Completion of phase I
January '86—Initiation of phase II
September '86—Phase II trial terminated
March '87—Retrovir approval

In March 1987, only 25 months later, the drug was approved by the FDA as the result of a unique collaboration between industry and public health agencies. This process involved substantive negotiations and clarifications on major issues. Some of these issues were: (1) public health responsibilities in the creation of policies; (2) the balancing of risk vs benefit in the treatment of a terminal disease; (3) the rapid approval of a drug, with no shortcuts in the regulatory review of the entire process; (4) the specification and monitoring of special postmarketing studies; and (5) the implementation of a limited drug distribution program. Other agencies involved besides the FDA included the National Institutes of Health, Centers for Disease Control, Health and Resources Service Administration and many state and local public health departments, with the overview of Congress and the very vocal AIDS patient advocate groups.

Phase I

Beginning in July 1985, 21 patients were enrolled in a six-month trial to determine the safety of short-term and chronic dosing. Some of the clinical responses were weight gain (16/21); resolution of oral ulcers or thrush (2/2); defervescence (3/3); and neurologic improvement (3/3): restored memory in 2 patients and peripheral neuropathy improvement in 1 patient. There were also improvements in immune function as manifested by increased T_4 cell counts and responses to skin test antigens. Significant adverse events were hematologic abnormalities in 60% of the patients which were reversible by reduced dosing. There were some reversible neurologic complaints in three patients, consisting of dystonia, anxiety, and headache. There were four deaths: two due to AIDS, one following a traffic accident, and one following surgery. Conclusions from the Phase I trial were that Retrovir had possible efficacy, but no direct attribution was possible without a control group, and further studies were warranted.

Phase II

Two hundred eighty-one patients, 144 treated with Retrovir and 137 with placebo, who were similar in clinical status and prognosis, were studied for an average of 18 weeks (February 1986 to June 1986) in 12 medical centers. The study subjects were patients with AIDS who had recently recovered from *Pneumocystis carinii* pneumonia or who suffered from severe AIDS-related complex (ARC):

- 160 patients with AIDS; all had recovered from their first episodes of PCP within four months prior to enrollment
- 121 patients with ARC; all had multiple signs of HIV infection (i.e., weight loss, thrush, lymphadenopathy, fever)
- two groups of patients based on T_4 cell number:
  - high = T_4 cells >100 cells/mm^3 but <500 cells/mm^3
  - low = T_4 cells <100 cells/mm^3

The trial was ended earlier than the planned 26 weeks on the recommendation of an independent Data and Safety Monitoring Board because of a significant difference in mortality between the Retrovir and placebo groups.

	Placebo	Retrovir
AIDS deaths	11	1
ARC deaths	5	0
Total	16	1

At the time of study termination, the number of deaths had increased to 19 in the placebo group and was still 1 in the Retrovir-treated group. All the differ-

Table 1. Summary of Phase II Results

Event	Retrovir (n = 144)	Placebo (n = 137)
Deaths	1	19
Survival at 24 weeks	0.98	0.78
OIs after 6 weeks		
AIDS	0.30	0.45
ARC	0	0.25
Positive skin tests	0.29	0.09
Hematology		
anemia	0.38	0.13
leukopenia	0.65	0.42
neutropenia	0.83	0.57

Note: Clinical outcomes: Increased functioning (Karnofsky); Weight gain; Decreased frequency of HIV symptoms.

ences shown in Table 1, which summarizes Phase II results, are statistically significant at the 95% confidence level. An update on the Phase II trials was published in July 1987 in two articles in the *New England Journal of Medicine*. After 36 weeks the mortality rate was 10.3% in the original Retrovir group and 39% in the placebo patients, who were switched at the end of the Phase II trial to Retrovir.

By the end of the Phase II trial, many important questions remained, such as the benefits and problems of long-term Retrovir therapy, the natural history and pathophysiology of HIV infections, predictive variables for toxicity or patient response, the management and avoidance of toxicity, and finally, how much testing should be performed before allowing use of the only available therapy for AIDS, since placebo studies were no longer reasonable or ethical.

TREATMENT INVESTIGATIONAL NEW DRUG STUDY

As indicated, an independent Data and Safety Monitoring Board determined that the excess mortality in the placebo group mandated that the clinical trials be terminated. At that time, because of the urgent need to make available therapy to patients with HIV infection, the Food and Drug Administration established criteria by which patients could receive Retrovir under an innovative Treatment IND, which operated under the old Treatment IND regulations. This IND was sponsored by Burroughs Wellcome Co. and was initially comanaged by Burroughs Wellcome Co. and the National Institutes of Health.

The FDA specified that patients who met certain criteria would be eligible for enrollment in Treatment IND 29,025. First, patients had to have a history of one or more episodes of histologically confirmed *Pneumocystis carinii* pneumonia and no current AIDS-defining conditions requiring chemotherapy. This had implications, obviously, for data analysis and interpretation. The population of AIDS patients who present with PCP at the time of AIDS diagnosis, as most of these patients probably did, encompass about 50% of the total AIDS population. The rest are diagnosed with other opportunistic infections or malignancies. Secondly, patients had to have a hemoglobin of 9.0 g/dL or greater and aspartate aminotransferase not more than 3 times the upper limit of normal, but this was changed three months after the trial began to 5 times the upper limit of normal. Other criteria included total granulocyte count ≥1000, a platelet count ≥50,000, normal serum creatinine, positive test for HIV antibody, and age of 12 years or older. The Karnofsky score (which describes a patient's ability to carry on normal daily activities) initially was required to be ≥60, but was changed later on to >20. A score of 60 would be equivalent to a patient being able to carry on about 50% of normal activity, while a score of 20 would apply to a patient who was bedridden. This change also had important implications for data analysis.

Definitions of moderate and severe toxicity were amended during the trial. Initially, for instance, a hemoglobin drop of 2–3 g/dL was considered a reason to decrease the dose. As data were evaluated, it became clear that a patient who enrolled with a hemoglobin of 15 g which subsequently dropped to 12 was not necessarily a candidate for reduced therapy, and so these criteria were amended as follows:

Initial dose	200 mg every 4 hours
Decreased dose	100 mg every 4 hours
for moderate toxicity	decrease in hemoglobin of 2–3 g/dL, or granulocyte count <750/mm^3 but >500/mm^3, or Grade III toxicity (hemoglobin ≤7 g/dL but >6 g/dL or absolute neutrophil count <750 but >500)
Discontinuation of therapy	
for severe toxicity	decrease in hemoglobin >3 g/dL or granulocyte count <500/mm^3, or Grade IV toxicity (hemoglobin <6 g/dL or absolute neutrophil count <500)
resumption of therapy	100 mg every 4 hours if hemoglobin ≥9 g/dL

Excluded from the trial were pregnant women, nursing mothers, and women of childbearing potential not employing barrier contraception or abstinence. The purpose of this Treatment IND was to make available, at no cost to patients with AIDS, a treatment which had been shown in clinical trials to prolong lives. The drug was provided to patients *gratis* by Burroughs Wellcome Co.

The process by which patients were enrolled in the Treatment IND was complicated—as shown in the following list—which also had implications for probable selection bias.

- Physician requests information packet.
- Physician completes FDA-1573 form and a patient registration form and submits to a registered pharmacy along with medical license number, state of license, and signed patient consent form.
- (Pharmacy must have submitted letters from the pharmacy director and appropriate hospital administrator requesting to participate in protocol. Letter is sent to Burroughs Wellcome AZT IND Coordinating Center—BW-AZTICC).
- Pharmacist forwards one copy of registration package to BW-AZTICC, keeping one copy of FDA-1573 on file.
- BW-AZTICC notifies both pharmacy and physician of review actions taken.
- Burroughs Wellcome Co. ships a one-month supply of 100 mg capsules for each patient directly to pharmacy.
- Physicians provide pharmacy with prescription renewal and patient follow-up form two weeks after patient begins monthly treatment cycle.
- Pharmacist forwards forms to BW-AZTICC.

It is important to note that physicians had to provide a monthly summary of relevant patient information. Approval to treat approximately 5000 patients was given during the course of the IND. Among these, just over 4800 actually received treatment, the rest either having withdrawn or died before they could actually start taking the drug.

Because of the nature of the Treatment IND, i.e., the submission of largely voluntary information, the data base was originally designed completely with all fields in text format. When Burroughs Wellcome Co. took over sole operation of this activity in February 1987 and attempted to analyze the data, it was quickly determined that although the data were there, they were not in any analyzable form. A wealth of data from about 1300 physicians and 4800 patients were available, but the data base had to be entirely reconfigured twice in order to get it into a manageable form. Because of the dedicated efforts of a contract group in Rockville, MD at the Retrovir Center and the data management capabilities of Peggy Doi at Burroughs Wellcome Co., it has been possible to extract a great deal of very important data from this trial. Some innovative techniques have been used to collect missing data. For instance, extensive use has been made of a toll-free telephone hotline to contact physicians and pharmacists for missing data. In addition, physicians were encouraged to use that hotline to report any adverse events or patient deaths or to discuss any problems relating to the conduct of the trial. Consequently, the number of missing data points was minimized, and the data are of much higher quality than might have been expected from a trial of this type. These data are extremely important because, in the millieu of fast-track approval for Retrovir due to the overwhelming urgency of trying to find some answer to the problem of AIDS, the preclinical and clinical evaluations of this drug were much shorter than for any drug ever approved previously. Because of a limited drug supply when the drug was marketed, a limited distribution system was put into place. Patients who had been enrolled in the Treatment IND retained their unique patient number. This number, along

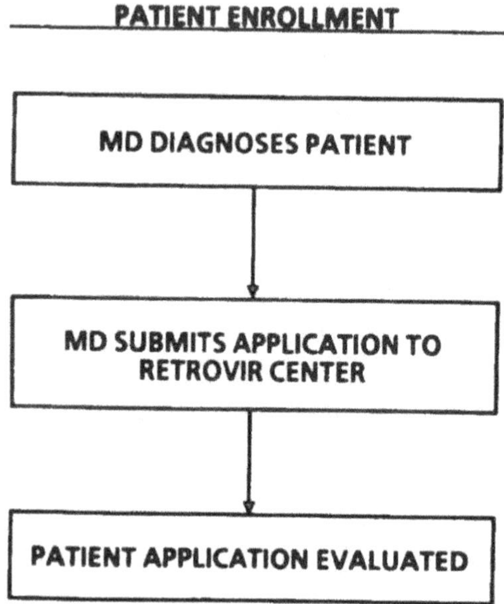

Figure 3. Retrovir distribution system for a new patient.

with the birthdate, was a patient's only identifier. No access to patient names was sought. The process by which patients enrolled in the distribution system is shown in Figure 3; patients who were in the Treatment IND were automatically enrolled. All patients who continued to receive Retrovir were identified through drug shipment records. These patients were assumed to be alive, and that information was considered in survival analysis.

Follow-up for patients was extended to a postmarketing protocol called ZVD-501. In September 1987, at least some information on patient status was available for all but 287 patients treated in the original Treatment IND. Although the data had limitations, some degree of confidence in carrying out survival analyses in this population was justified.

The overall survival at 36 weeks of treatment remained about 85% in this patient group. In Figure 4, the solid line represents the survival analysis, while the dotted lines represent the confidence limits. However, in the patients most comparable to those treated in the original double-blind placebo-controlled study, i.e., patients with entry hemoglobin of >9 and a diagnosis data <90 days prior to treatment, survival remained at approximately 90%. This was comparable to what was seen in the patients who were treated in the original clinical trial. When survival was stratified into patient groups treated less than 90 days prior to diagnosis of their *Pneumocystis carinii* pneumonia and those treated greater than 90 days after this PCP episode, the differences in survival were striking (Figure 5), and the confidence limits do not overlap. Several caveats must be considered in viewing these data. First, the PCP episode required for entry into this trial had to be histologically confirmed. Although

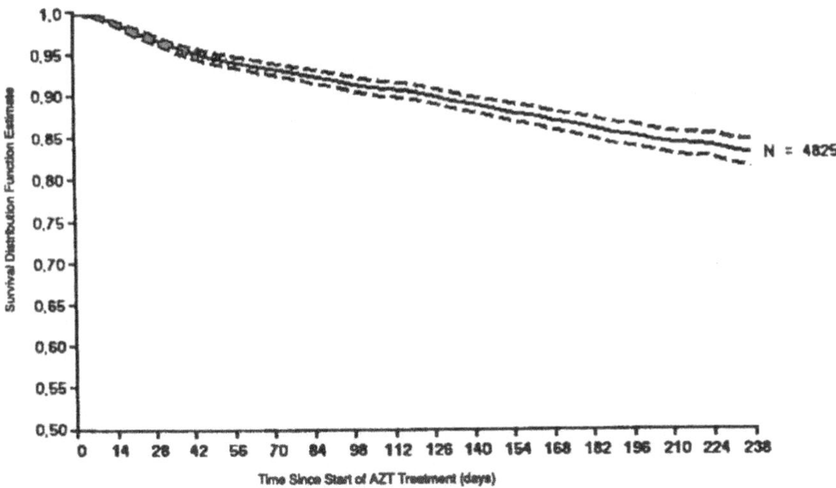

Figure 4. Survival after start of AZT treatment (days).

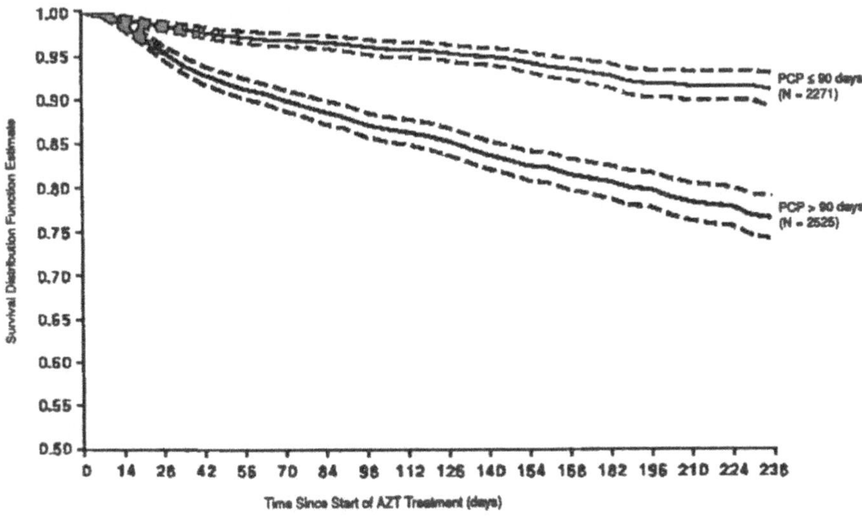

Figure 5. Survival according to time since *Pneumocystis carinii* pneumonia diagnosis.

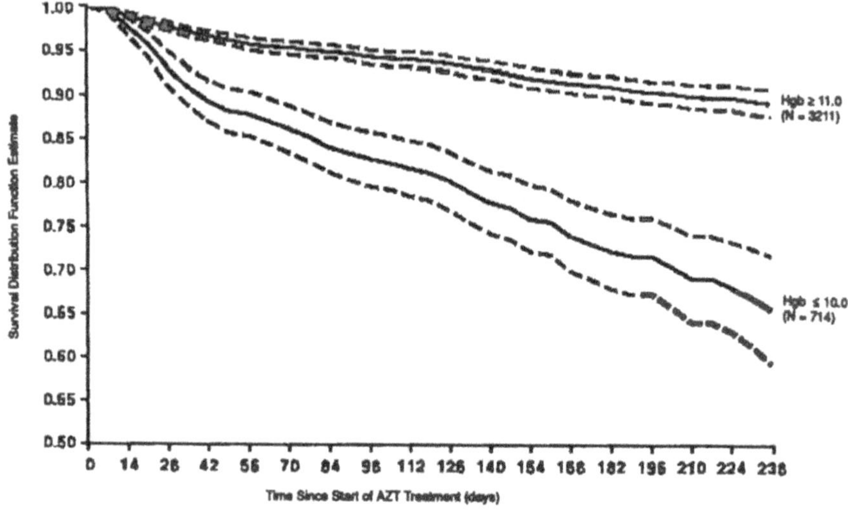

Figure 6. Survival according to hemoglobin level at start of treatment.

it did not necessarily have to be the diagnostic episode for AIDS, it is likely that the diagnostic episode would be the episode that was histologically confirmed. Second, it is likely that patients entering the trial earlier in the course of the disease would survive longer without treatment. What is not clear is whether the differences would be this striking in the absence of drug therapy. In the controlled clinical trial, differences in mortality between drug and placebo groups forced an end to the study on ethical grounds.

When patients were stratified according to whether the pretreatment hemoglobin was ≥ 11 or ≤ 10, again, striking differences in survival are seen (Figure 6). As previously, the confidence limits do not overlap. Additionally, there were no missing entry hemoglobin values for patients enrolled in the study. Thus, the data were not in any way influenced by missing values for any subgroup of patients. Again, survival in the group whose hemoglobin was ≥ 11 at enrollment was $>90\%$.

These analyses are preliminary and have been shown only to indicate what can be done in analyzing a data base of this nature. This is probably the largest cohort of AIDS patients being followed in the world. We feel that we have been able to extract some very important data from the study, with a number of caveats and biases, of course, which we have to always keep in mind. These patients will continue to be monitored through Protocol ZVD-501. Additionally, another protocol, ZVD-502, designed to intensively monitor 1500 patients being treated with Retrovir, was due to start in October 1987. We also have in place an intensive postmarketing surveillance program for spontaneous adverse events being reported to Burroughs Wellcome.

POSTMARKETING SURVEILLANCE

The Retrovir postmarketing surveillance program consists of the three different types of ongoing studies:

- extended monitoring program (ZVD-501)
- intensive monitoring program (ZVD-502)
- spontaneous monitoring program

The first is the ZVD-501 program, which follows the former Treatment IND patients for a minimum of two years or until the death of each patient (Figure 7). Follow-up data are obtained from a mailed questionnaire to the treating physicians every two months. There is a toll-free number at the Retrovir Center which continues to be used for reporting interim adverse events or critical events in the treatment of the patients. Limitations are shown; some of them are fairly obvious. It is an entirely voluntary system since there is no incentive either to the patient or to the provider at this time. There is minimal baseline information depending upon the data we originally obtained on each patient. There is no validation of ongoing medical data. We have no concurrent unexposed cohort, and there are obvious problems linked to confidentiality and expected patient attrition over the two- to three-year period.

The second postmarketing program is ZVD-502 (Figure 8), in which 1500 patients, divided into three risk groups, are being followed at 12 major medical centers, similarly for a minimum of two years or until the death of each patient. This is an observational chart abstraction study with a principal investigator and monitor at each site. All data are analyzed at the Johns Hopkins Hospital, where Dr. Craig Smith is the coordinating investigator. The limitations are known, and again most of them are fairly obvious. One of the critical issues is that we have to be careful not to interfere with medical care by requiring the provider to perform additional tests or requesting information that would cause procedures to be performed on a more frequent basis than in the normal mode of practice for *that* provider.

The third postmarketing surveillance program is the standard spontaneous monitoring program (Figure 9) which we perform on all marketed drugs. This is worldwide and ongoing as long as the drug is marketed. All reports from this voluntary reporting system are reviewed at Burroughs Wellcome Co. and reported to the FDA on a periodic basis, with increased frequency analyses as required. Limitations again are that it is completely voluntary, we do not have baseline information for the patients, the criteria probably will be changing over time, and we have no access to primary medical records.

CONCLUSIONS

These are some of the approaches to data collection, data base linkage, and information management which will help ensure an effective, coordinated

RETROVIR POST-APPROVAL EPIDEMIOLOGIC PROGRAM

Extended Monitoring Program (ZVD-501)

Objectives:

- describe and quantify survival time - particularly for specific risk groups
- better understand and quantitate known adverse and beneficial effects
- discover rarer but important effects and effects of long-term therapy

Scope:

- all surviving patients from U.S. pre-approval compassionate release (Treatment IND)
- two years or until death

Methods:

- mailed follow-up survey on treated patients; no untreated controls
- cohort "assembled" at end of Treatment IND
- status check on all registered IND patients for uniform baseline (May/June 1987)
- mailed status report form to each M.D. for each patient every two months, starting July 1987
- toll-free number at The RETROVIR Center for reporting major interim events

Limitations:

- voluntary reporting
- minimal baseline information
- no validation of medical data
- lack of a concurrent, unexposed cohort
- confidentiality concerns
  - limited database linkages
  - complicated medical provider monitoring

Figure 7. Extended monitoring program (ZVD-501), part of the Retrovir postapproval epidemiologic program.

RETROVIR POST-APPROVAL EPIDEMIOLOGIC PROGRAM

Intensive Monitoring Program (ZVD-502)

Objectives:
- estimation of survival time by risk group status and drug-related covariates
- identification of factors which may predispose patients to serious toxicity
- identification and estimation of significant new positive or negative medical events under long-term therapy

Scope:
- 1500 patients
  - 500 severe ARC (T4<200)
  - 500 AIDS with recent initial PCP
  - 500 non-PCP AIDS
- 10-12 geographically-distributed major treatment centers
- 2-3 year follow-up

Methods:
- observational chart abstraction follow-up study
- multicenter, protocol-driven, collaborative
- principal investigator and monitor at each site
- all charts abstracted every two months
- all data analyzed at central site (Johns Hopkins)

Limitations:
- Unknown attrition rate
  - Losses to follow-up
  - Competitive studies
- Variable data availability
- Lack of influence on medical care

Figure 8. Intensive monitoring program (ZVD-502), part of the Retrovir postapproval epidemiologic program.

response to the most significant public health problem in the modern era. There are now real prospects for improved patient care and survival through the collaborative efforts of Burroughs Wellcome Co. and the front-line public health agencies in the effort to control the AIDS epidemic while research proceeds on a cure for the disease.

RETROVIR POST-APPROVAL EPIDEMIOLOGIC PROGRAM

Spontaneous Monitoring Program

Objectives:

- generation of signals regarding possible adverse drug reactions
- case documentation of sentinel events

Scope:

- all "non-study" treatments
- all literature reports
- alert reports from all structured studies
- worldwide
- ongoing

Methods:

- spontaneous, voluntary reports monitoring
- ADE's received, reviewed, reported
  - BW standard follow-up
- coordination and cross-referral with The RETROVIR Center (TRC)/toll-free number 1-800-843-9388
- "increased frequency" analyses quarterly

Limitations:

- Voluntary reports
- Minimal eligibility criteria
- Unavailable primary medical records

Figure 9. Spontaneous monitoring program, part of the Retrovir postapproval epidemiologic program.

REFERENCES

1. *Morbidity and Mortality Weekly Report, 36*(31), 522.

24. *Differences in Psychotropic Medications Reported Used by Blacks and Whites*

SHARYN R. BATEY
HARRY H. WRIGHT
ELISABETH A. COLE
BRIAN BUTLER

INTRODUCTION

Since the prescribing of psychotropic medications usually proceeds from a psychiatric diagnosis or problem, any discussion of the differences in the use of psychotropic medications in blacks and whites must address the issue of the diagnosis and misdiagnosis of psychiatric disorders in blacks, a topic which has been discussed by several authors.[1-5]

It has been consistently reported that a larger percentage of blacks are diagnosed as schizophrenic than are whites, and blacks are less frequently diagnosed as having affective disorders than whites.[1,6-8] Mukherjee et al,[3] reported 68% of 76 bipolar patients had previously been diagnosed as schizophrenic. Of these bipolar patients, Hispanics and blacks were more frequently ($p < 0.01$) misdiagnosed as schizophrenic than whites. This certainly has implications in terms of prescribing medications, because psychotropic medications are the most frequently prescribed treatment for schizophrenic and affective disorders.

Mayo[9] reported that black males with generalized anxiety disorders were more frequently diagnosed as schizophrenic than white males. She postulated that this difference was due to their environmental upbringing which compelled them to mask their anxiety and exhibit hostility, machoism, and false pride. For black males to admit they were depressed or anxious was to admit they were weak and had failed.

The physicians' interpretation of the symptomatology of a patient's illness can affect not only the assignment of the psychiatric diagnosis but also the prescribing of psychotropic medications. In addition to the extensive discussion of misdiagnosis of psychiatric disorders in blacks, there is also an emerging literature on racial and ethnic differences regarding response to psychotropic medications.[10-13] Nearly all reports on the possible biological differences in response to psychotropic medications have been comparisons between Asian and white patients. There are no similar data available on black and Hispanic patients. The apparent racial and ethnic differences in drug effects may be the result of differences in metabolizing capacity on a genetic or environmental basis.[14] Cultural factors may also be involved.[15] Significantly more research needs to be done in this area before any firm conclusions can be made.

Because there is limited information available about the differences or similarities in prescribing psychotropic medications to blacks and whites, this study was conceived to investigate the use of prescription psychotropic medications by blacks and whites. Patients were studied during the year prior to admission to a psychiatric hospital and during hospitalization, and the findings were related to sociodemographic and psychological variables of the population.

METHODOLOGY

The study consisted of a retrospective review of the closed charts of 659 patients aged 18–65 years who were admitted to a Southern state department of mental health facility over a four-year period and who had a pharmacy-conducted medication history taken during the hospitalization. Each chart was reviewed using a standard data collection form to obtain sociodemographic data, psychological variables, and medications prescribed during hospitalization.

The frequency and percentage distribution of the medications used were reported by sociodemographic and psychological variables. The data were compared using chi-square analysis with a minimum level of significance set at $p < 0.05$.

The study was limited by the patient's recall and/or the patients' willingness to disclose information about medications they used during the year prior to admission. The reliability might also be limited due the self-reporting of medication histories by a psychiatric population. As a retrospective study, only data recorded in the charts were obtained.

RESULTS

The study population (Table 1) included 659 patients between the ages of 18 and 65 years of whom 359 (54%) were male and 300 (46%) were female. The population included 129 blacks (20%) and 530 whites (80%). An age gradient was present, with almost half the population represented by the youngest group, 18–24 year olds (47%), followed in decreasing order by the 25–34 year olds (30%), 35–49 year olds (15%), and 50–65 year olds (8%). Only 32% of the patients were married; the majority of the patients were single/never mar-

Table 1. Composite of Sociodemographic Variables

Variable	Race: Black (n = 129) No.	%	White (n = 530) No.	%	Total (n = 659) No.	%
Gender						
Male	74	57	285	54	359	54
Female	55	43	245	46	300	46
Age (years)						
18–24	65	51	246	46	311	47
25–34	42	33	157	30	199	30
35–49	15	12	83	16	98	15
50–65	6	5	44	8	50	8
Marital status						
Single	66	51	196	37	262	40
Married	32	25	177	33	209	32
Divorced	7	5	92	17	99	15
Separated	20	16	44	8	64	10
Widowed	4	3	21	4	25	4
Educational level						
Less than high school	29	23	68	13	97	15
Some high school	40	31	116	22	156	24
High school graduate	36	28	155	29	191	29
Some college	19	15	120	23	139	21
Bachelor's degree or more	5	4	70	13	75	11

ried (40%), divorced (15%), separated (10%), or widowed (4%). The majority of patients obtained at least a high school education. Fifteen percent had less than a high school education, 24% attended some high school but did not graduate, 29% received a high school diploma, 21% obtained some post-high school training but less than a bachelor's degree, and 11% completed a bachelor's degree or higher education.

When the psychiatric variables were examined (Table 2), it was determined that 66% of the patients received a final primary diagnosis of either affective disorder (43%) or schizophrenia (24%). Patients reported having been hos-

Table 2. Composite of Psychiatric Variables

Variable	Race: Black (n = 129) No.	%	White (n = 530) No.	%	Total (n = 659) No.	%
Diagnosis						
Affective disorder	18	14	265	52	283	43
Schizophrenia	72	56	83	16	155	24
Number of prior psychiatric admissions						
0	33	26	124	23	157	24
1–2	44	34	211	40	255	39
3–4	29	22	104	20	133	20
5 or more	23	18	91	17	144	17

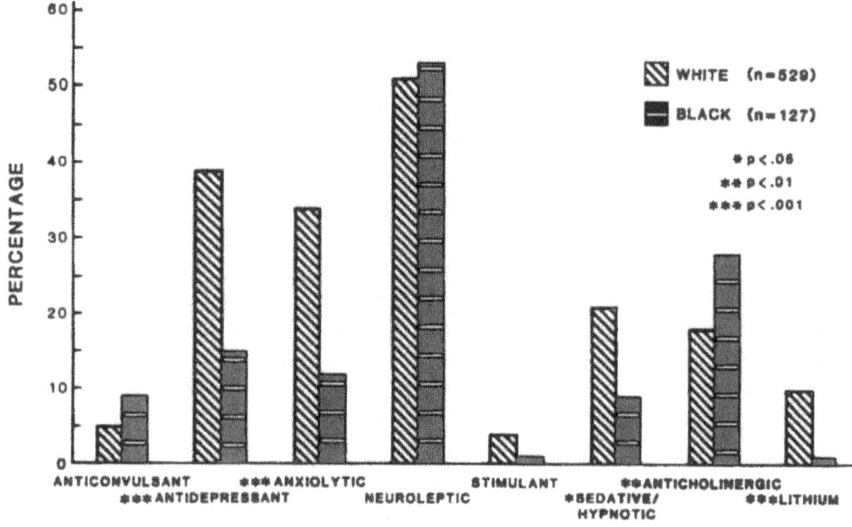

Figure 1. Prescribed psychotropic medication use by race prior to admission to the hospital.

pitalized previously from zero to 11 times for psychiatric problems. Twenty-four percent of the population reported no previous psychiatric hospitalizations; 17% reported that they had had five or more prior psychiatric hospitalizations.

ANALYSIS OF MEDICATIONS USE DATA

For analysis, the psychotropic medications were divided into eight categories: anticonvulsants, antidepressants, anxiolytics, neuroleptics, psychostimulants, sedatives/hypnotics, anticholinergics, and lithium. Approximately 82% of the population reported taking some type of psychotropic medication during the year prior to admission. During admission to the psychiatric hospital, 99% of the patients were prescribed psychotropic medications.

Figure 1 displays the use of prescribed psychotropic medications by race prior to hospitalization. The use of psychostimulants and anticonvulsants will not be discussed since the overall usage of these agents was small. The racial differences in the use of antidepressants, anxiolytics, and lithium were statistically significant at $p < 0.001$; the use of sedatives/hypnotics was statistically significant at $p < 0.05$. Whites were prescribed these four categories of medications more frequently than blacks. Antidepressants were reported by 40% of whites and 15% of blacks, anxiolytics by 35% of whites and 8% of blacks, lithium by 10% of whites and 1% of blacks, and sedatives/hypnotics by 20% of whites and 10% of blacks. The difference in the use of anticholinergics was statistically significant at $p < 0.01$, with blacks (28%) reporting using these

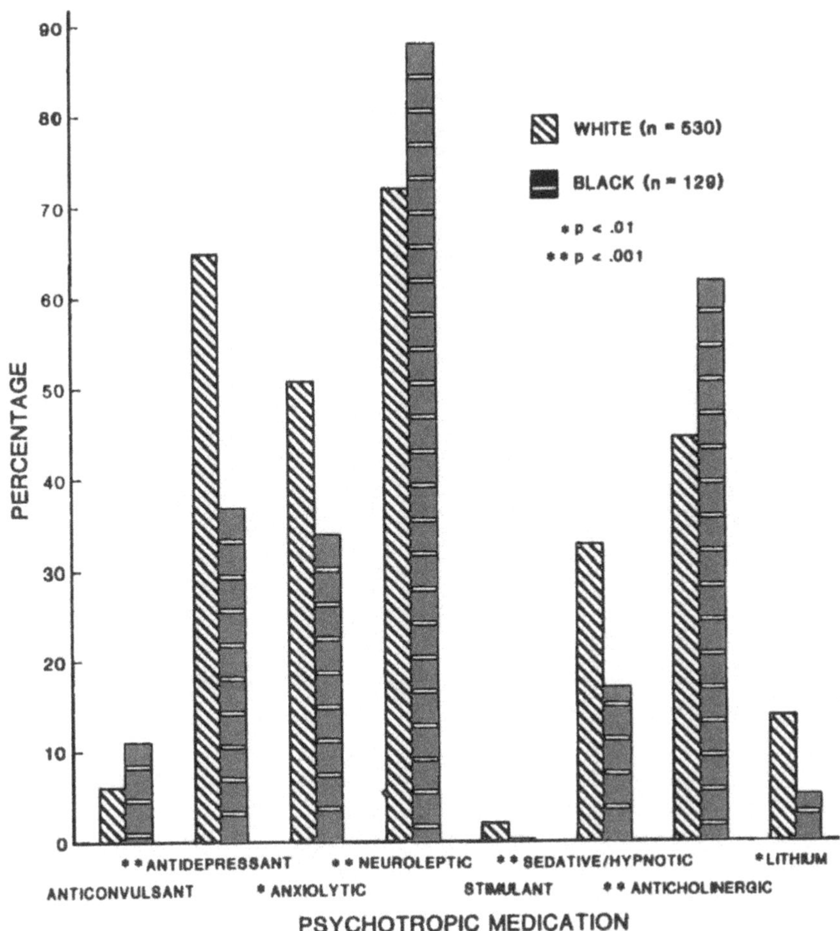

Figure 2. Prescribed psychotropic medication use by race during admission to the hospital.

agents more frequently than whites (15%). The difference in the use of neuroleptics was not statistically significant, with 50% of whites and 53% of blacks reporting these agents.

Figure 2 shows the prescribing of psychotropic medications by race during hospitalization. The differences in prescribing antidepressants, neuroleptics, sedatives/hypnotics, and anticholinergics were statistically significant at $p < 0.001$, while differences in the use of anxiolytics and lithium were statistically significant at the $p < 0.01$ level. As was observed with psychotropic medications prior to admission, whites more frequently than blacks were prescribed antidepressants (65% versus 32%), anxiolytics 51% versus 34%), sedatives/hypnotics (33% versus 17%), and lithium (14% versus 5%). Blacks were more

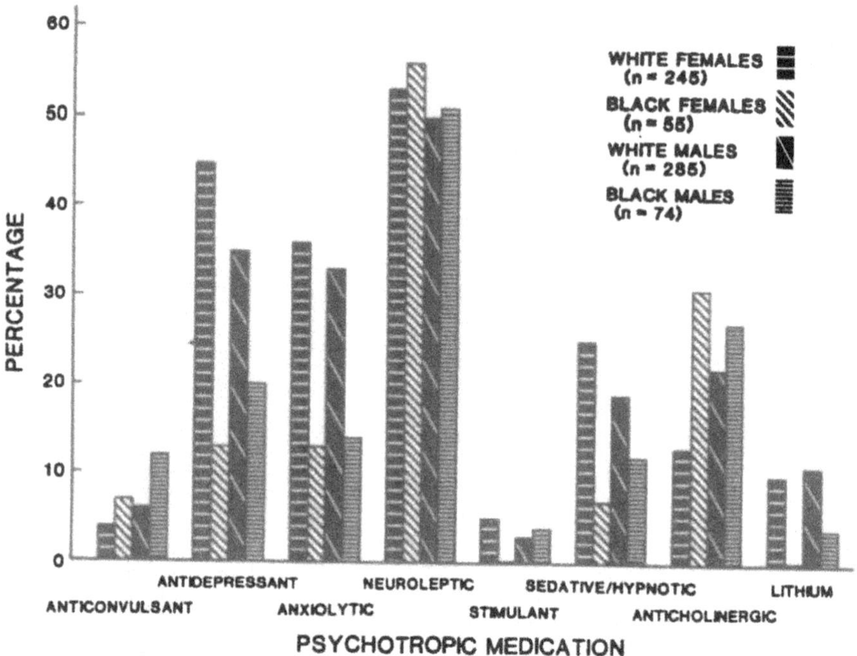

Figure 3. Prescribed psychotropic medication use by sex and race prior to admission to the hospital.

frequently prescribed neuroleptics (88% versus 72%) and anticholinergics (62% versus 44%) than were whites during hospitalization.

Figure 3 presents the use of psychotropic medications by gender and race during the year prior to admission to the hospital. More white than black females reported using antidepressants (45% versus 13%), anxiolytics (36% versus 13%), sedatives/hypnotics (25% versus 7%), and lithium (10% versus 0%); only neuroleptics (56% versus 53%) and anticholinergics (31% versus 13%) were used by more black than white females. The differences in psychotropic medication use between black and white females were statistically significant for antidepressants ($p < 0.001$), anxiolytics ($p < 0.01$), sedatives/hypnotics ($p < 0.01$), anticholinergics ($p < 0.01$), and lithium ($p < 0.05$).

Similar trends in the use of psychotropic medications were reported for males as for females. White more often than black males reported using antidepressants (35% versus 20%), anxiolytics (33% versus 14%), sedatives/hypnotics (19% versus 12%), and lithium (11% versus 4%). Black males reported using neuroleptics (51% versus 50%) and anticholinergics (27% versus 22%) more frequently than white males. The differences between white and black males were statistically significant for anxiolytics ($p < 0.01$) and antidepressants ($p < 0.05$).

Figure 4 shows the prescribing of psychotropic medications during hospitalization by gender and race. The same trends in prescribing psychotropic medi-

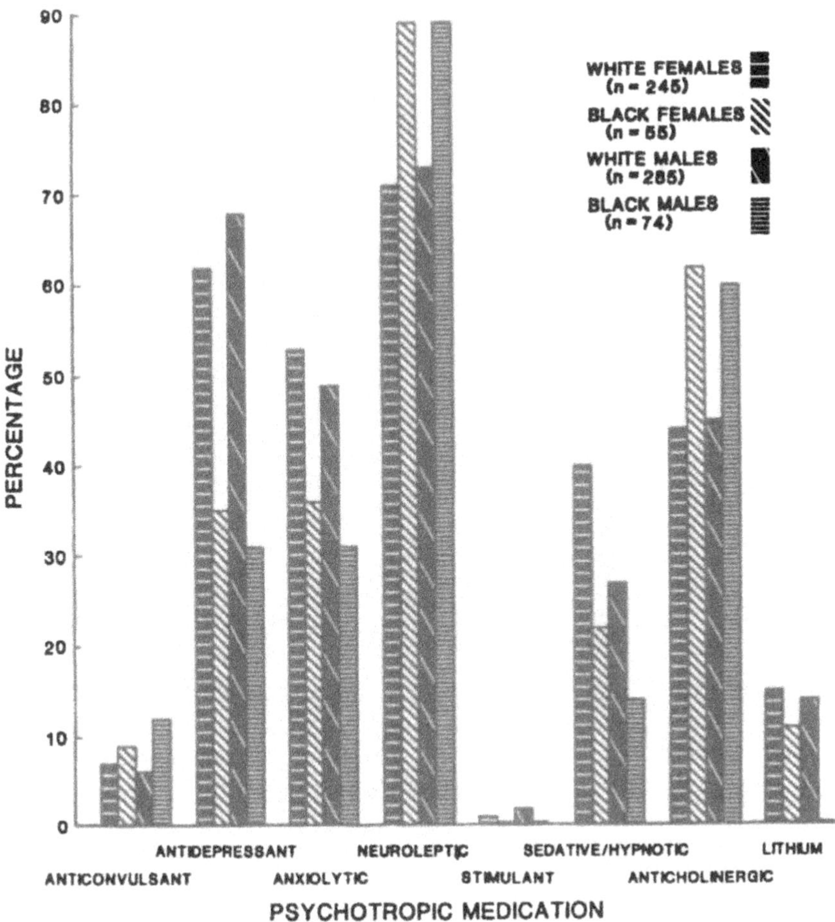

Figure 4. Prescribed psychotropic medication use by sex and race during admission to the hospital.

cations were observed during hospitalization as were reported prior to admission. White females were more frequently prescribed antidepressants (62% versus 35%), anxiolytics (53% versus 36%), sedatives/hypnotics (40% versus 22%), and lithium (15% versus 11%) than black females. Black females were more frequently prescribed neuroleptics (89% versus 71%) and anticholinergics (62% versus 44%) than white females. The differences in psychotropic medication use between white and black females during hospitalization were statistically significant for antidepressants ($p < 0.001$), anxiolytics ($p < 0.05$), neuroleptics ($p < 0.01$), sedatives/hypnotics ($p < 0.05$), and anticholinergics ($p < 0.05$). White males were more frequently prescribed antidepressants (68% versus 31%), anxiolytics (49% versus 31%), sedatives/hypnotics (27%

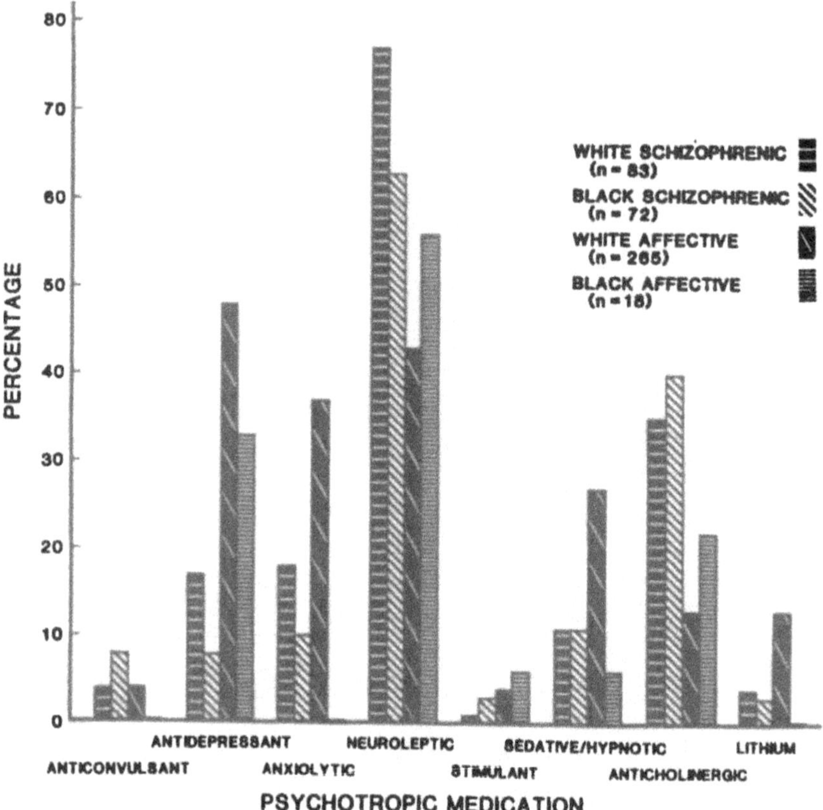

Figure 5. Prescribed psychotropic medication use by illness and race prior to admission to the hospital.

versus 14%), and lithium (14% versus 0%) than black males. Black males were more frequently prescribed neuroleptics (89% versus 73%) and anticholinergics (60% versus 45%) than white males. The differences in psychotropic medication use between white and black males were statistically significant for antidepressants ($p < 0.001$), anxiolytics ($p < 0.01$), neuroleptics ($p < 0.01$), lithium ($p < 0.01$), sedatives/hypnotics ($p < 0.05$), and anticholinergics ($p < 0.05$).

In looking at Figure 5, the medications prescribed to blacks and whites by diagnosis prior to admission, several differences are apparent. Whites with schizophrenic disorders were almost twice as frequently prescribed antidepressants (17% versus 8%) and anxiolytics (18% versus 10%) as were blacks. Although white patients with a schizophrenic diagnosis were more frequently prescribed neuroleptics (77% versus 63%), blacks were more frequently prescribed anticholinergic agents (40% versus 35%). The use of sedative/hypnotics (11% versus 11%) and lithium (4% versus 3%) was similar between white and black schizophrenics prior to admission to the hospital. The differences in psychotropic medication use between white and black schizophrenics prior to admissions were statistically significant for neuroleptics ($p < 0.05$).

Prior to admission, white patients with affective disorders were more frequently prescribed antidepressants (48% versus 33%), anxiolytics (37% versus 0%), sedative/hypnotics (27% versus 6%), and lithium (13% versus 0%) than were blacks. Blacks with affective disorders, however, were more frequently prescribed neuroleptics (56% versus 43%) and anticholinergics (22% versus 13%) than were whites. Significant differences were observed for anxiolytics and sedatives/hypnotics at $p < 0.01$ and $p < 0.05$, respectively.

During admission to the hospital, one can again see the differences in prescribing psychotropics in black and white patients by psychiatric diagnosis (Figure 6). White patients with schizophrenia were more frequently prescribed antidepressants (36% versus 18%), anxiolytics (28% versus 21%), neuroleptics (98% versus 96%), sedatives/hypnotics (22% versus 17%), anticholinergics (75% versus 72%) and lithium (10% versus 3%) than were blacks. There were no significant differences in the reported use of psychotropic medications by race for schizophrenics during hospitalization.

In reviewing by race the prescribing of psychotropic medications during hospitalization for patients with an affective disorder, again white patients were more frequently prescribed antidepressants (36% versus 18%), anxiolytics (58% versus 50%), sedatives/hypnotics (37% versus 17%), and lithium (20% versus 11%) than black patients similarly diagnosed. Black affective disorder patients were more frequently prescribed neuroleptics (72% versus 60%) and anticholinergics (44% versus 34%) than were white patients. There were no significant differences in the prescribing of psychotropic medications by race for patients with affective disorders during hospitalization.

DISCUSSION

The trends found in the data are supported by other authors who found that white and black patients were prescribed psychotropic medications differently. The trends in prescribing psychotropic medications were similar whether patients were in the community or in the hospital except when the specific diagnoses of schizophrenia and affective disorders were examined. White patients were more frequently prescribed antidepressants, anxiolytics, sedatives/hypnotics, and lithium; black patients were more frequently prescribed neuroleptics and anticholinergics.

The disparity between the percentage of black and white patients diagnosed as having schizophrenia or an affective disorder certainly is supported by other authors.[3,6-8,16] The extensive prescribing of neuroleptics and anticholinergics for black patients is consistent with their more frequent diagnoses of schizophrenia. More than half of the black population in the study were diagnosed as

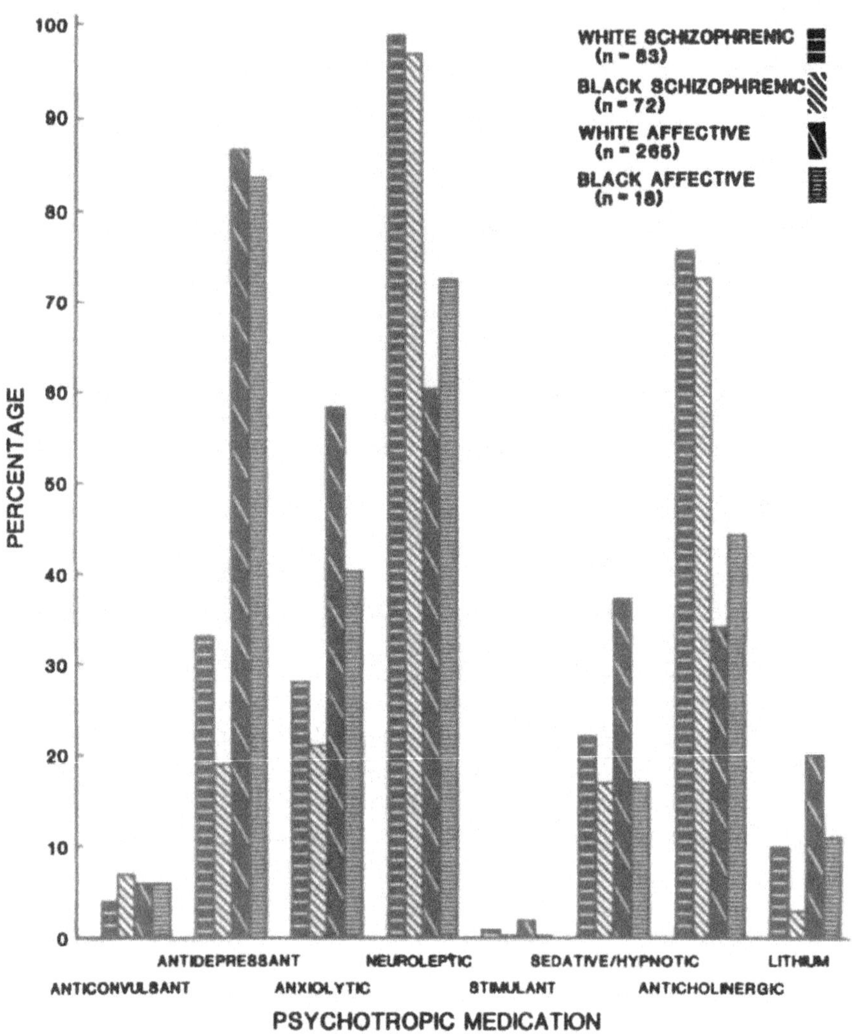

Figure 6. Prescribed psychotropic medication use by illness and race during admission to the hospital.

schizophrenic, while half of the white population were diagnosed as having an affective disorder.

Most of the published reports on the differences in mental health interventions with black or white patients have focused on psychotherapeutic interventions.[3,6,16,17] There is very little published information on the differences in psychopharmaceutical intervention with black and white patients.[2] Although several factors may account for the difference in the use of the psychotropic medications by black and white patients, the misdiagnosis of black psychiatric patients has emerged in nearly all discussions. In addition to misdiagnosis, overestimation, underestimation, or neglect of psychopathology are frequent problems when clinicians and patients are from different cultural or subcultural groups.[18]

Since most studies have focused on the overdiagnosis of schizophrenia and the underdiagnosis of affective disorder in blacks, this study has also focused on these two diagnoses.* Despite the fact that the prevalence of most major psychiatric disorders does not differ between whites and blacks when standard diagnostic protocols are used,[2,4-5] the data in this study indicate that the medications most often used to treat affective disorders were used at a higher frequency by blacks prior to admission to the hospital.

The same trends appear in prescribing medications for black and white patients with affective disorders and schizophrenia before and during hospitalization except for the prescribing of sedatives/hypnotics and anxiolytics for affectively ill patients prior to hospitalization. In contrast to the other data reported in this chapter, we believe the nonsignificant difference in psychoactive medication use by black and white patients diagnosed with schizophrenia and affective disorder during hospitalization was due to the strict adherence to specific criteria for making these diagnoses in the teaching hospital setting.

If the prescribing of anxiolytics is related to recognizing anxiety symptoms, black patients are identified at a much lower frequency than white patients. This agrees with the problems of diagnosing reported by Westermeyer[18] and the cultural variation in the presentation of anxiety and affective disorders in black patients.[9]

Obviously, there is a need for more research on the differences in prescribing of psychoactive medications in black and white psychiatric patients to help sort out the relative contributions of diagnostic problems, biological differences in response to medications, and cultural factors.

REFERENCES

1. Jones BE, Gray BA, Parson, EB: Manic-depressive illness among poor urban blacks. *Am J Psychiatry* 1981;138:654–657.
2. Lawson WB. Racial and ethnic factors in psychiatric research. *Hosp Comm Psychiatry* 1986;37:50–54.
3. Mukherjee S, Shukla S, Woodle K, et al: Misdiagnosis of schizophrenia in biopolar patients: A multiethnic comparison. *Am J Psychiatry* 1983; 140:1571–1574.
4. Adebimpe VR: Overview white norms on psychiatric diagnosis of black patients. *Am J Psychiatry* 1981;138:279–285.
5. Abramson RK, Wright HH: Diagnosis of black patients. *Am J Psychiatry* 1981;138:1515.
6. Collins, JL, Rickman LE, Mathura CB: Frequency of schizophrenia and depression in a black inpatient population. *J Nat Med Assoc* 1980; 72:851–856.

7. Simon RJ, Fleiss JL, Garland BJ, et al: Depression and schizophrenia in hospitalized black and white mental patients. *Arch Gen Psychiatry* 1973;28:509–512.
8. Adebimpe VR, Hedlund JL, Cho Dw, et al: Symptomatology of depression in black and white patients. *J Nat Med Assoc* 1982;74:185–190.
9. Mayo AJ: The concept of masked anxiety in young black males, in Klein DK, Rabkin J (eds): *Anxiety: New Research and Changing Concepts*. New York, Raven Press, 1981.
10. Rudorfor MV, Lane EA, Chaney WH, et al: Desipramine pharmacokinetics in Chinese and Caucasian volunteers. *Brit J Clin Pharm* 1984; 17:433–440.
11. Lin KM, Finder E: Neuroleptic dosage for Asians. *Am J Psychiatry* 1983; 140:490–491.
12. Ziegler VE, Briggs J: Tricyclic plasma levels effect of age, race, sex, and smoking. *JAMA* 1982;238:457–460.
13. Overall JA, Hollister LE, Kimball I, et al: Extrinsic factors influencing responses to psychotherapeutic drugs. *Arch Gen Psychiatry* 1969;21:89–94.
14. Kalow W: Ethnic differences in drug metabolism. *Clin Pharmacokinet* 1982;7:373–400.
15. Tung JM: Psychiatric care for Southeast Asians: How different is different? In Owen TC (ed): *Southeast Asians Mental Health: Treatment, Prevention, Services, Training and Research*. Bethesda, MD, NIMH, 1985.
16. Jones BE, Gray BA: Problems in diagnosing schizophrenic and affective disorder among blacks. *Hosp Comm Psychiatry* 1986;37:61–65.
17. Wilkerson CB, Spurlock J: The mental health of black Americans, in Wilkerson CB (ed): *Ethnic Psychiatry*. New York, Plenum, 1986.
18. Westermeyer J: Cultural factors in clinical assessment. *J Consul Clinical Psychol* 1987;55:471–478.

25. *The Dunedin Program: A Longitudinal Study of Aging*

RONALD B. STEWART
WILLIAM E. HALE
RONALD G. MARKS

INTRODUCTION

Persons over 65 years of age represent about 12% of the population in the United States, but account for almost 30% of the health care expenditures and receive 31% of all prescribed medications.[1,2] Health care professionals of the future will undoubtedly be confronted with an ever-increasing array of problems related to older persons. In order to provide appropriate care for the elderly there is a need for more accurate information concerning the normal aging process, including the incidence and prevalence of diseases and symptoms, value of and response to treatment and health care practices, and beliefs of the elderly.

In 1975 there were few ongoing studies to collect information in the elderly population.[3-5] With those needs in mind, a program was designed and implemented to screen ambulatory elderly persons for previously undetected disorders and utilize information collected for research on aging. The purpose of this chapter is to describe the background, objectives, methods, and initial findings of this epidemiologic program.

THE DUNEDIN PROGRAM

The Dunedin Program began in July 1975 to provide health screening to ambulatory elderly residents of Dunedin, Florida on an annual basis.[6] Dunedin is located on the midwest coast of Florida, and at the time the program began the community had a population of 23,288 residents with 6826 persons over 65 years of age.

The program was designed to evaluate participants annually for previously undetected medical disorders and to refer these persons to private physicians for follow-up care. No treatment is provided by Dunedin Program staff. In addition to the screening service it was believed that data collected in the program would provide answers to health questions regarding the elderly such as:

- Will the frequency of detected disorders cost justify a screening program?
- Which laboratory tests are the most valuable for routine screening?
- Will patients seek follow-up care for detected disorders?
- What are normal laboratory values in this age group?
- What is the extent of prescribed and nonprescribed medication use in this population?
- What is the prevalence of common diseases and symptoms in this population?
- Can epidemiologic information on drug use be used to identify drug-induced disease?

The James Hilton and Emma Austin Manning Foundation agreed to fund the program for one year and then reassess the results. The success of the program was evident after one year and the Foundation agreed to fund the project on a long-term basis.

Dunedin Program personnel include a physician director with specialty training in internal medicine, a registered nurse, and a technician. A civic organization consisting of outstanding women in the community assumed responsibility for scheduling groups of volunteers to perform tasks such as typing, filing, answering telephones, and calling participants to remind them of their appointments. A small five-room frame house was renovated to serve as the clinic facility, and in 1980 a larger clinic facility was occupied.

METHODS

Program participants are scheduled for clinic appointment by telephone or personal visit about 12 months in advance of their visit. A week prior to the scheduled visit, a letter is mailed to remind subjects of their appointment and a detailed health questionnaire is enclosed. Information collected on the questionnaire is listed below:

family history
previous illnesses
present illnesses
current symptoms
drug history
alcohol intake
coffee consumption
diet habits
frequency of medical exams
social activities
exercise habits
sleep habits
perceived value of screening program
attitude toward current health care
hair color
eye color

A form is included which asks the participant to list all prescribed and nonprescribed medications used regularly. For each medication, the participant is asked to specify the intended therapeutic use, how frequently the product is used, and how long the product has been used. Medications were coded using a

Table 1. Laboratory Measurements in the Dunedin Program

BIOCHEMICAL DETERMINATIONS		HEMOGRAM
Glucose	Total protein	Leukocyte count
Sodium	Albumin	Erythrocyte count
Potassium	Globulin	Hemoglobin
Chloride	A/G ratio	Hematocrit
Carbon dioxide	Alkaline phosphatase	Mean corpuscular volume
Blood urea nitrogen (BUN)	Lactate dehydrogenase (LDH)	Mean corpuscular hemoglobin
	SGOT (transaminase)	Mean corpuscular hemoglobin concentration
BUN/Creatinine ratio	SGPT (transaminase)	
Uric acid	Cholesterol	**URINALYSIS**
Calcium	Triglycerides	Blood
Phosphorus	Iron	Protein
		Glucose

modification of the therapeutic and pharmacologic classification of the World Health Organization.[7] Drugs were coded to permit identification of all ingredients used in the population. Information on the questionnaire and drug history form is reviewed with each participant by a nurse when the person arrives for the appointment.

When a participant arrives at the clinic, the name of a close friend or living relative is obtained to facilitate follow-up. The subject is then taken into an examining room where a nurse or technician reviews the questionnaire information supplied by the participant. Then the nurse administers the Folstein Mini-Mental Status Examination and a Beck Depression Inventory.

Blood pressure (BP) determinations are obtained in both arms and several reevaluations are made throughout the visit. An electrocardiogram (ECG) is obtained, and venipuncture is performed. Hemogram and SMAC-23 biochemical determinations are subsequently performed on the blood sample (Table 1). A urine sample is tested for glucose, protein, and blood. Carotid arteries are auscultated. After all data have been reviewed by the director, the participant is notified of any important abnormalities and urged to see his/her physician for evaluation. The entire examination process requires about one hour.

Health questionnaire, laboratory, and electrocardiographic information has been collected since the program's inception in 1975. In addition, death certificates have been collected, whenever possible, on all participants since 1975. Although limited information on drug use has been collected since 1975, complete drug use information has been recorded since 1979. Cognitive function evaluation and the Beck Depression Inventory were initiated for all participants in 1987. The time frame for all information collected is shown in Figure 1.

RESULTS AND DISCUSSION

Since the program began in 1975, over 5000 subjects have been screened for the first visit, while over one-third of the original 2983 subjects have been

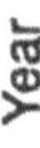

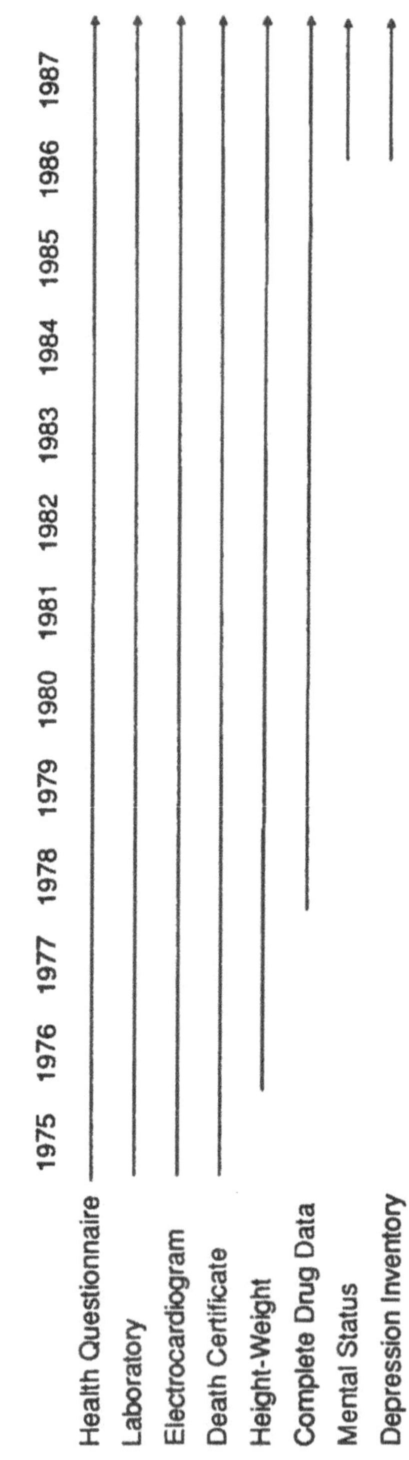

Figure 1. Dunedin data base.

Table 2. Most Common Therapeutic Indications for All Drugs

	Participants Using	
Therapeutic Indication	**No.**	**%**
Antihypertensives	1082	38.2
Analgesics (nonnarcotic)	637	22.5
Antirheumatics	532	18.8
Multivitamins	521	18.4
Vitamin E	435	15.3
Cathartics	430	15.2
Vitamin C	408	14.4
Coronary vasodilators	385	13.6
Nutritional supplements	342	12.1
Multiple vitamins with minerals	302	10.7

screened for all 12 visits. A follow-up program was conducted to determine the reasons for participants' failure to return to the screening program. Information obtained on subjects who have not returned revealed that about 25% moved from the area, 25% failed to keep their appointment due to physical illness, transportation, or other reasons, and 50% have died.

Information collected in the Dunedin Program has been used to study a wide range of questions relating to the aging process. Initially, the information was used to study overall drug use patterns in the elderly and their specific therapeutic categories of drugs. Studies have also been conducted to evaluate laboratory values in the elderly, symptom complexes, and adverse effects of medications used by this population. Results of several of these studies will be described to illustrate how this epidemiologic data base has been used.

Drug usage was studied in Dunedin participants who completed at least one visit to the program during the period July 1983 to June 1985. There were 2834 subjects included in this analysis.[8] Drug histories were obtained on 1842 (65%) women and 992 (35.0%) men. The mean age for women was 76.8 years compared to a mean age for men of 77.6 years. The average number of drugs used by these participants was 3.71 including 3.88 for women and 3.40 for men ($p < 0.0001$). In a study conducted in this population five years earlier, the average number of drugs used was 3.2 (3.5 for women and 2.8 for men). Therefore, it appears that the number of medications used by this population has increased over the past five years; however, it should also be noted that the mean age of the population has increased.

The most common therapeutic indication for drugs used by participants were antihypertensives, analgesics, antirheumatics, cathartics, and multiple vitamins (Table 2). The most common prescription medications used are shown in Table 3. Hydrochlorothiazide-triamterene was the most frequently used prescribed medication. Interestingly, of the 10 most frequently prescribed medications, 8 are used primarily for cardiovascular disease and 1, potassium chloride, is used to prevent hypokalemia resulting from diuretic use.

After we had described general patterns of drug use in the population, several classes of drugs were studied in more detail. Patterns of diuretic use

Table 3. Most Common Prescription Drugs

Drug	Participants Using	
	No.	%
Hydrochlorothiazide-triamterene	383	13.5
Digoxin	273	9.6
Hydrochlorothiazide	237	8.4
Nitroglycerin (sublingual)	214	7.6
Potassium chloride	201	7.1
Furosemide	198	7.0
Propranolol	197	7.0
Dipyridamole	126	4.4
Isosorbide dinitrate	114	4.0
Diazepam	92	3.2

and their effects on laboratory values were analyzed.[9] Over 40% of women and 29% of men used at least one diuretic. Mean biochemical test values for subjects using diuretics were compared to a control group that did not use diuretics. The mean serum potassium concentration was lowest in participants using chlorthalidone (3.47 mEq/L) followed by thiazide (3.74 mEq/L), furosemide (4.05 mEq/L), and hydrochlorothiazide-triamterene (3.99). This suggests that use of potassium-retaining diuretics may be a useful method of maintaining potassium balance in the elderly. Similar studies were conducted on laxatives, nutritional supplements, psychotropic drugs, analgesic drugs, and antacids.[10]

Vitamin E is a nutritional supplement widely used by the elderly. There are few documented beneficial effects of this vitamin, but some clinicians have attributed numerous clinical disorders to its use.[11] The Dunedin data base was used to evaluate the effect of vitamin E use on medical disorders and laboratory parameters.

There were 369 participants using vitamin E, and 1861 subjects in the nonusers group.[12] Eleven clinical disorders that had possibly been associated with vitamin E use, such as hypertension, headache, shortness of breath, vaginal bleeding, diarrhea, and angina, were studied to determine whether the prevalence of these disorders was increased in vitamin E users. The only difference observed was that men using vitamin E reported a greater prevalence of shortness of breath and angina compared with controls. No difference in hematologic values were found in the vitamin E group when compared to controls. Of the 21 biochemical parameters studied, men using vitamin E had higher SGOT concentrations compared to controls, although both were within the accepted range for normal. In summary, no clinical disorder resulting from the use of vitamin E could be documented, and the use of this vitamin appeared to have little influence on hematologic or biochemical parameters.

Hematological and biochemical test results of 2242 participants completing the screening process were used to study normal ranges for these values.[13] A large percentage of white blood cell, red blood cell counts, and hemoglobin and hematocrit values were below the reference range of the laboratory per-

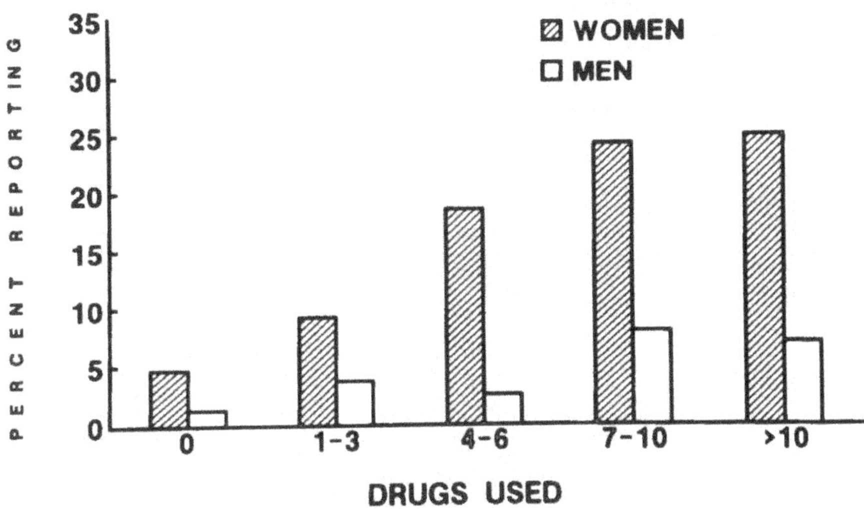

Figure 2. Relationship of headaches to the number of medications used as reported by Dunedin participants. Reprinted with permission from the American Geriatrics Society, "Symptom Prevalence in the Elderly: An Evaluation of Age, Sex, Disease, and Medication Use," by W.E. Hale, L.L. Perkins, F.E. May, et al., *J Am Geriatr Soc* 1986;34(5):337.

forming the test. Over 25% of erythrocyte counts were below the lower limit of normal. Many biochemical values were altered in this population, e.g., serum potassium and serum phosphorus were shifted downward, and blood urea nitrogen and serum creatinine were shifted upward. Only five persons had bilirubin concentrations above the upper limit of normal, making the value of this screening test in the elderly of little value.

The prevalence of 28 symptoms reported by 1927 participants in the program was studied to determine the effect of age, sex, disease, and medication.[14] Women reported a mean of 3.99 symptoms compared with 3.22 reported by men ($p < 0.0001$). The five most common symptoms reported by women were nocturia (80.4%), swollen feet and ankles (30.5%), cold feet and legs (28.6%), constipation (23.7%), and irregular heartbeat (23.6%). Men complained most often of nocturia (79.8%), irregular heartbeat (24.8%), cold feet and legs (23.6%), tinnitus (23.1%), and dyspnea (23.0%). A multiple regression model was used to determine if the number of symptoms was related to age, sex, and their interactions. It was found that the number of symptoms was most strongly related to the number of disease states, followed by the number of drugs used, and then age. Figure 2 shows the relationship of headache to the increasing number of medications used by participants.

The prevalence of headache was studied in 1284 participants to determine the association between this symptom and risk factors, including age, sex, number of reported symptoms and diseases, drug use, and physical characteristics.[15] Eleven percent of women and 5% of men reported frequent headache. There was no relation between age and reported headache in this population. For women there was a significant correlation between headache and the total number of other diseases and symptoms reported ($p < 0.0001$). Subjects who reported sleeping less than seven hours a day reported a greater prevalence of headache (13.5%) than those who slept more than seven hours (8.1%) ($p < 0.01$). No correlation of headache was found with systolic or diastolic blood pressure, or coffee, alcohol, or tobacco use. As is found in younger populations, headache in elderly subjects can result from numerous medical and psychological causes.

SUMMARY

The Dunedin Program is an example of a health screening program that can also be used to collect useful epidemiologic information about the elderly. The authors are unaware of another data base with such complete longitudinal information on ambulatory elderly subjects. The program has already generated useful information on drug utilization patterns, normal laboratory values, and symptom prevalence patterns. We would encourage development of similar programs in other parts of the United States and in other countries.

ACKNOWLEDGMENT

This study was supported in part by AARP Andrus Foundation, Mease Health Care, and SmithKline Clinical Laboratories.

REFERENCES

1. Lamy PP: Patterns of prescribing and drug use, in Butler RN, Bearn AG (eds): *The Aging Process, Therapeutic Implications*. New York, Raven Press, 1985, p. 57.
2. Rowe JW: Health care of the elderly. *N Engl J Med* 1985;312:827–835.
3. Shock NW, Greulich RC, Andres RA, et al: *Normal Human Aging: The Baltimore Longitudinal Study of Aging*, publication No. 84–2450. Bethesda, MD, National Institutes of Health, 1984.
4. Kannel WB, Gordon T: *The Framingham Study: An Epidemiologic Investigation of Cardiovascular Disease*. US Department of Health, Education, and Welfare publication No. (NIH) 74–478. Government Printing Office, 1973.
5. Busse EW, Maddox GL: *The Duke Longitudinal Studies of Normal Aging 1955–1980*. New York; Springer Publishing Co, 1985.

6. Hale WE, Marks RG, Stewart RB: The Dunedin Program, a Florida geriatric screening process: Design and initial data. *J Am Geriatr Soc* 1980;27:377–380.
7. Helling M, Venulet J: Drug recording and classification by the World Health Organization Research Center for international monitoring of adverse reactions to drugs. *Methods Inf Med* 1974;13:169–178.
8. Hale WE, May FE, Marks RG, et al: Drug use in an ambulatory elderly population: A five year update. *Drug Intell Clin Pharm* 1987;21:530–531.
9. Stewart RB, Hale WE, Marks RG: Diuretic use in an ambulatory elderly population. *Am J Hosp Pharm* 1983;40:409–413.
10. Stewart RB, Hale WE, Marks RG: Drug use and adverse drug reactions in an ambulatory elderly population: A review of the Dunedin Program. *Pharm Int* 1984;5:149–152.
11. Roberts HJ: Perspective on vitamin E as therapy. *JAMA* 1981;246:129.
12. Hale WE, Perkins LL, May FE, et al: Vitamin E effect on symptoms and laboratory values in the elderly. *J Am Diet Assoc* 1986;86:625–629.
13. Hale WE, Stewart RB, Marks RG: Haematological and biochemical laboratory values in an ambulatory elderly population: An analysis of the effects of age, sex, and drugs. *Age and Ageing* 1983;12:275–184.
14. Hale WE, Perkins LL, May FE, et al: Symptom prevalence in the elderly: An evaluation of age, sex, disease, and medication use. *J Am Geriatr Soc.* 1986;34:333–340.
15. Hale WE, May FE, Marks RG, et al: Headache in the elderly: An evaluation of risk factors. *Headache* 1987;27:272–276.

26. *Psychotropic Drug Use and Health Outcomes in Nursing Homes*

ELIZABETH A. CHRISCHILLES
MARY NDUAGUBA
ROBERT B. WALLACE
TODD P. SEMLA

INTRODUCTION

The Iowa 65+ Rural Health Study is a prospective cohort study of all persons aged 65 and older residing in two rural Iowa counties. It is one of four components of the National Institute on Aging's "Established Populations for Epidemiologic Studies of the Elderly" (EPESE).[1] This chapter describes the first analysis of the nursing home portion of this data and first investigation of associations between drug use and health outcome in this cohort of nursing home residents. It is the first of several planned investigations of drug use and health outcomes in this elderly population on whom comprehensive health data are collected annually.

The principal objectives of this study were (1) to characterize psychotropic drug use in a population of nursing home residents and (2) to determine whether psychotropic drug use, present at the time of a baseline survey of these residents, is associated with altered mortality rates within three years of that survey. An additional implicit objective was to gain some insight by working with the data base, identifying any problems and determining possible solutions to them.

Certain patient characteristics such as advanced age, male sex, type of physical illness, and functional status have been associated with mortality. It is quite logical to expect that some or all of these characteristics might also be associated with a greater or lesser likelihood of being prescribed psychotropic drugs, and thus potentially confound an epidemiologic study of psychotropic drug use and mortality. Other potential confounding factors are aberrant behaviors, which increase the likelihood of psychotropic drug use and might also be associated with mortality. Also, the number of prescription drugs a patient takes may be related to both mortality and psychotropic drug use if for no other reason than serving as a proxy for severe and complex patient medical problems. Thus the question to be answered is: Once potential confounding factors are controlled for, does an association remain between psychotropic drug use and mortality in these nursing home residents?

METHODS

The Iowa study is the only one of the four EPESE studies that includes a nursing home cohort, comprised of all 647 persons aged 65 years and older residing in the 11 chronic care facilities within the study area. This cohort was initially surveyed in 1982 and continues to be followed with an annual survey. Both the baseline survey and the annual follow-up survey are obtained from nursing home staff who are familiar with the patient and who are asked to complete a nursing home staff report. In addition, the vital status of all patients is established at each annual contact. Mortality surveillance involves continuous monitoring of death certificates, newspaper obituaries, and hospitalization records.

The data collected that are relevant to this chapter include demographic variables, ambulatory status, functional status, existing disease conditions, behavioral status, and medication usage. To establish drug use, the staff member was asked to record drug name, strength, and directions for all prescribed drugs, whether legend or nonlegend. For those drugs prescribed to be used only as needed, the staff member recorded the number of times the patient received the drug yesterday and whether the patient received it in the past two weeks. For this study, only drugs that were used in the past two weeks were considered in designating drug use.

The following definition of psychotropic drug use was employed. Psychotropic drugs consisted of antipsychotics, antidepressants, and sedative-hypnotics. Lithium was excluded because it is so different pharmacologically from the rest of the class. Monoamine oxidase inhibitors were not actually excluded; however, there were no patients taking these drugs. Phenobarbital was excluded because it is frequently prescribed for seizure disorders. Diphenhydramine and hydroxyzine were included as sedative-hypnotics.

RESULTS

One or more antipsychotics were used by 112 (17.3%) of the study population (136 drugs); 59 (9.1%) were using one or more antidepressants (64 drugs); and 103 (15.9%) were using one or more sedative-hypnotic. Overall, 242 persons (37.4%) were taking at least one psychotropic drug. The majority of users were taking only one drug. However, 56 people (8.7%) were using two, seven (1.1%) were using three, and one person was using five psychotropic drugs. In descending order of frequency, haloperidol, chlorpromazine, and thioridazine

Table 1. Distribution of Psychotropic Drug Use, by Age

Age Group	Users	Total in Age Group	% of Sample
65–69	15 (60.00)	25	3.89
70–79	51 (36.96)	138	21.33
80–89	120 (37.74)	318	49.15
90+	56 (33.73)	166	25.66
Total	242 (37.40)	647	100.00

were the most frequently used antipsychotics; amitriptyline, doxepin, and imipramine were the most commonly used antidepressants; flurazepam, diazepam, chloral hydrate, and diphenhydramine were the most commonly used sedative-hypnotics.

When psychotropic drug use is stratified by age as in Table 1, there appears to be decreasing use of psychotropic drug use with advancing age. The National Nursing Home Survey[2] detected a similar negative trend, which was attributed to a greater number of patients with mental retardation in the youngest age group, a finding that was true of this population as well.

Table 2 displays psychotropic drug use by the various disease conditions in persons without a diagnosis of depression or dementia. The entries in the table are not independent, since subjects frequently had more than one of the listed conditions. Inspection of this table reveals that, in persons without dementia or depression, there was a considerable degree of psychotropic drug use, regardless of disease condition. Of interest also was the finding that 32% of subjects with dementia and 49% of subjects with depression took psychotropic drugs. These figures are not substantially different from the figures in Table 2 for other disease conditions in persons *without* dementia or depression.

Further elucidation of this somewhat surprising finding is expressed in Table 3. When the proportions of persons with dementia or depression who took the three types of psychotropic drugs are compared with those for subjects with *neither* depression nor dementia, two observations can be made. First, depressed and/or demented persons did not have impressively different rates of psychotropic drug use than persons with neither condition. Second, the proportions of persons with depression who were taking antidepressants and

Table 2. Psychotropic Drug Use, by Disease Condition in Persons Without Dementia or Depression

Condition	% Users	Condition	% Users
Diabetes	45.9	Hypertension	40.9
Heart trouble	39.6	Angina	31.6
Cancer	24.3	Cataracts	46.6
Glaucoma	37.9	Parkinson's disease	48.3
Arthritis	42.2	Emphysema	41.7
Peptic ulcer	50.0	Hardening of arteries	41.7
Osteoporosis	43.3	Blindness	36.4
Hearing loss	36.6	History of stroke	46.8
History of heart attack	37.0	History of hip fracture	32.1

Table 3. Psychotropic Drug Use In Patients With and Without Depression or Dementia

	Type of Psychotropic Drug Use		
Condition	Antipsychotic	Antidepressant	Sedative-hypnotic
Depression (N = 53)	10 (18.9)	11 (20.7)	7 (13.2)
Dementia (N = 188)	38 (20.2)	10 (5.3)	19 (10.1)
Neither (N = 430)	67 (15.6)	43 (10.0)	78 (18.1)

demented people taking antipsychotics were strikingly low. This suggests that misclassification of these disease conditions might have occurred. Presence of disease conditions was determined by asking the staff members whether a physician had determined if that the patient currently had any of these conditions. Infrequent documentation by physicians of diagnoses in the medical record could have resulted in misclassification, since resolution or initiation of conditions might not have been apparent from the medical record.

When psychotropic drug use is stratified by the nursing home staff member's assessment of whether the resident displayed aberrant behavior (Table 4), it can be seen that patients with depressive symptomatology and symptomatology consistent with organic brain syndrome did appear to use more psychotropic drugs that those without these symptoms. Thus, whereas disease conditions (obtained by the staff member from physician documentation in the medical record) did not discriminate between users and nonusers of psychotropic drugs, psychotropic drug use did vary by staff assessment of resident behavioral symptoms.

Psychotropic drug use rates appeared to be consistent, regardless of ambulatory status. Psychotropic drug use was reported for 57 of 166 persons (34.4%) who could not walk at all; 114 of 297 persons (38.4%) who could walk with help only; and 70 of 182 persons (38.5%) who walked without help. It is of interest that patients who may be of most concern when these drugs are prescribed, i.e., those who require help to ambulate and are perhaps most susceptible to falls, are receiving just as many psychotropic drugs as lower risk individuals.

Functional status, as an indicator of severity of illness which summarizes

Table 4. Psychotropic Drug Use, by Behavior Status

Behavior Status	Users	Total in Category	% of Sample
Depressed for days at a time	63 (56.25%)	112	17.31
Abusive toward staff	16 (51.61%)	31	4.79
Abusive toward patients	2 (25.00%)	8	1.24
Confused or disoriented	103 (43.46%)	237	36.63
Wander at night	4 (57.14%)	7	1.08
No behavior problem	126 (33.60%)	375	57.96

Table 5. Psychotropic Drug Use, by Activities of Daily Living (ADL) Score

ADL Score	Users	Total in Category	% of Sample
0 (independent)	46 (36.80%)	125	19.32
1	37 (33.33%)	111	17.16
2–4	57 (43.18%)	132	20.41
5	43 (32.09%)	134	20.71
6 (total dependence)	59 (40.69%)	145	22.41

Table 6. Psychotropic Drug Use, by Number of Other Drugs Used

No. of Other Drugs*	Users	Total in Category	% of Sample
0	27 (25.71%)	105	16.2
1	44 (36.07%)	122	18.9
2	51 (38.93%)	131	20.2
3	54 (40.30%)	134	20.7
4	34 (42.50%)	80	12.4
5+	32 (42.67%)	75	11.7

* Other drugs = all drugs prescribed in addition to psychotropic drugs.

across conditions, was considered to be a potential confounder of a relation between psychotropic drug use and mortality. However, Table 5 shows no impressive association between psychotropic drug use and functional status. This was borne out in logistic models in which the Activities of Daily Living score was added to the model containing age, sex, and number of psychotropic drugs, and the odds ratio did not change.

It appeared that those patients who used other drugs with central nervous system (CNS) activity (narcotic analgesics, anticonvulsants, and skeletal muscle relaxants) were also somewhat more likely to use psychotropic drugs (40.9% of 115 users of CNS drugs) than were nonusers (36.7% of 532 nonusers). Similarly, the more drugs in addition to psychotropics that persons were taking, the more likely they were to also take a psychotropic drug (Table 6).

The overall three-year mortality rate for this nursing home cohort was 50.7%. As expected, mortality rates increased with age, and males had higher mortality than females (Table 7).

The relation between number of psychotropic drugs and three-year mortality is presented in Table 8, a two-way table unadjusted for covariates. No

Table 7. Three-Year Mortality, by Age and Sex

	Males			Females		
Age Group	No. Dead	%	Total	No. Dead	%	Total
65–69	2	(15.38)	13	4	(33.33)	12
70–79	20	(41.69)	48	27	(30.00)	90
80–89	58	(66.67)	87	108	(46.75)	231
90+	31	(81.58)	38	78	(60.94)	128
Total	111	(59.67)	186	217	(47.07)	461

Table 8. Three-Year Mortality, by Psychotropic Drug Use

No. of Psychotropic Drugs	Alive (%)	Dead (%)	Total
0	192 (47.4)	213 (52.6)	405
1	95 (53.4)	83 (46.6)	178
2+	32 (50.0)	32 (50.0)	64

obvious association was apparent. However, because of the need to address the issue of potential confounding, multivariate logistic regression analysis was used. Table 9 presents the results of this analysis. As expected, advancing age, male sex, poor functional status, and inability to ambulate were all associated with increased mortality, as indicated by the odds ratios and the approximate 95% confidence intervals, none of which include 1. Heart trouble, cancer, and emphysema were the disease conditions significantly associated with mortality. Although dementia, osteoporosis, and history of stroke appeared to be associated with mortality when only age and sex were controlled for, this no longer was apparent after addition of the other model variables. Similarly, numbers of CNS and other drugs were not significantly associated with three-year mortality, nor were any of the behavioral variables. Finally, the number of psychotropic drugs was not associated with three-year mortality (odds ratio

Table 9. Logistic Regression Model

Model Variables*	Odds Ratio	(95% CI)
Age	1.07	(1.04, 1.10)
Sex (0 = M, 1 = F)	0.39	(0.25, 0.60)
ADL score (0 = independent, 6 = dependent in all six areas)	1.23	(1.10, 1.36)
Ambulatory status (0 = can't walk, 1 = walks alone or with help)	0.35	(0.20, 0.59)
Disease variables (0 = absent, 1 = present)		
Heart trouble	2.60	(1.75, 3.86)
Cancer	2.27	(1.11, 4.65)
Emphysema	4.92	(1.69,14.36)
Dementia	1.01	(0.62, 1.65)
Osteoporosis	1.34	(0.67, 2.68)
History of stroke	1.03	(0.65, 1.64)
Behavioral variables (0 = absent, 1 = present)		
Depressed for days at a time	1.38	(0.78, 2.42)
Abusive toward staff	0.94	(0.34, 2.55)
Confused or disoriented	1.11	(0.67, 1.85)
No. of other CNS drugs	1.18	(0.77, 1.79)
No. of other drugs	0.99	(0.89, 1.11)
No. of psychotropic drugs	1.09	(0.82, 1.44)

Note: Model chi-square: 157.75, 16 d.f.

* 0 = alive; 1 = dead.

1.09, 95% confidence interval from 0.82 to 1.44) after controlling for other variables.

CONCLUSION

In conclusion, these data do not support an association between use of psychotropic drugs and three-year mortality in nursing home residents 65 years of age and older. Perhaps as important as this conclusion is the insight that has been gained into the nursing home data base. We continue to be excited about the advantages this data base offers in terms of allowing the consideration of a wide variety of personal characteristics in drug-health outcome studies. However, some potential limitations should be addressed.

First, since this study began as a *prevalence* survey, short-term and terminal care patients, i.e., the extremes of the case-mix spectrum, are underrepresented. Second, the independent variables were measured at a single point in time. Psychotropic drug users at baseline may not have continued to use them and nonusers may have started to use them. This potential misclassification of exposure status could bias our findings toward the null. In the future we will make use of the annual follow-up surveys to ascertain the extent to which this might have occurred. Third, the three-year mortality in this nursing home cohort was high, thus making it difficult to detect a small increase in risk that may have been posed by psychotropic drug use. Finally, serious questions have been raised about the quality of physician documentation of disease conditions in medical records of these nursing home patients. Use of nursing home staff assessment of certain characteristics may more accurately reflect the patient's condition.

ACKNOWLEDGMENT

This work has been supported by contract no. NO1A6–2106 from the National Institute on Aging.

REFERENCES

1. Cornoni-Huntley J, Brock DB, Ostfeld AM, et al (eds): *Established Populations for Epidemiologic Studies of the Elderly: The Resource Data Book*, National Institute on Aging, NIH publication No. 86–2443.
2. Hing E: *Characteristics of Nursing Home Residents, Health Status, and Care Received: 1977 Nursing Home Survey*, DHHS publication No. (PHS) 81–1712 (Vital and health statistics; series 13; no. 51), Government Printing Office, 1981.

27. *What is the Cost of Nephrotoxicity Associated with Aminoglycosides?*

JOHN M. EISENBERG
HARRIS KOFFER
HENRY A. GLICK
MARGARET L. CONNELL
LARRYE E. LOSS
GEORGE H. TALBOT
NEIL H. SHUSTERMAN
BRIAN L. STROM

We measured the economic impact of aminoglycoside-associated nephrotoxicity in a nested case-control study at six Philadelphia area hospitals. From the charts of 1756 patients who received aminoglycosides and met entry criteria, we collected data on patient demographics, clinical characteristics, and resource utilization for all patients with nephrotoxicity and for a sample of patients without nephrotoxicity. Of the 1756 patients, 129 (7.3%) developed aminoglycoside-associated nephrotoxicity. The component costs of nephrotoxicity were calculated by hospital accounting methods; room and board costs were enumerated with per diem rates. The additional cost of hospital ancillary services per case of nephrotoxicity was $446 ($p < 0.001$); the additional cost of hospital stay was $825 for additional routine days (2.74 days) ($p < 0.02$) and $1152 for intensive care days (1.50 days) ($p < 0.001$). Additional consultations were $78 per patient. Therefore, the mean total additional cost of aminoglycoside-associated nephrotoxicity was $2501. The average additional cost per patient receiving aminoglycosides was $183.

[MeSH terms: amikacin; aminoglycosides; cost benefit analysis; costs and cost analysis; creatinine; gentamicins; hospitalization; intensive care units; kidney

[1] From the Department of Medicine (Sections of General Medicine, Infectious Diseases, and Renal-Electrolyte), Clinical Epidemiology Unit, and Leonard Davis Institute of Health Economics, University of Pennsylvania; and the Philadelphia Association for Clinical Trials; Philadelphia, Pennsylvania. Requests for reprints should be addressed to John M. Eisenberg, M.D., M.B.A.; Box 624, Hospital of the University of Pennsylvania, 3400 Spruce Street; Philadelphia, PA 19104.

Reproduced, with permission, from Eisenberg, JM, Koffer, H, Glick MA, et al. What is the cost of nephrotoxicity associated with aminoglycosides? *Ann Intern Med.* 1987;107:900–909.

failure, acute; length of stay; ototoxicity; tobramycin. Other indexing term: nephrotoxocity]

Nephrotoxicity is a well-recognized adverse event associated with the use of aminoglycoside antibiotics. Estimates of the frequency of nephrotoxicity range between 0% and 63%; studies that have used well-defined measures of nephrotoxicity suggest a rate in the range of 10% to 25%.[1-8] Although the occurrence of aminoglycoside-associated nephrotoxicity is well established, its impact on clinical care of the patient and the cost of medical care is not. One study[9] used a simulation to estimate the costs of hospital care associated with aminoglycoside use, but there are no published studies that have measured resources consumed in the treatment of nephrotoxicity.

New antibiotics without a known risk of nephrotoxity have been developed as alternatives to aminoglycosides. One such class of antibiotics, the monobactams, have solely a gram-negative spectrum of activity; their use may have a substantial impact on the cost of medical care by eliminating the economic consequences of nephrotoxicity. This study was done to evaluate these potential savings. We measured the consumption of hospital resources associated with nephrotoxicity and calculated the cost to the hospital and to the payer of aminoglycoside-associated nephrotoxicity. By comparing 111 patients who had nephrotoxicity with 149 patients who did not, drawn from a sample of 1756 patients who met our entry criteria and received aminoglycoside antibiotics at six Philadelphia area hospitals, we show the hidden cost of aminoglycoside use.

METHODS

Study Design

In a case-control study nested within an historical cohort study, we compared patients who had nephrotoxicity with patients who did not from a cohort of patients treated with aminoglycoside antibiotics. The hospital records of study patients were reviewed to determine other clinical factors that might be associated with high use of hospital resources, as well as to determine the use of hospital and physician services related to nephrotoxicity. The economic analysis was done from the perspective of the hospital with the exception of the cost for physician services. In this study, physician consultations represent a cost to the payer (individual or insurer) rather than the hospital, and are reported as an economic effect of aminoglycoside-associated nephrotoxicity.

Hospitals of different sizes and types of governance frequently have distinct styles of operation that may affect the cost of medical care. Therefore, we selected six hospitals in the Philadelphia metropolitan area for study: two

Table 1. Hospital Demographics and Rates of Nephrotoxicity

	Hospital						
	1	2	3	4	5	6	Total
Hospital size (beds), *n*	687	372	308	428	188	370	...
Hospital type*	UT	UT	CT	CT	CH	CH	...
Patients meeting criteria for inclusion, *n*	658	211	365	93	103	326	1756
Nephrotoxic patients, *n*	55	9	23	6	8	28	129
Percentage of patients who developed nephrotoxicity, %	8.4	4.3	6.3	6.5	7.8	8.6	7.3

*UT = university teaching hospital; CT = community teaching hospital; CH = community hospital.

university-based teaching hospitals (372 and 687 beds); two community-based teaching hospitals (308 and 428 beds); and two community-based nonteaching hospitals (188 and 370 beds). These six hospitals are described in Table 1.

Patient Population

Patients receiving at least 72 hours of continuous treatment with gentamicin, tobramycin, or amikacin, who were at least 18 years old, and who were discharged between 1 July 1984 and 30 June 1985 were eligible for inclusion. Patients were excluded if they had amphotericin B administration during hospitalization, renal failure requiring dialysis or transplantation before aminoglycoside therapy, shock (two consecutive systolic measurements of less than 80 mm Hg or a decrease of 50 mm Hg from a baseline systolic pressure of 150 mm Hg or greater) within 72 hours before the start of or during aminoglycoside therapy, amyloidosis, or multiple myeloma.

Patients were divided into two groups according to changes in serum creatinine levels. Patients with nephrotoxicity were defined as those with an increase in serum creatinine of 0.5 mg/dL (40 μmol/L) or more when the baseline value was less than 3.0 mg/dL (270 μmol/L), or an increase of 1.0 mg/dL (90 μmol/L) or more when the baseline value was 3.0 mg/dL (270 μmol/L) or more. All other patients were considered not to have nephrotoxicity. Baseline serum creatinine values were defined as the mean of the last available measurements (up to three stable values) obtained within 7 days before the initiation of aminoglycoside therapy.

The serum creatinine levels must have begun to increase during aminoglycoside treatment or within 48 hours after the termination of therapy and remained elevated for two consecutive determinations in order to define the patient as having nephrotoxicity. The highest value obtained during and up to 48 hours after antibiotic therapy was defined as the peak; this value was used to calculate the absolute change from baseline. In patients for whom creatinine values were rising but did not reach a peak within 48 hours after discontinuation of antibiotic therapy, the level was observed until it reached its zenith, which was considered the peak value.

All patients with nephrotoxicity were included in the study. For each patient with nephrotoxicity identified, the next available patient treated with

Table 2. Demographic and Clinical Characteristics of Study Subjects*

Characteristics	Patients with Nephrotoxicity (n = 111)	Patients without Nephrotoxicity (n = 149)
Age, *yrs*	67 ± 14†	58 ± 20
Gender, *n (%)*		
Male	57(51)	81(54)
Female	54(49)	68(46)
Race, *n (%)*		
White	78(70)	91(61)
Black	32(29)	57(38)
Other	1(1)	1(1)
Baseline creatinine level, *mg/dL*	1.3 ± 0.6	1.2 ± 0.7
Infection with, *n (%) Pseudomonas aeruginosa*	20(18)	27(18)
Total aminoglycoside dosage, *mg*	1978 ± 1577†	1593 ± 1237
Days of aminoglycoside treatment	11.4 ± 8.7†	7.6 ± 5.4
Secondary diagnoses	5.5 ± 2.3†	4.1 ± 2.4
Sites of infection	1.4 ± 1.1†	0.9 ± 0.9
Diagnosis-related group weight	2.23 ± 1.48†	1.48 ± 0.87
Diagnosis-related group mean length of stay, *d*	13.8 ± 5.3†	11.0 ± 4.6
Patient status, *n (%)*		
Discharged alive	77(69)‡	140(94)
Death before mean length of stay (23 days)	19(17)‡	2(1)
Death after mean length of stay (23 days)	15(14)‡	7(5)

* Values are mean ± SD.

† Student's *t*-test, $p < 0.05$, comparing patients who had nephrotoxicity with those who did not.

‡ Chi square, $p < 0.05$, comparing patients who had nephrotoxicity with those who did not.

aminoglycosides who did not develop nephrotoxicity was selected as a control. We also reviewed 37 randomly drawn charts of patients without nephrotoxicity. Patients' charts were reviewed by trained data collectors at each study site, and information was collected on variables that may be associated with the development of nephrotoxicity, variables that may be monitored to detect nephrotoxicity in patients who are receiving aminoglycosides, and other demographic and clinical variables (Table 2).

Data Collected

Data were collected on the following variables: length of stay in the medical intensive care unit after the start of aminoglycoside therapy; length of stay in the surgical intensive care unit after the start of aminoglycoside therapy; length of stay in a routine care unit after the start of aminoglycoside therapy; costs of ancillary services and consultations related to aminoglycoside use or nephrotoxicity; total hospital charges; variables to control for severity of illness before the start of aminoglycoside therapy, including length of stay in a routine care unit before start of aminoglycoside therapy, length of stay in the intensive care unit before the start of aminoglycoside therapy, laboratory tests before the start of aminoglycoside therapy, patient age, nephrology consultations before the start of aminoglycoside therapy, and infectious disease consultations before the start of aminoglycoside therapy; variables to control for other indicators of severity of illness during the hospitalization, including total parenteral nutrition, death, number of infection sites, and *Pseudomonas aeruginosa* infection; variables to control for underlying illness including diagnosis-related group weight, arithmetic mean length of stay for diagnosis-related group, and number of secondary diagnoses (independent of renal diagnoses); a variable to indicate the degree of nephrotoxicity (measured as the absolute change in serum creatinine level); and variables to control for case-mix and practice patterns, characterized as a set of 0/1 dummy variables representing the six study hospitals.

Costs

Two methods were used to assess the cost of resources consumed in association with aminoglycoside-related nephrotoxicity. First, the costs of ancillary services and consultations associated with the treatment of nephrotoxicity were calculated; additional days of hospitalization associated with nephrotoxicity were determined and the per diem costs for these days were added. The costs of ancillary services were calculated using cost-to-charge ratios applied to actual charges, a hospital accounting mechanism to convert charges to estimates of the actual cost of providing care. Charge information for each ancillary service was obtained from the billing office at each hospital. Cost-to-charge ratios were procured from the Medicare intermediary for each hospital. Charges for consultative services were obtained from the Medicare prevailing charge profile by medical specialty (nephrology, infectious diseases, and general medicine). Routine and intensive care costs were obtained from the per diem rates reported in the hospitals' Medicare cost reports. From these data, the cost of incremental days in medical intensive care units and days in routine care units was calculated, using a weighted average cost of $768 per day for medical intensive care unit days and $301 per day for routine care unit days. A weighted average cost per episode of nephrotoxicity and per patient treated with aminoglycosides was then calculated based on the number of patients at each study site.

Second, total patient charges were obtained directly from hospital billing records. Professional charges for consultative services are not billed by the hospital and thus were excluded from the analysis from the hospital's perspective, but these charges are reported as a cost to payers.

Finally, to estimate the economic impact of aminoglycoside-associated nephrotoxicity on all patients who received aminoglycosides, including both those who developed nephrotoxicity and those who did not, we calculated an average cost per patient adjusted for the observed percentage of patients developing nephrotoxicity (per hospitalization for patients exposed to aminoglycosides).

Analysis

Univariate analyses were done to explore the relationship between each variable and the presence or absence of nephrotoxicity. Student's *t*-tests and chi-squared tests were used to assess differences. A two-tailed *p* value of ≤ 0.05 was necessary for rejection of null hypotheses.

Multiple regression analyses were used to control for potential confounding variables that might be associated with higher hospital costs. As with the univariate statistics, a two-tailed *p* value of ≤ 0.05 was necessary for rejection of null hypotheses. The *R*-square and *R*-bar-square statistics are also reported. The *R*-square represents the proportion of explained variation captured by the regression, independent of the number of explanatory variables. The *R*-bar-square accounts for the number of explanatory variables used in the regression equation, correcting the *R*-square statistic for degrees of freedom. Unlike *R*-square, *R*-bar-square can decrease as the number of explanatory variables increases. Ninety-five percent confidence intervals (95% CI) were calculated for the nephrotoxicity coefficients.

Regressions were done using nephrotoxicity both as a continuous variable (reported as mg/dL increase in creatinine) and as a discrete, dummy variable (reported as nephrotoxic or not). These regressions enabled us to evaluate both the dose and exposure effect of nephrotoxicity. Because the regression models using nephrotoxicity as a continuous variable were more consistent with clinical practice, explained more variance, and did not change the study results, we report the regressions using nephrotoxicity as a continuous variable.

The regression analyses were first done on the entire sample of nephrotoxic patients. In order to assess the impact of the dialysis on the cost of nephrotoxicity, we reestimated these costs excluding the patients who underwent dialysis. These results are reported separately.

In addition, in order to evaluate the impact of outlier points on the outcome of the regression analyses, we identified influential observations in the data and reestimated the regressions excluding these points. These observations have independent variables that are generally all larger or all smaller than the mean of the independent variables. The observations also have standardized residuals that are statistically significantly larger than the mean of the standardized residuals.

By collecting data solely on those services that were assumed to be associated with nephrotoxicity, we risked not capturing other services that might be added to or withdrawn from the patient due to this complication. Total charges represent the sum of hospital charges for services provided to the patient during the entire course of hospitalization and comprise the measured component costs plus other costs that we did not tabulate. Although charges generally do not provide a precise measure of actual resources consumed during a hospitalization, analysis of total charges may provide insight into whether services associated with nephrotoxicity are substituted for other services during hospitalization (that is, offset one another). To evaluate the question of substitution, we did two separate regressions for both the component cost and total charge data. In the first set of regressions, we excluded days attributable to nephrotoxicity (as predicted by the length-of-stay regressions) from the length-of-stay variables predicting cost or charges. By making this exclusion we transferred all of nephrotoxicity's explanatory power (in terms of its effect on both length of stay and intensity of ancillary services) to the variable that explicitly measures nephrotoxicity (creatinine). In the second set of regressions, we included the days attributable to nephrotoxicity in the length-of-stay variables predicting cost and charges. We thus split the explanatory power of nephrotoxicity into its effect on length of stay (captured by the length-of-stay variables) and its effect on the intensity of services (captured by the nephrotoxicity variable). We then saw whether or not the nephrotoxicity variable was statistically significant in the different regressions.

RESULTS

From the records of 4700 patients who received aminoglycoside antibiotics at the study hospitals, we identified 1756 who met our criteria for inclusion. Of these, 129 (7.3%) patients met our criteria for nephrotoxicity. Table 1 shows the characteristics of the six hospitals and their rates of nephrotoxicity. In addition, we collected data from the records of 166 patients who received aminoglycosides but did not develop nephrotoxicity. Thirty-five patients (18 with nephrotoxicity, 17 without) from the total group were omitted from analyses because of insufficient information about their diagnoses, including their diagnosis-related groups. This left 111 patients with nephrotoxicity and 149 controls. Another 18 patients (5 with nephrotoxicity, 13 without) were omitted only from the total charge regression analyses because of missing charge data.

Patient and Infection Characteristics

The patients' characteristics are shown in Table 2. Univariate analyses showed that these two groups of patients were not significantly different in gender, race, mean baseline creatinine value, and proportion with *Pseudomonas aeruginosa* infections. Patients having nephrotoxicity were older and received larger doses of aminoglycosides for a longer duration. Other differences also suggested that the patients with nephrotoxicity were more seriously ill: fewer were discharged from the hospital alive; their mean number of secondary diagnoses was 5.5, compared with 4.1 for controls; and their mean number of sites of infection was higher, as was the mean weight of their diagnosis-related groups.

Table 3. Total Length of Stay and Length of Stay in Intensive Care Unit*

	Length of Stay	
	Patients with Nephrotoxicity (n = 111)	Patients without Nephrotoxicity (n = 149)
	← d →	
Overall length of stay	30.6 ± 21.1†	17.5 ± 12.6
Overall length of stay in routine care units	24.2 ± 20.9†	16.2 ± 11.8
Overall length of stay in medical intensive care unit	4.7 ± 8.2†	0.9 ± 2.9
Overall length of stay in surgical intensive care unit	1.7 ± 4.8†	0.4 ± 1.3
Length of stay before		
Aminoglycoside therapy		
Overall	6.7 ± 9.1†	4.6 ± 8.3
Routine care unit length of stay	5.4 ± 8.5	4.2 ± 7.7
Medical intensive care unit length of stay	0.6 ± 1.9	0.3 ± 1.3
Surgical intensive care unit length of stay	0.7 ± 2.4†	0.1 ± 0.5
Length of stay after intitation of		
Aminoglycoside therapy		
Overall	23.9 ± 17.4†‡	12.9 ± 7.5
Routine care unit length of stay	19.1 ± 17.6†	12.1 ± 7.3
Medical intensive care unit length of stay	4.0 ± 7.3	0.6 ± 2.3
Surgical intensive care unit length of stay	0.7 ± 2.5	0.3 ± 1.1

* Values expressed as mean ± SD.

† Student's t-test, $p < 0.05$, comparing patients who had nephrotoxocity with those who did not.

‡ The difference in the overall length of stay after initiation of aminoglycoside and the sum of its component parts is due to rounding error.

Length of Stay, Serum Creatinine Level, and Cost

Table 3 shows that the length of stay was longer for patients with nephrotoxicity (30.6 days compared with 17.5 days). Both the length of stay before initiation of aminoglycoside therapy and that after were longer for the patients having nephrotoxicity.

The absolute change in serum creatinine values was used to measure the degree of nephrotoxicity. Mean ± SD baseline creatinine values were similar in the two groups: 1.3 ± 0.6 mg/dL (110 ± 50 μmol/L) in patients with nephrotoxicity and 1.2 ± 0.7 (110 ± 50 μmol/L) in controls. However, the peak determinations and absolute change for patients with nephrotoxicity (3.3 ± 1.9 mg/dL [290 ± 170 μmol/L] and 2.0 ± 1.6 mg/dL [180 ± 140 μmol/L, respectively) were significantly different ($p < 0.001$, Student's t-test) from results for controls (1.3 ± 0.7 mg/dL [110 ± 50] μmol/L] and 0.1 ± 0.3 mg/dL [10 ± 30 μmol/L]).

Table 4 shows the differences in component costs and total charges for the two groups. Comparisons of the component costs, both including and excluding physician consultations, show that the costs incurred by patients with nephrotoxicity ($1396 and $1163, respectively) were significantly greater than those borne by controls ($620 and $529) ($p < 0.001$). These component costs do not include the cost of prolonged hospital stay. Mean total charges per

Table 4. Component Costs and Total Charges*

	Patients with Nephrotoxicity	Patients without Nephrotoxicity
	←— $ —→	
Component costs (including consultations)†	1396 ± 1404‡	620 ± 482
Component costs (excluding consultations)	1163 ± 1203‡	529 ± 381
Total charges	41 185 ± 28 155‡	21 463 ± 20 768

* Values expressed as mean ± SD.

† Component costs included consultations (infectious disease, general medicine, renal, dietary and nutritional support, and pharmacokinetic monitoring services); serum creatinine determinations; serum aminoglycoside levels; other related laboratory tests (electrolytes, urine creatinine, urine protein); other diagnostic tests (renal scan, ultrasound, computed tomography, intravenous pyelogram, renal biopsy); and other services (special diets, hyperalimentation, urinary catheterization).

‡ Student's *t*-test, $p < 0.05$, comparing patients who had nephrotoxicity with those who did not.

patient were also higher for patients with nephrotoxicity ($41 185) than for controls ($21 463) ($p < 0.001$).

Increases in resource utilization could be caused by nephrotoxicity but also may have occurred among patients with nephrotoxicity due to their underlying diseases. Regression analysis was used to estimate the resources consumed in association with nephrotoxicity and to control for variables that suggest more severe disease.

The results of regressions for length of stay are shown in Table 5. The regression model for medical intensive care unit length of stay captured 47% of the variation in this variable and was significant (*R*-bar-square = 0.43; $p < 0.001$). The nephrotoxicity variable (defined by absolute change in creatinine) was positive and statistically significant ($p < 0.001$). The coefficient of this variable showed that every 1-mg/dL (90-μmol/L) absolute change in creatinine level between baseline and peak added 0.75 days (95% CI, 0.35 to 1.15) to patient's stay in the medical intensive care unit after the initiation of drug therapy. Because the average absolute change in creatinine values for patients with nephrotoxicity equaled 2.0 mg/dL (180 μmol/L), the average patient with nephrotoxicity would have stayed in the medical intensive care unit 1.50 days longer, when other variables associated with severity of disease were controlled.

Unlike the regression for medical intensive care unit, the model describing the surgical intensive care unit stay after the initiation of drug therapy explained only 18% of the observed variation in this stay (*R*-bar-square = 0.12). The nephrotoxicity variable was not a statistically significant predictor.

The estimated model for routine care unit length of stay captured 33% of the variation in this variable (*R*-bar-square = 0.28; $p < 0.001$). The nephrotoxicity variable was positive and statistically significant ($p < 0.02$); a 1-mg/dL (90-μmol/L) absolute change in creatinine values between baseline and the peak value added 1.37 days (95% CI, 0.26 to 2.48) to the patients' length of

Table 5. Length of Stay Regressions

Independent Variables*	Medical Intensive Care Unit Length of Stay Coefficients†	Routine Care Unit Length of Stay Coefficients‡
Intercept	−0.61	3.91
Absolute change in creatinine	0.75§	1.37§
Length of stay before aminoglycosides	−0.13§	0.30§
Length of stay in medical intensive care unit before aminoglycosides‖	...	−1.60§
Length of stay in medical intensive care unit before aminoglycosides¶	6.38§	...
Length of stay in surgical intensive care unit before aminoglycosides	...	1.01§
Diagnosis-related group weight	0.35	...
Diagnosis-related group arithmetic mean length of stay	...	0.49§
Age	−0.03	0.06
Hospital 2	−0.73	−5.75§
Hospital 3	2.55§	−2.88
Hospital 4	0.64	−5.63
Hospital 5	3.12§	−2.83
Hospital 6	0.24	−3.08
Number of infected sites	0.46	1.85§
Number of secondary diagnoses	0.40§	−0.03
Death later than 23rd day	3.91§	−3.77
Death on or before 23rd day	−0.67	−12.41§
Infectious disease consultations before aminoglycosides	−1.94	8.80§
Nephrology consultation before aminoglycosides	...	−10.23
Parenteral nutrition	...	36.40§
Infection with *Pseudomonas aeruginosa*	−1.09	...
Number of observations	260	259
R-square	0.47	0.33
R-bar-square	0.43	0.28
F-statistic	13.41§	6.53§

* Hospital 1 is not depicted because it was the base case to which the other hospitals were compared.
† Dependent variable: stay in medical intensive care unit after initiation of aminoglycoside therapy.
‡ Dependent variable: stay in routine care unit after the initiation of aminoglycoside therapy
§ $p < 0.05$, Student's *t*-test.
‖ Length of stay as a continuous variable.
¶ Length of stay as a discrete (0 = absent, 1 = present) variable.

stay in routine care units after the initiation of aminoglycoside therapy. Because patients with nephrotoxicity had an average absolute change in creatinine values of 2.0 mg/dL (180 μmol/L), the expected additional hospitalization in a routine care unit for the average patient with nephrotoxicity would be 2.74 days when controlling for other variables with severity of disease.

The regression model for the cost of the components of care (ancillary services and consultations) that might increase with the presence of nephrotoxicity captured 66% of variation in this dependent variable (*R*-bar-square =

Table 6. Variable and Coefficients of Component Cost and Total Charge Regressions

Independent Variables	Component Costs Coefficients*	Total Charges Coefficients†
Intercept	262	−2514
Absolute change in creatinine	262‡	2649‡
Length of stay in routine care units§	...	901‡
Length of stay in medical intensive care unit§	...	1546‡
Length of stay in surgical intensive care unit	...	2251‡
Length of stay in routine care units after aminoglycosides§	37‡	...
Length of stay in medical intensive care unit after aminoglycosides§	111‡	...
Length of stay in surgical intensive care unit after aminoglycosides	89‡	...
Diagnosis-related group weight	46	3944‡
Age	−4	− 73
Hospital 2	−229	− 89
Hospital 3	−255	−3638
Hospital 4	−249	−10 956‡
Hospital 5	30	−5115‡
Hospital 6	−101	4461‡
Number of secondary diagnoses	...	823‡
Death later than 23rd day	305	4026
Death on or before 23rd day	−248	4816
Days of total parenteral nutrition	−16‡	192
Infection with *Pseudomonas aeruginosa*	...	3087
Laboratory tests/day before aminoglycosides	37	1236‡
Number of observations	260	242
R-square	0.66	0.84
R-bar-square	0.64	0.83
F-statistic	31.06‡	68.22‡

* Dependent variable: component costs.
† Dependent variable: total charges.
‡ $p<0.05$, Student's *t*-test.
§ Excludes days attributable to nephrotoxicity (determined by length of stay regressions). Hospital 1 is not depicted because it was the base case to which the other hospitals were compared.

0.64; $p < 0.001$) (Table 6). The regression indicated an increase of \$262 (95% CI, 201 to 323; $p < 0.001$) in component costs per 1-mg/dL (90-μmol/L) change in creatinine value. Therefore, the additional total calculated component costs for the average patient with nephrotoxicity, based on the mean absolute change in creatinine (2.0 mg/dL [180 μmol/L]), was \$524 (\$446 plus \$78 for physician consultations).

In this regression we excluded the length of stay attributable to nephrotoxicity from the length-of-stay independent variable. We also did a second regression that included the entire length of stay in the length-of-stay variables (whether it was due to nephrotoxicity or not). The nephrotoxicity variable remained statistically significant in this second analysis, even though the explanatory power of nephrotoxicity itself was split between the length-of-stay variables and the creatinine variable.

The regression model for total charges captured 84% of variation in this variable (*R*-bar-square = 0.83; $p < 0.001$) (Table 6). This analysis was based on 242 patients: 106 with nephrotoxicity and 136 without. Five patients with nephrotoxicity and 13 without were excluded from this analysis because of missing charge information. When the absolute change in creatinine was used to define nephrotoxicity and days attributable to nephrotoxicity were excluded from the length-of-stay measures, a 1-mg/dL (90-μmol/L) absolute change in creatinine level was related to a $2649 (95% CI, 1558 to 3740; $p < 0.001$) increase in total charges. This figure represented an increase in total charges of $5298, based on an absolute change in creatinine of 2.0 mg/dL (180 μmol/L) for the 106 patients with nephrotoxicity included in this analysis. The cost to payers combines hospital charges as well as consultation fees, and equals $5376.

As with the analysis of component costs, the independent variables in this regression excluded length of stay attributable to nephrotoxicity. This exclusion attributed the additional charges arising from nephrotoxicity-associated changes in length of stay to the nephrotoxicity variable. In addition, a second regression that included total length of stay was done. This analysis split the explanatory power attributable to nephrotoxicity between the nephrotoxicity and length-of-stay variables. In this case, the nephrotoxicity measure lost its statistical significance.

Cost estimates were reevaluated after excluding from the analysis the three patients with nephrotoxicity who underwent dialysis. The exclusion of dialysis patients reduced the mean absolute change in creatinine to 1.9 mg/dL (170 μmol/L). The coefficient for the effect of nephrotoxicity on days in the medical intensive care unit decreased from 0.75 to 0.42 (95% CI, 0.02 to 0.82; $p = 0.036$), and the coefficient for days in a routine care unit increased from 1.37 to 1.74 days (95% CI, 0.56 to 2.92; $p = 0.004$). These changes yielded an average increment in medical intensive care unit length of stay of 0.80 days (which is 0.7 days less than the estimated increment when patients with dialysis were included) and an increment in stays in routine care units of 3.31 days (which is 0.57 days more than the estimated increment when patients with dialysis were included).

Excluding patients who required dialysis decreased the component cost estimate from $262 to $142 (95% CI, 100 to 184; $p < 0.001$) per 1-mg/dL (90-μmol/L) increase in creatinine and shifted the total charge estimate from $2649 to $2591 (95% CI, 1425 to 3757; $p < 0.001$) per 1-mg/dL (90-μmol/L) increase in creatinine. Thus, exclusion of patients requiring dialysis yielded an average increase in component costs due to nephrotoxicity of $270 ($254 less than the estimate with dialysis patients included) and an average increase in charges due to nephrotoxicity of $4923 ($375 less than the estimate with dialysis patients included).

Similarly, cost estimates were reevaluated after excluding outlier observations from the analysis. In all cases, the regression models remained statistically significant ($p < 0.001$). The exclusion of outlier observations reduced the mean absolute change in creatinine to 1.9 mg/dL (170 μmol/L) for the medical intensive care unit length of stay and component cost regressions. The coefficient for the effect of nephrotoxicity on days in the medical intensive care unit decreased from 0.75 to 0.67 (95% CI, 0.27 to 1.07) and the coefficient for days in a routine care unit increased from 1.37 to 1.39 days (95% CI, 0.36 to 2.42). These changes yielded an average increment in medical intensive care unit length of stay of 1.27 days (which is 0.23 days less than the estimated increment when all observations are included) and an increment in stays in routine care units of 2.78 days (which is 0.04 days greater than the estimated increment when all observations are included).

When outlier observations were excluded, the component cost estimate decreased from $262 to $194 (95% CI, 153 to 235) per 1-mg/dL (90-μmol/L) increase in creatinine and the total charge estimate increased from $2649 to $2872 (95% CI, 2107 to 3637) per 1-mg/dL (90-μmol/L) increase in creatinine. Therefore, exclusion of outlier observations resulted in an average increase in component costs due to nephrotoxicity of $369 ($155 less than the estimate with outlier observations included) and an average increase in charges due to nephrotoxicity of $5744 ($446 greater than the estimate with outlier observations included).

After we examined the residuals of our predictive models, it appeared that the models tended to underpredict longer lengths of stay and higher costs and charges, and that the residuals appeared to correlate with the predictions of the dependent variable (a demonstration of heteroscedasticity). To correct these problems, we analyzed several respecifications of the models, including log and root transformations of the dependent variables and of the nephrotoxicity measures. Because the explanatory power of the component cost and total charge regressions was decreased when these transformations were made, we concluded that these transformations were inferior to the nontransformed regressions.

Cost of Nephrotoxicity

The total cost of nephrotoxicity was calculated by adding the results of the regressions for component costs, medical intensive care unit length of stay, and length of stay in routine care units. Each of these three types of hospital cost was affected by nephrotoxicity and represents an important element in the cost of hospital care. The additional cost of medical intensive care unit days attributable to nephrotoxicity was $1152 (1.50 days × $768 per day). The attributable cost of days in a routine care unit was $825 (2.74 days × $301 per day), and the costs of the additional components of care were $524 (including consultations). Therefore, the total additional cost associated with nephrotoxicity averaged $2501 per patient with nephrotoxicity. As expected (because costs are generally less than reported charges), this estimated additional cost was substantially less than the estimate of $5376 based on the regression analysis of total charges. Because 7.3% of patients exposed to aminoglycosides at the six study hospitals developed nephrotoxicity, the average cost per patient exposed to aminoglycoside antibiotics was $183 (0.073 × $2501).

Sensitivity Analysis

Because the estimates of the length of hospital stay and component costs due to aminoglycoside-associated nephrotoxicity are dependent on whether outlier observations and patients undergoing dialysis are included in the sample and whether the dependent variables are represented by log or root transformations, we did a sensitivity analysis of the cost of nephrotoxicity. This analysis was particularly important because some investigators have suggested that aminoglycoside-associated nephrotoxicity rarely, if ever, requires dialysis.[9] By using the estimates derived from the model when dialysis patients were excluded from the analysis, and summing the medical intensive care unit cost, the cost of care in a routine care unit and component costs, we calculated the average additional cost associated with nephrotoxicity: (0.8 days × $768 per day) + (3.31 days × $301 per day) + $270 = $1881. In a second calculation, we substituted the cost estimates for medical intensive care unit and routine care unit derived from the respecified models (using log or root transformations of the dependent variables): (0.92 days × $768 per day) + (2.90 days × $301 per day) + $524 = $2103. Finally, we calculated the average additional cost associated with nephrotoxicity when outlier observations were excluded from the analysis: (1.27 days × $768 per day) + (2.78 days × $301 per day) + $369 = $2181. Therefore, our estimate of the cost of nephrotoxicity as $2501 per nephrotoxic episode should be considered in light of these lower estimates. Using these cost figures and the 7.3% incidence figure, we estimate that the lower bound of average cost per patient of aminoglycoside-associated nephrotoxicity ranges from $137 to $159.

Because the published literature suggests various frequencies for aminoglycoside-associated nephrotoxicity, our results are also dependent on the rate of nephrotoxicity. Assuming an average cost per episode of nephrotoxicity of $2501, Figure 1 shows how the average cost per patient exposed to aminoglycosides would change as the frequency of aminoglycoside-associated nephrotoxicity changes. This analysis assumes a linear relationship between cost and frequency of nephrotoxicity.

An additional potential cost of nephrotoxicity is that incurred when a patient is switched from less expensive aminoglycoside antibiotics to considerably more expensive alternative antibiotics because of a continued decline in renal function. We examined the potential impact of this switch in drug therapy on the total cost of aminoglycoside-associated nephrotoxicity in a small cohort of patients at one of the six study hospitals. The results suggest that such a switch occurred infrequently and did not substantially affect the total cost of nephrotoxicity. Often, when a decline in renal function was seen, the prescribing physician modified the dosing regimen or duration of therapy instead of discontinuing therapy with an effective drug.

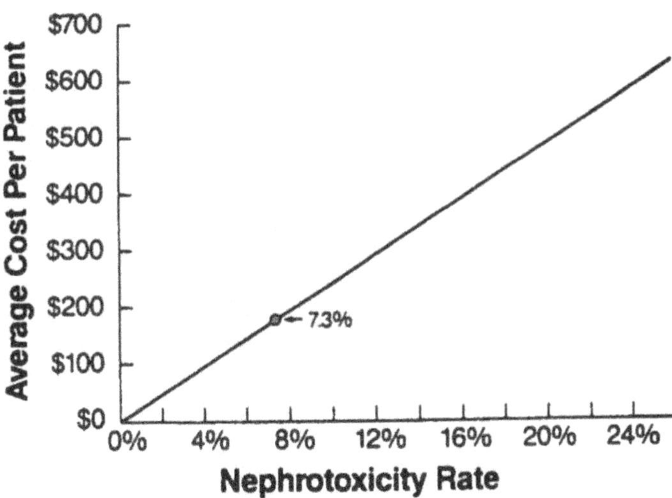

Figure 1. Sensitivity analysis showing the average expected cost of aminoglycoside-associated nephrotoxicity per patient exposed to aminoglycosides. Based on the 7.3% incidence of nephrotoxicity in our study, the average cost per patient exposed to aminoglycoside antibiotics was $183.

DISCUSSION

The potential but undocumented cost of nephrotoxicity related to aminoglycosides is important in assessing the value of an alternative drug. Therefore, we carried out a case-control study nested in an historical cohort study to determine the frequency and economic consequences of aminoglycoside-associated nephrotoxicity. We used the perspectives of both the hospital and the payer for medical care in this analysis. Therefore, we estimated the cost of nephrotoxicity based on both the cost to the hospital of resources consumed in caring for patients with nephrotoxicity as well as charges to the payer.

Among the 1756 patients eligible for our study, 7.3% met our criteria for aminoglycoside-associated nephrotoxicity; they had a mean 2.0 mg/dL (180 μmol/L) increase in creatinine value. We compared the costs incurred by these patients with costs incurred by a sample of patients without nephrotoxicity. Our analysis of the costs induced by nephrotoxicity included $1152 for 1.50 days of prolonged medical intensive care unit stay, $825 for 2.74 days of prolonged hospital stay in a routine care unit, and $446 for additional components of care (ancillary services). When the additional $78 cost of physician consultations was included (it is not usually a cost to the hospital, but rather to the patient or third party payer), the total average additional cost of aminoglycoside-associated nephrotoxicity was $2501. The additional charge to the payer (as expected, a higher figure than estimated cost) was $5376. When we excluded 3 patients undergoing dialysis, these additional costs were $1881 and additional charges were $4923. Based on the incidence of nephrotoxicity of

7.3% and the cost of $2501 per episode of nephrotoxicity, the average cost of nephrotoxicity per patient exposed to aminoglycosides was $183.

Aminoglycoside exposure is one of the five principal causes of hospital-acquired acute renal failure, along with volume depletion, congestive heart failure, shock, and radiocontrast media exposure.[10] (Shusterman, NH. Unpublished data). Although other risk factors have been suggested, few have been shown to be significant in clinical trials.[11]

Various investigators have reported rates of gentamicin nephrotoxicity ranging between 4% and 63%;[1-3,5,6] for tobramycin, the reported rates have ranged from 0% to 44%.[3-7] Other aminoglycosides are also associated with nephrotoxicity.[4,11-14] When measures of nephrotoxicity more sensitive than serum creatinine concentration are used (such as urinary lysosomal enzyme excretion, which indicates proximal tubular damage), estimates of the frequency of aminoglycoside nephrotoxicity are higher. [5,6]

Although most estimates of the frequency of aminoglycoside-associated nephrotoxicity are in the 10% to 25% range (with one large clinical series suggesting the rate to be 4.1%),[8] it is unclear how often nephrotoxicity is of clinical importance. Even less evident is the impact of aminoglycoside-associated nephrotoxicity on the cost of hospital care. One study[9] of the cost effectiveness of gentamicin and tobramycin used a simulated model of hospital care to estimate hospital expenses due to nephrotoxicity and concluded that the cost per case of nephrotoxicity would be $238. However, this study did not measure the costs of actual episodes of nephrotoxicity, but instead enumerated the charges for laboratory tests, diagnostic procedures, and consultations that expert opinion considered appropriate for three strata (mild, moderate, and severe) of renal failure; second, it assumed that the length of hospital stay would not be increased due to nephrotoxicity and that no patients would require dialysis; and third, it did not consider the effect on resource utilization of the patients' underlying diseases and severity at the time of admission. In contrast to this experience, we have found that the development of hospital-acquired renal failure may substantially increase length of stay (Shusterman NH. Unpublished data).

The component cost regressions in our study indicated that nephrotoxicity increases the cost of medical care because it lengthens patient stay and thus the time period in which these services are needed, and because during each day of the patient's stay, it increases the relative intensity of the resources consumed. We drew this latter conclusion from the fact that the nephrotoxicity variable remained a statistically significant predictor of component costs even when the days attributable to nephrotoxicity were included in the length-of-stay variables.

The results of the total charge regressions indicated that substitution of services may have occurred; the increased intensity in measured component costs may have been matched by decreased intensity in other services that we did not tabulate. Charges were increased due to prolonged length of stay for patients with nephrotoxicity. However, during each day of the hospitalization (excluding the effect of length of stay) charges were not increased due to nephrotoxicity, as was shown by the loss of statistical significance of the nephrotoxicity variable in the regression when the days attributable to nephrotoxicity were included. There may be reasons other than substitution of services that explain this lack of statistical significance for cost per day when changes in length of stay are excluded, including the insensitivity of charges to actual changes in resource utilization and problems in statistical power due to sample size. However, this result suggests an important methodologic implication: investigators should be cautious when analyzing costs of only a small subset of services related to economic consequences of a complication.

Investigators must also be cautious when using charge data rather than cost data to represent the economic impact of a clinical outcome. Although additional hospital services represent increases in both costs and charges, charges overstate the actual cost of these services to the hospital. In our study, using charges as a proxy for costs would have overstated the "cost" of nephrotoxicity by 100%. For this reason, investigators should be careful to specify whether their results are expressed in charge or cost measurements.

Conventional evaluation of new drugs focuses on their safety and efficacy. With increasing concern on the cost of medical care, the economic consequences of new drugs have also become important. The purchase price of a drug represents only one of its economic costs. The sometimes hidden costs of drug administration, laboratory tests to monitor for serum levels and complications, the management of these complications when they occur, and the treatment of other clinical consequences (such as the development of resistant organisms) also deserve attention. One potential hidden cost of antibiotic administration is the increased resources used because of the occurrence of aminoglycoside-associated nephrotoxicity.

Because the clinical and economic impacts of aminoglycoside-associated nephrotoxicity have not been fully evaluated, it is important to determine the advantages of new antibiotics that could replace the aminoglycosides without causing nephrotoxicity. For example, recent reports suggest that aztreonam can be combined with antistaphylococcal, antistreptococcal, or antianaerobic agents for use as an alternative to aminoglycosides without the risk of nephrotoxicity or other important adverse effects.[2,15]

The total cost of nephrotoxicity enumerated in our study did not incorporate the cost of monitoring for nephrotoxicity, which includes the periodic measurement of serum creatinine and aminoglycoside levels during therapy. Because most patients who receive aminoglycoside antibiotics are monitored closely for signs of impending renal dysfunction, the resultant cost of this monitoring may be substantial. These data would be useful in assessing the economic impact of the newer, less toxic alternatives to aminoglycosides that would avoid many of the monitoring costs.

Costs and benefits can be calculated with respect to the point of view of society, the patient, the payer, or the provider. A study's perspective influences what is counted as a cost or benefit. Our analysis took the perspectives of the hospital and by including physician consultations, the payer. However, if one adopts the societal or patient's perspective, additional costs would become important. For example, indirect costs of morbidity might occur because the patient remains in the hospital longer and thus misses work or is unable to resume employment. Patients who require long-term dialysis certainly incur these additional indirect costs as well as the direct costs of dialysis. In addition, the intangible costs of nephrotoxicity, such as pain, suffering, and grief, are substantial. We enumerated only the direct medical costs of nephrotoxicity and thus have excluded these indirect and intangible costs that may add significantly to the overall cost of nephrotoxicity.

Finally, we only measured the cost of nephrotoxicity associated with aminoglycoside use. However, other complications of this therapy may also add significantly to the economic burden of aminoglycoside antibiotics. Vestibular and auditory ototoxicity occur in 10% to 30% of patients.[16-22] The development of ototoxicity frequently is unrecognized in the hospital, in part because monitoring for vestibular and auditory damage is done infrequently at many hospitals. Therefore, the economic burden of ototoxicity is not often encountered in the hospital. For these reasons, we did not attempt to calculate the cost of this complication, although it may be significant from nonhospital perspectives.

A common limitation in previous studies that have attempted to estimate the costs of medical complications has been their failure to account for the initial severity of illness in the patients in the study (because those who have the complications may be more severely ill before receiving the drug than those who do not). For example, patients who developed nephtrotoxicity in the present study tended to be older, have higher diagnosis-related group weights and more secondary diagnoses, and have longer hospital stays than did patients who remained free of nephrotoxicity during aminoglycoside therapy. Additionally, in measuring the cost of infectious disease, many studies fail to account for the severity of infection. We have attempted to overcome these limitations by incorporating indicators of severity into our regression models. Thus, we were able to explain a significant amount of the observed variation due to these confounding variables in our model and still show a strong positive association between the nephrotoxicity variables and the dependent variables of length of stay and ancillary services.

It is important to note that we studied aminoglycoside-associated nephrotoxicity and have carefully avoided using the term aminoglycoside-induced nephrotoxicity. No single measure of renal function can provide conclusive evidence that the nephrotoxicity was caused by the aminoglycoside antibiotics. To eliminate other potential causes of renal failure that can confound the effect of aminoglycosides but occur too rarely to adjust for, we excluded those patients known to have received other nephrotoxic agents as well as those patients found to be at risk for nephrotoxicity from other causes. In addition, we excluded patients who received very short courses of aminoglycosides.

Therefore, we may have underestimated the frequency of nephrotoxicity caused by aminoglycosides.

This case-control study nested in an historical cohort study enumerated the costs of aminoglycoside-associated nephrotoxicity. The average cost of nephrotoxicity in those patients who developed it was $2501, which corresponded to a charge of $5376 to the payer. The average cost per patient exposed to aminoglycoside antibiotics was $183. From the perspective of the hospital and the payer, aminoglycoside use imposes a significant economic burden on the health care system.

ACKNOWLEDGMENTS

Grant support: in part by a contract from E. R. Squibb & Sons, Inc., to the Philadelphia Association for Clinical Trials.

REFERENCES

1. Lerner SA, Schmitt BA, Seligsohn R, Matz GJ. Comparative study of ototoxicity and nephrotoxicity in patients randomly assigned to treatment with amikacin and gentamicin. *Am J Med.* 1986;**80** (suppl 6B):98–104.
2. Henry SA, Bendush CB. Aztreonam: worldwide overview of the treatment of patients with gram negative infections. *Am J Med.* 1985;**78** (suppl 2A):57–64.
3. Tablan OC, Reyes MP, Rintelmann WF, Lerner AM. Renal and auditory toxicity of high-dose, prolonged therapy with gentamicin and tobramycin in pseudomonas endocarditis. *J Infect Dis.* 1984;**149**:257–63.
4. Gatell JM, San Miguel JG, Zamora L, et al. Comparison of nephrotoxicity and auditory toxicity of tobramycin and amikacin. *Antimicrob Agents Chemother.* 1983;**23**:897–901.
5. Kumin GD. Clinical nephrotoxicity of tobramycin and gentamicin: a prospective study, *JAMA.* 1980;**244**:1808–10.
6. Smith CR, Lipsky JJ, Laskin OL, et al. Double-blind comparison of the nephrotoxicity and auditory toxicity of gentamicin and tobramycin. *N Engl J Med.* 1980;**302**:1106–9.
7. Bendush CL, Senior SL, Wooller HO. Evaluation of nephrotoxic and ototoxic effects of tobramycin in world-wide study. *Med J Aust.* 1977;**2**:22–6.
8. Hewitt WL. Reflections on the clinical pharmacology of gentamicin. *Acta Pathol Microbiol Immunol Scand [B].* 1973;**82** (suppl 241):151–6.
9. Holloway JJ, Smith CR, Moore RD, Feroli ER Jr, Leitman PS. Comparative cost effectiveness of gentamicin and tobramycin. *Ann Intern Med.* 1984;**101**:764–9.
10. Hou SH, Bushinsky DA, Wish JB, Cohen JJ, Harrington JT. Hospital-acquired renal insufficiency: a prospective study. *Am J Med.* 1983:**74**:243–8.

11. Meyer RD. Risk factors and comparisons of clinical nephrotoxicity of aminoglycosides. *Am J Med.* 1986;**80** (suppl 6B):119–25.
12. Bergeron MG, Lessard C, Ronald A, Stiver G, Van Rooyen CE, Chadwick P. Three to eight weeks of therapy with netilmicin: toxicity in normal and diabetic patients. *J Antimicrob Chemother.* 1983;**12**:245–8.
13. Lane AZ, Wright GE, Blair DC. Ototoxicity and nephrotoxicity of amikacin: an overview phase II and phase III experience in the United States. *Am J Med.* 1977;**62**:911–8.
14. Nicot G, Merle L, Valette JP, Charmes JP, Lachatre G. Gentamicin and sisomicin-induced renal tubular damage. *Eur J Clin Pharm.* 1982;**23**:161–6.
15. Scully BE, Neu HC. Use of aztreonam in the treatment of serious infections due to multiresistant gram-negative organisms, including *Pseudomonas aeruginosa. Am J Med.* 1985;**78**:251–61.
16. Dayal VS, Smith EL, McCain WG. Cochlear and vestibular gentamicin toxicity: a clinical study of systemic and topical usage. *Arch Otolaryngol.* 1974;**100**:338–40.
17. Meyers RM. Ototoxic effects of gentamicin. *Arch Otolaryngol.* 1970;**92**:160–2.
18. Banck G, Belfrage S, Juhlin I, Nordstrom L, Tjernstrom O, Toremalm NG. Retrospective study of the ototoxicity of gentamicin. *Acta Pathol Microbiol Scand* [B]. 1973;**81** (suppl 241):54–7.
19. Fee WE JR, Vierra V, Lathrop GR. Clinical evaluation of aminoglycoside toxicity: tobramycin versus gentamicin, a preliminary report. *J Antimicrob Chemother.* 1978;**4** (suppl A):31–6.
20. Dayal VS, Chait GE, Fenton SS. Gentamicin vestibulotoxicity: long term disability. *Ann Otol Rhinol Laryngol.* 1979;**88**:36–9.
21. Barza M, Lauermann NW, Tally FP, Gorbach SL. Prospective, randomized trial of netlmicin and amikacin, with emphasis on eighth-nerve toxicity. *Antimicrob Agents Chemother.* 1980;**17**:707–14.
22. Moore RD, Smith CR, Leitman PS. Risk factors for the development of auditory toxicity in patients receiving aminoglycosides. *J Infect Dis.* 1984;**149**:23–30.

Appendix

3RD INTERNATIONAL CONFERENCE ON PHARMACOEPIDEMIOLOGY

PROGRAM COMMITTEE

Stanley A. Edlavitch, PhD, University of Minnesota, Conference Chairman
Jerry Avorn, MD, Harvard University Medical School
Thomas Choi, PhD, University of Minnesota
Linda Cottler, MPH, Washington University School of Medicine
Lael Gatewood, PhD, University of Minnesota
David Lilienfeld, MD, MS Engin, MPH, Mt Sinai Medical School
Joseph Mariano, MD, The Upjohn Company
Michael Murray, PharmD, Purdue and Indiana Universities
Robert Pocelinko, MD, Stuart Pharmaceuticals
Todd Semla, MS, PharmD, University of Illinois at Chicago
Craig Smith, MD, Johns Hopkins University
Andy Stergachis, PhD, Group Health Cooperative of Puget Sound
Brian Strom, MD, MPH, University of Pennsylvania School of Medicine
Hugh Tilson, MD, DrPH, Burroughs Wellcome Company
John Urquhart, MD, University of Limberg and Aprex Corporation
Alexander Walker, MD, MPH, Boston University School of Medicine
Robert Wallace, MD, MSc, University of Iowa
Albert Wertheimer, PhD, University of Minnesota
Bengt-Erik Wiholm, MD, Swedish National Board of Drugs

CONTRIBUTING COMPANIES

Ayerst Laboratories
Boehringer Ingleheim, Ltd.
Burroughs Wellcome Company
Eli Lilly and Company Glaxo, Inc.
Lederle Laboratories
Marion Laboratories, Inc.
Merck Sharp & Dohme Research Laboratories
Norwich Eaton Pharmaceuticals, Inc.
The Procter & Gamble Company
Riker Laboratories/3M
The Upjohn Company

Index

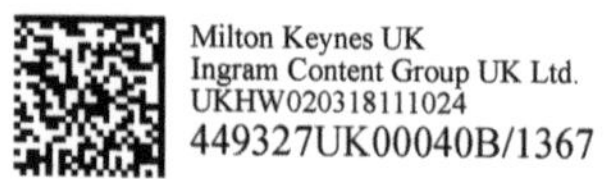

Milton Keynes UK
Ingram Content Group UK Ltd.
UKHW020318111024
449327UK00040B/1367